Hormones and Behavior

CONTRIBUTORS

JACK D. BARCHAS

H. KEITH H. BRODIE

ROLAND D. CIARANELLO

R. L. CONNER

JULIAN M. DAVIDSON

VICTOR H. DENENBERG

D. DE WIED

E. ENDRÖCZI

W. H. GISPEN

DAVID A. HAMBURG

SEYMOUR LEVINE

BENJAMIN D. SACHS

JON M. STOLK

A. M. L. van DELFT

TJ. B. van WIMERSMA GREIDANUS

JOAN VERNIKOS-DANELLIS

J. A. W. M. WEIJNEN

M. X. ZARROW

Hormones and Behavior

Edited by SEYMOUR LEVINE

Department of Psychiatry
Stanford University School of Medicine
Stanford, California

 1972

ACADEMIC PRESS *New York and London*

ACADEMIC PRESS, INC.
111 Fifth Avenue, New York, New York 10003

United Kingdom Edition published by
ACADEMIC PRESS, INC. (LONDON) LTD.
24/28 Oval Road, London NW1

LIBRARY OF CONGRESS CATALOG CARD NUMBER: 78-187245

PRINTED IN THE UNITED STATES OF AMERICA

Contents

1. Introduction and Basic Concepts

Seymour Levine

2. Effects of Hormones on the Central Nervous System

Joan Vernikos-Danellis

3. Hormones and Reproductive Behavior

Julian M. Davidson

4. Hormones and Maternal Behavior in Mammals

M. X. Zarrow, Victor H. Denenberg, and Benjamin D. Sachs

5. The Role of Pituitary-Adrenal System Hormones in Active Avoidance Conditioning

D. De Wied, A. M. L. van Delft, W. H. Gispen,
J. A. W. M. Weijnen, and Tj. B. van Wimersma Greidanus

6. Pavlovian Conditioning and Adaptive Hormones

E. Endröczi

7. Hormones, Biogenic Amines, and Aggression

R. L. Conner

8. Biogenic Amines and Behavior

Jack D. Barchas, Roland D. Ciaranello, Jon M. Stolk,
H. Keith H. Brodie, and David A. Hamburg

List of Contributors

Numbers in parentheses indicate the pages on which the authors' contributions begin.

JACK D. BARCHAS (235), Department of Psychiatry, Stanford University, School of Medicine, Stanford, California

H. KEITH H. BRODIE (235), Department of Psychiatry, Stanford University, School of Medicine, Stanford, California

ROLAND D. CIARANELLO (235), Department of Psychiatry, Stanford University, School of Medicine, Stanford, California

R. L. CONNER* (209), Department of Psychiatry, Stanford University, School of Medicine, Stanford, California

JULIAN M. DAVIDSON (63), Department of Physiology, Stanford University, School of Medicine, Stanford University, Stanford, California

VICTOR H. DENENBERG (105), Departments of Biobehavioral Sciences and Psychology, The University of Connecticut, Storrs, Connecticut

D. DE WIED (135), Rudolf Magnus Institute for Pharmacology, Medical Faculty, University of Utrecht, Utrecht, The Netherlands

E. ENDRÖCZI (173), Central Research Division, Postgraduate Medical School, Budapest, Hungary

W. H. GISPEN (135), Rudolf Magnus Institute for Pharmacology, Medical Faculty, University of Utrecht, Utrecht, The Netherlands

DAVID A. HAMBURG (235), Department of Psychiatry, Stanford University, School of Medicine, Stanford, California

SEYMOUR LEVINE (1), Department of Psychiatry, Stanford University, School of Medicine, Stanford, California

BENJAMIN D. SACHS (105), Department of Psychology, The University of Connecticut, Storrs, Connecticut

* Present address: Department of Psychology, Bowling Green State University, Bowling Green, Ohio.

JON M STOLK* (235), Department of Psychiatry, Stanford University, School of Medicine, Stanford, California

A. M. L. van DELFT† (135), Rudolf Magnus Institute for Pharmacology, Medical Faculty, University of Utrecht, Utrecht, The Netherlands

Tj. B. van WIMERSMA GREIDANUS (135), Rudolf Magnus Institute for Pharmacology, Medical Faculty, University of Utrecht, Utrecht, The Netherlands

JOAN VERNIKOS-DANELLIS‡ (11), Department of Pharmacology, The Ohio State University, School of Medicine, Columbus, Ohio

J. A. W. M. WEIJNEN (135), Rudolf Magnus Institute for Pharmacology, Medical Faculty, University of Utrecht, Utrecht, The Netherlands

M. X. ZARROW (105), Department of Biobehavioral Sciences, The University of Connecticut, Storrs, Connecticut

*Present address: Department of Pharmacology and Psychiatry, Dartmouth Medical School, Hanover, New Hampshire.

†Present address: Department of Pharmacology, Medical Faculty, Free University, Amsterdam, The Netherlands.

‡Present address: Environmental Biology Division, Ames Research Center, NASA, Moffett Field, California.

Preface

In 1948, Dr. Frank Beach wrote a book entitled "Hormones and Behavior." In the ensuing years this area of research has grown extensively. In one sense, therefore, this book represents a progress report in the area of hormonal control, not only of sexual behavior but of many other behaviors which have now been shown to be influenced in some way by a multitude of hormonal determinants. In this volume we deal primarily with the action of two major hormonal systems on behavior—the pituitary-gonadal system and the pituitary-adrenal system. The control and modulation of sex behavior, maternal behavior, learning and conditioning, and aggressive behavior are discussed by the contributors. The authors of these chapters have made salient contributions to the fund of accumulating knowledge concerning the hormonal control and modulation of behavior and are continuously engaged in the study of the phenomena within the scope of this area.

Our principal objective in assembling and editing these papers was to juxtapose material covering a wide spectrum of species, procedures, processes, and interpretations to facilitate a broad and integrated understanding of the role of hormones in behavior. This volume is intended for advanced students and specialists of physiological psychology, neuroendocrinology, and psychiatry, but should prove of value to individuals interested in understanding the biological bases of behavior.

To the contributors, each of whom I hold in the highest esteem both personally and professionally, I wish to express my gratitude. I also wish to acknowledge my debt to many persons who have so generously aided me in one or more phases of the preparation of this volume; in particular the efforts of Mrs. Rosemary Gutt, Mrs. Renée Sonderman, and Miss Mary Erskine are deeply appreciated.

This book was prepared with the support of USPHS Research Scientist Award 1-K05-MH-19936 from the National Institute of Mental Health and the Leslie Fund, Chicago.

Seymour Levine

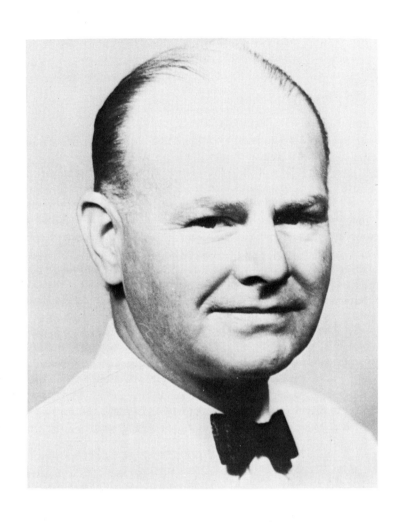

Geoffrey W. Harris

(1913–1971)

This volume is dedicated to Professor Geoffrey Harris who was the Professor of Anatomy at Oxford University. It is an acknowledgment of his contributions to the understanding of the relationships between the brain and endocrine system and of his profound insights in neuroendocrinology which have provided a conceptual framework for much of the research that is reported. It is also a personal expression of appreciation—Geoffrey Harris was not only my teacher but my dear and personal friend. His untimely death in December of 1971 was a shock and loss to all of us in the field. Though it is always difficult to assess the loss of an individual in terms of what future insights and scientific revelations may have emerged from his work, it is not difficult to assess the loss of a friend. It is always tempting when writing a memorial dedication to idolatrize an individual, but I can pay no greater tribute to Professor Harris than to say that he was infinitely human and profoundly affected many of us. He leaves us a legacy of accomplishments almost too numerous to cite. It was through his vision, creativity, and devotion that the field of neuroendocrinology advanced to its present state—a fully recognized scientific discipline encompassing a range of research interests from molecular biology through behavior. His historic monograph on the neural control of the pituitary written in 1950 remains a landmark, and many of the hypotheses contained within that volume have proved highly significant. There is no question that what has already been accomplished in neuroendocrinology has had important influence on the solutions to many of the problems plaguing mankind.

There is no way to truly honor a man of the stature of Geoffrey Harris. Giants among men are rare, as he indeed was, and his death at any time would have been untimely.

Seymour Levine

1

Introduction and Basic Concepts

Seymour Levine

For as long as man has been concerned with the attempt to understand his behavior, there has been a long-standing belief in the chemical control of behavior. Galen's postulation of the four humors—blood, phlegm, yellow bile, and black bile—formed the basis of one of the first chemical theories of behavior, and in fact the basis for a whole system of medicine which lasted for centuries. The ancients observed that castrating bulls pacified them as well as improving the quality of their meat. The ancient Chinese alchemists not only administered testicular tissue for sexual debility and impotence but also developed some skills in fractionating human urine to obtain partially purified steroids for this purpose (Needham and Gwei-Djen, 1968). Perhaps the first experimental verification of the role of hormones in behavior, however, derived from Berthold's (1849) classic observation on castration and testicular transplants in fowls, which included observations on behavioral changes. However, the experimental study of the influence of hormones on behavior is due primarily to the efforts of one man, Dr. Frank Beach, who in the late 1930's and early 1940's pioneered in the experimental investigation of the physiological control of sexual behavior and unequivocally demonstrated the important role of the gonadal hormones in the regulation of such behaviors. In 1948 Dr. Beach published a volume entitled *Hormones and Behavior.* In one sense this book represents a 25-year progress report in the area of hormonal control of not only sexual behavior but many other behaviors which have now been shown to be influenced, in some way or another, by a multitude of hormonal determinants.

1

At the time Dr. Beach published his book research in experimental psychology and neuroendocrinology was in its most primitive and infantile state. The past two decades have seen an enormous growth in experimental techniques and understanding of the regulation and control of behavior and a whole new field of neuroendocrinology, which has been involved in attempting to elucidate the relationships between the central nervous system and the regulation of endocrine function.

In this volume we deal primarily with the action of two major hormonal systems on various aspects of behavior. These are the pituitary-gonadal system and the pituitary-adrenal system. Unfortunately, the chapter which was to have been written concerning the influence of thyroid on behavior was terminated by the accidental death of Dr. Shawn Schapiro.

The primary purpose of this brief introductory chapter is to familiarize the reader with some of the very basic concepts in the endocrinology and neuroendocrinology of the two major hormonal systems which will be discussed by the various authors in this volume.

I. PITUITARY-GONADAL SYSTEM

The endocrine control of reproduction must be viewed as one of the major adaptive systems in almost all living organisms, for, in terms of evolutionary theory, one of the primary functions of each member of any species is to reproduce the species. Perhaps one of the most dramatic changes in evolution was when organisms changed from autosexual reproduction to heterosexual reproduction, for once heterosexual reproduction became the predominant mode of replicating the species, it also became necessary to bring sex behavior under the regulation of those systems which regulate the physiological aspects of reproduction. In the mammalian species the principal glands to be considered are the ovary in the female, the testes in the male, as well as the pituitary and central nervous system (CNS) structures. If we examine the major distinction between females and males, in most species of mammals the female has a cyclic pattern of ovulation, the human female ovulating about every 28 days, the rat every 4 or 5 days, and the guinea pig every 15 days, etc. This process is dominated by the CNS and the anterior pituitary peptide hormones. Thus, in a cyclic fashion the anterior pituitary delivers to the ovary a follicle-stimulating hormone (FSH) which promotes the growth of the Graafian follicles and a luteinizing hormone (LH) which induces the formation of the corpora lutea and triggers ovulation. Figure 1 presents a schematic of the interplay of the sex hormones, both in the female and in the male (Levine, 1966). In the cyclic system the pituitary initially releases FSH that induces the ovary to produce estrogen from the Graafian follicles. The estrogen then presumably acts both on

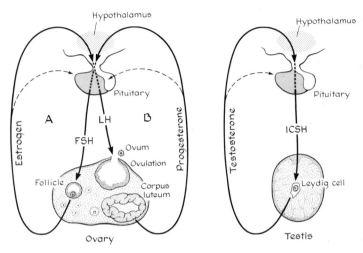

Fig. 1. Interplay of sex hormones.

the hypothalamus and pituitary to inhibit further release of FSH by the pituitary and to stimulate the release of LH. The initial surge of LH triggers ovulation and induces the ovary to produce yet another hormone, progesterone. Once again when progesterone is seen by the hypothalamus or pituitary, this hormone inhibits further pituitary release of LH, thereby completing the cycle.

In the male this system is noncyclic and the pituitary more or less continually releases LH, which in the male is called interstitial cell stimulation hormone (ICSH), that induces the testes to produce testosterone and other testicular hormones. Testosterone acts upon the CNS to inhibit the release of ICSH by the pituitary. It is further assumed, and there is a large body of information to indicate, that there are humoral substances synthesized and secreted by the hypothalamus which control the secretions of the anterior pituitary. These hormones are called releasing factors. The general class of hormones related to the regulation of FSH and LH is called gonadotropin-releasing factors. [For a general review of the releasing factors see Geschwind (1969).] The number of reviews concerned with the control of gonadotropin secretion is legion and only a select few will be presented here (Davidson, 1969; Everett, 1964; Flerkó, 1966; Harris and Campbell, 1966; Sawyer et al., 1966).

II. PITUITARY-ADRENAL SYSTEM

The essentials of the pituitary-adrenal system are presented in Fig. 2 (Levine, 1971). In response to a variety of environmental variables, the pituitary-adrenal system is activated. Thus information concerning the environmental change,

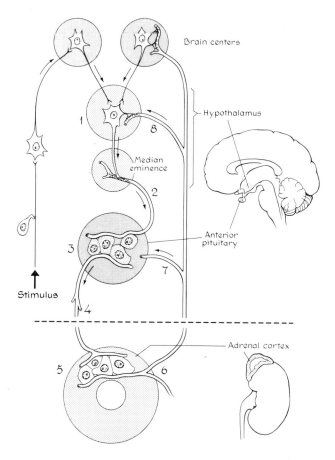

Fig. 2. Pituitary-adrenal system involves nerve cells and hormones in a feedback loop. A stress stimulus reaching neurosecretory cells of the hypothalamus in the base of the brain (1) stimulates them to release corticotropin-releasing factor (CRF), which moves through short blood vessels (2) to the anterior lobe of the pituitary gland (3). Pituitary cells thereupon release adrenocorticotropic hormone (ACTH) into the circulation (4). The ACTH stimulates cells of the adrenal cortex (5) to secrete glucocorticoid hormones (primarily hydrocortisone in man) into the circulation (6). When glucocorticoids reach neurosecretory cells or other brain cells (it is not clear which), they modulate CRF production (7).

coming either from external sources in the sensory system or from internal sources such as changes in body temperature or blood composition, is received and integrated by the CNS. The hypothalamus secretes corticotropin-releasing factor (CRF) (Guillemin and Schally, 1963), which induces the pituitary to secrete adrenocorticotropic hormone (ACTH). In response to ACTH the adrenal cortex synthesizes and releases its hormones, predominantly glucocorticoids. In man the predominant glucocorticoid is hydrocortisone and in many lower animals the predominant adrenal corticoid is corticosterone. There is a large body of information indicating that there is, as in the case of the pituitary-gonadal system, feedback regulation of ACTH. The site of the feedback action of the adrenocortical hormones for the regulation of the secretion of ACTH is still controversial. There is evidence which indicates that both the CNS and the pituitary may indeed be feedback sites for the adrenal corticoids. The fact that the brain is a receptor site for hormones and particularly adrenal corticoids, has been very amply demonstrated (see Chapter 2). The action of the glucocorticoids on the pituitary is only in relationship to the feedback regulation of ACTH. [For more extensive reviews of the control and regulation of corticotropin ACTH, see Fortier (1966); Ganong (1963), Saffran (1966).]

III. THE HYPOTHALAMUS

"It is clear that the central nervous system is largely responsible for correlating endocrine activity with that of other systems of the body." Thus in his now classic volume on the neural control of the pituitary gland, Harris postulated (1955) that the hypothalamus and anterior pituitary function together as an integrated unit and that the major controls on the pituitary were predominantly CNS in origin, with the final common pathway being hypothalamus. The control of the anterior pituitary by the hypothalamus is predominantly chemical since the only anatomical link of significance between these two structures is the pituitary portal vessels (Fig. 3). Thus when the communication between hypothalamus and pituitary is severed by means of pituitary stalk section the pituitary, although *in situ*, essentially becomes nonfunctional. It is not the purpose of this section to review in detail the hypothalamic control of

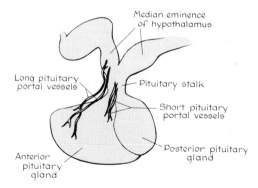

Fig. 3. Relationship of hypothalamus and anterior pituitary gland (after Sawin).

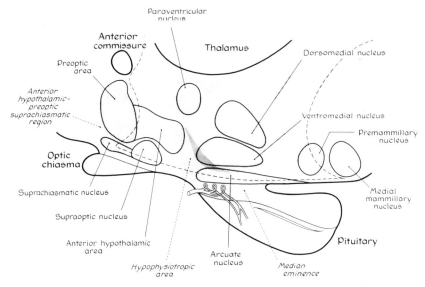

Fig. 4. Schematic diagram of hypothalamus showing major nuclei.

the pituitary gland, since this has been the subject of several volumes including the volume by Harris and a subsequent volume by Szentágothai *et al.* (1962).

Figure 4 presents the major nuclei of the hypothalamus which appear to be involved in one way or another in the control of anterior pituitary function. There have been three principal techniques which have been utilized to examine the role of the hypothalamus. These techniques have included lesions or ablation of specific nuclei in the hypothalamus, electrical stimulation of these nuclei, and the implantation of chemicals, predominantly hormones, into specific areas of the hypothalamus. It has now been clearly demonstrated that with regard to reproductive function, certain specific nuclei are involved. In particular, the hypothalamic preoptic suprachiasmatic region appears to control cyclic LH release. This area also appears to be the site for the stimulatory action of steroids on endocrine activity and female sex behavior. The arcuate nucleus also appears to be intimately involved in the maintenance of male sexual behavior. In general, the median eminence appears to be rich in all of the releasing factors, including FSHRF, LHRF, and CRF. In fact all of the known releasing factors appear to be synthesized at present only within hypothalamic tissue.

IV. THE LIMBIC SYSTEM

Although there appears to be little question that the final common pathway with regard to regulation of anterior pituitary function is via the hypothalamus,

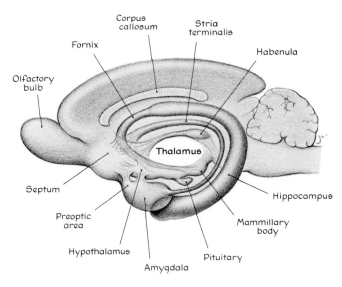

Fig. 5. Schematic diagram of limbic system (after de Groot).

there is an abundance of information which indicates that other CNS structures are involved in regulation and modulation of hypothalamic function. These structures are principally subcortical and predominantly within the system which was elucidated by Papez in 1937 and called the limbic system. The major structures of the limbic system are presented in Fig. 5.

There is extensive evidence of the influence of the limbic system on pituitary function in relationship to reproduction [see de Groot (1965)] and of the limbic system involvement in the regulation of the pituitary-adrenal system (Schadé, 1970). Many of the details concerning the manner in which the limbic system regulates hypothalamic function and subsequently anterior pituitary function, have by no means been worked out. Sawyer *et al.* (1966) have presented a model showing the relationships between the brain, anterior pituitary, and the gonadal system. This model implicates two major neural systems that are involved with hypothalamic function, these being the limbic hypothalamic system and the reticular hypothalamic system. He presents evidence which clearly indicates that both of these systems are in some way modulators of the hypothalamus.

V. CONCLUSIONS

In this brief discussion we have presented a profoundly oversimplified view of those physiological systems which are involved in the synthesis and release of the chemical compounds known as hormones which we know now to have a major role in the regulation of many behavioral functions. My primary purpose, however, is to give the reader some frame of reference and to visualize some of these systems so that in subsequent detailed descriptions of the role of these hormones and behavior, at least a rudimentary knowledge of the physiology is available.

Many years ago I was privileged to attend a lecture by the famous reproductive physiologist, A. S. Parks. It was about the time that there was a tremendous flurry about the explorations of outer space. Parks concluded his lecture by applauding all the major technological advances which had made outer space exploration possible but indicated that as far as he was concerned the explorations of inner space still had for him profound significance and intense excitement. I must express my concurrence with this view and that the contributors to this volume have indeed led us through many facets of the exploration of inner space. I hope the reader will enjoy following these explorations with us.

Acknowledgment

This research was supported by USPHS Research Scientist Award 1-K05-MH-19, 936-01 from the National Institute of Mental Health and the Leslie Fund, Chicago.

References

Beach, F. A. (1948). "Hormones and Behavior." Harper (Hoeber), New York.
Berthold, A. A. (1849). *Arch. Anat. Physiol.* **16**, 42.
Davidson, J. M. (1969). *In* "Frontiers in Neuroendocrinology, 1969" (W. F. Ganong and L. Martini, eds.), pp. 343-388. Oxford Univ. Press, London and New York.
de Groot, J. (1965). *In* "Sex and Behavior" (F. A. Beach, ed.), pp. 496-511. Wiley, New York.
Everett, J. W. (1964). *Physiol. Rev.* **44**, 373.
Flerkó, B. (1966). *In* "Neuroendocrinology" (L. Martini and W. F. Ganong, eds.), Vol. I, pp. 613-653. Academic Press, New York.
Fortier, C. (1966). *In* "The Pituitary Gland" (G. W. Harris and B. T. Donovan, eds.), Vol. 2, pp. 195-234. Univ. of California Press, Berkeley.
Ganong, W. F. (1963). *Advan. Neuroendocrinol. Proc. Symp. 1961* pp. 92-157.
Geschwind, I. I. (1969). *In* "Frontiers in Neuroendocrinology, 1969" (W. F. Ganong and L. Martini, eds.), pp. 389-431. Oxford Univ. Press, London and New York.
Guillemin, R., and Schally, A. V. (1963). *Advan. Neuroendocrinol. Proc. Symp. 1961* pp. 314-344.
Harris, G. W. (1955). "Neural Control of the Pituitary Gland." Arnold, London.
Harris, G. W., and Campbell, H. J. (1966). *In* "The Pituitary Gland" (G. W. Harris and B. T. Donovan, eds.), Vol. 2, pp. 99-165, Univ. of California Press, Berkeley.
Levine, S. (1966). *Sci. Amer.* **214**, 84.
Levine, S. (1971). *Sci. Amer.* **224**, 26.
Needham, J., and Gwei-Djen, L. (1968). *Endeavor*, **27**, 130.
Papez, J. W. (1937). *Arch. Neurol. Psychiat.* **38**, 725.
Saffran, M. (1966). *In* "Endocrines and the Central Nervous System" (R. Levine, ed.), Vol. XLIII, pp. 36-46, A.R.N.M.D. Williams & Wilkins, Baltimore, Maryland.

Sawin, C. T. (1969). "The Hormones. Endocrine Physiology." Little, Brown, Boston, Massachusetts.

Sawyer, C. H., Kawakami, M., and Kanematsu, S. (1966). *In* "Endocrines and the Central Nervous System" (R. Levine, ed.), Vol. XLIII, pp. 59-85, A.R.N.M.D. Williams & Wilkins, Baltimore, Maryland.

Schadé, J. O. (1970). *In* "Progress in Brain Research, Vol. 32, Pituitary, Adrenal and the Brain" (D. de Wied and J. A. W. M. Weijnen, eds.), pp. 2-11. Elsevier Publishing Co., Amsterdam.

Szentágothai, J., Flerkó, B., Mess, B., and Halász, B. (1962). "Hypothalamic Control of the Anterior Pituitary." Akademiai Kiado, Budapest.

2

Effects of Hormones on the Central Nervous System

Joan Vernikos-Danellis

I. INTRODUCTION

There is little doubt that hormones affect behavior by an action mediated by the central nervous system (CNS). The remaining chapters of this book provide evidence of the numerous and varied ways by which they do this. In fact, behavior has been increasingly used as an index of the actions of hormones upon nervous tissues. Yet little is known of the anatomic, physiological, and biochemical pathways involved in their action. Considerable evidence has accumulated in recent years to describe the neural mechanisms involved in the control of hormone secretion and the site and mechanisms of action of feedback regulation of hypothalamic-pituitary secretions by target organ products. Excellent symposia, reports, and reviews have appeared in the literature to cover this aspect of hormonal action on the CNS. Specifically, they include those by

Davidson (1969), Martini *et al* (1968), Davidson *et al.,* (1967), Motta *et al.* (1968), Mess and Martini (1968), and others.

Considerably less information exists about the way that hormones influence the activity of nervous tissues. For instance, some endocrine secretions are concerned with metabolic processes that affect the brain as well as the body as a whole (e.g., thyroid), while others appear to exert a significant and often specific part in regulating the growth and activity of the brain. With the exception of the brief, but informative, review of Campbell and Eayrs (1965), the subject of the effects of hormones on so-called "nonendocrine CNS mechanisms" has been covered by fragmented surveys of specific groups of hormones, among which, by far the most comprehensive and thorough on the adrenal cortex, is the excellent work of Woodbury (1958) and that by Beyer and Sawyer (1969) on the gonadal hormones. In fact, covering the literature in this field, one cannot but conclude that either certain hormones have been particularly popular or that a considerable volume of negative results must exist in academic archives to compensate for the gaps in information about particular hormones or aspects of their action on the CNS. For example, the hormones of the parathyroid and growth hormone seem to have entirely escaped attention. It is also rather interesting that the effects of oxytocin on neural processes have been studied to some extent, whereas this is not true for vasopressin. This review will, therefore, attempt to present examples of the variety of ways in which hormones may affect the CNS and perhaps indicate those gaps in knowledge of this most fundamental step between the secretion of a hormone and its end product, namely, alteration of behavior.

II. EFFECTS OF HORMONES ON BRAIN DEVELOPMENT, MORPHOLOGY, AND DIFFERENTIATION

Rapid growth during the embryonic fetal and early postnatal periods makes the developing brain more vulnerable to changes in its total environment. Factors such as nutrition, training, sensory stimulation or deprivation, and hormones and other drugs are but a few that are known to affect the morphological, physiological, and biochemical development of the CNS (Timiras and Vernadakis, 1967; Held, 1965; Miller, 1968). As a result of work done, particularly during the past couple of decades, the concept of "critical" periods in the regulatory influences of hormones on the CNS has emerged. This is particularly true for events concerned with sexual, thyroid, and adrenocortical hormones. It would appear that following exposure of the brain during these periods to certain kinds of hormonal influences, a powerful imprinting process occurs on cells involved in complex regulatory circuits so that both behavior and endocrine function may be profoundly modified in the adult animal (Levine and

Mullins, 1966). It should be emphasized that "critical periods" will differ for different species. The bulk of the information in the literature is based on experimental procedures using the rat—a species in which the state of cerebral development at birth resembles that of man during the early part of pregnancy.

Little is known about the role of hormones on CNS development before birth. Most studies have been concerned with the prenatal development of endocrine functions, with the interrelationship between the pituitary gland and other endocrines in fetuses, and with the effects of fetal endocrines on fetal growth. Hormones administered to animals during pregnancy have yielded little information on brain development. However, organ tissue culture studies have shown that estradiol and hydrocortisone in the culture medium improve the maintenance and growth of cerebellar explants removed from chick embryos (Vernadakis and Timiras, 1967). Similarly, these hormones have been reported to accelerate brain myelinogenesis of chick embryos *in vivo* (Granich and Timiras, 1967). In the human fetus the thyroid gland is active as early as the twelfth week of life. A limited amount of thyroid hormone may pass through the placenta from the maternal circulation, but there is evidence that in cretinism due to congenital aplasia of the thyroid the brain is histologically abnormal at the time of birth (Wilkins, 1957).

Certainly the thyroid is needed for the further growth and maturation of the brain after birth (Eayrs, 1967). The influence of this gland is clearly evident by the essential part it plays in the regulation of metamorphosis in amphibia (Allen 1938; Etkin, 1955). The administration of thyroid hormones has been found to promote general growth of the frog brain, specifically involving maturation of visual, olfactory, and locomotor apparatus (Tusques, 1956), and Weiss and Rossetti (1951) report a regression of Mauthner's cells and a proliferation of integrative neurons believed to be involved with the movements of the newly acquired limbs. Anatomical studies in the rat have shown that following thyroidectomy at birth there is a significant reduction in the weight and linear dimensions of the brain, more densely packed and smaller cortical neurons (Eayrs and Taylor, 1951; Hamburgh *et al.*, 1964), a decrease in cortical and axonal networks, dendritic lengths and branchings (Eayrs, 1955; Eayrs and Horn, 1955), as well as changes in cortical vascularity (Eayrs, 1954). It is not surprising, therefore, that these changes are accompanied by a corresponding failure in the maturation of behavior and of the electrical activity of the brain (Eayrs, 1960).

On the other hand, Kollros (1943) reported that local application of thyroxine on one side of the brain stem stimulated the maturation of reflexes on the same side. Thyroxine injection on postnatal days 2, 3, and 4 accelerated by approximately 2-3 days the maturation of evoked responses to visual, auditory, and sciatic nerve stimulation (Salas and Schapiro, 1969).

In contrast to the ubiquitous effect of thyroid hormone deficiency, early hypophysectomy (1 6 days of age) in the rat was found to have no effect on brain growth and development as measured by weight, although it delayed the growth and development of somatic and visceral structures similar to that following early thyroidectomy (Taurog et al., 1958; Trojanova and Mourek, 1966; Gregory and Diamond, 1968). It would, therefore, appear that sufficient thyroid hormone activity is available to the hypophysectomized rat to maintain normal brain growth in the absence of growth hormone and other pituitary tropic hormones. Similarly, morphological development of the hypophysec- tomized rat's brain is obviously not dependent on growth hormone (Gregory and Diamond, 1968), although growth hormone has been found to influence brain morphology when administered prenatally (Clendinnen and Eayrs, 1961; Walker et al., 1950, 1952; Zamenhof, 1942; Zamenhof et al., 1966) and postnatally (Eayrs, 1961b).

The administration of hydrocortisone on postnatal day 1 is reported to retard the development of the evoked responses to the visual cortex and to a lesser extent those elicited by auditory and sciatic nerve stimulation (Salas and Schapiro, 1969). However, hydrocortisone administered between day 8 and 16 is said to increase the development of neural activity as assessed by electroshock seizure thresholds (Vernadakis and Woodbury, 1963), whereas deoxycor- ticosterone (DOC) is without effect (Vernadakis and Woodbury, 1960). Estradiol has a similar effect to hydrocortisone on "neural maturation" only if administered on postnatal day 4-8 (Heim, 1966; Heim and Timiras, 1963). The myelination of hypothalamic centers is also accelerated by estradiol (Curry and Heim, 1966). Treatment of adult adrenalectomized rats with adrenocor- ticotropic hormone (ACTH) has been shown to result in marked changes in the nuclear size of hypothalamic cells (Ifft, 1966) and in an increased storage of neurosecretory material (Peczely, 1966).

The role of neonatal androgens on the differentiation of the hypothalamus provides a prime example of critical age and hormone specificity. It was generally held until recently that the patterns of nervous activity mediating sexual behavior were laid down independently of hormonal influence but triggered into activity by rising levels of appropriate sex hormones (Beach, 1948). The experiments of Pfeiffer (1936) transplanting gonads into newborn rats have now been confirmed by several laboratories using administration of androgen during a critical stage of development (Barraclough, 1961; Phoenix et al., 1959). This results in hypothalamic changes which permanently suppress the manifestations of female cyclic activity and a condition of permanent estrus and sterility develops with loss of mating behavior (Harris and Levine, 1962). Barraclough and Gorski (1962) have demonstrated that the effects of neonatal androgens on reproductive organs and on behavior are differentially influenced by the amount of androgen administered.

Analysis by means of lesions or electrical stimulation of various CNS areas has suggested that the androgen-sensitive centers are in the preoptic and suprachiasmatic regions of the hypothalamus (Barraclough and Gorski, 1961). It would appear that, administered during critical stages of development, hormones can play a major role in determining the rate of maturation and differentiation of the CNS. It is, however, not unlikely that some of these effects may be attributable to general metabolic phenomena.

III. HORMONAL UPTAKE, DISTRIBUTION, AND BINDING

The brain constitutes about 2% of the body weight, yet receives approximately 16% of the cardiac output. It is the most richly supplied with blood of all the body tissues. The average blood flow is about 0.5 ml/gm/min, compared with approximately 0.05 in resting muscles. It might be expected, therefore, that hormones would equilibrate very rapidly between blood and brain; however, many substances enter brain tissue only very slowly and some practically not at all.

A hormone may gain access to the tissues of the CNS by two distinct routes: the capillary circulation and the cerebrospinal fluid (CSF).

A. Brain-Blood Flow Distribution and Blood-Brain Barrier. Blood flow rates to various parts of the brain have been estimated by measuring the rate of transfer of radioactive krypton (^{79}Kr) from blood to tissues in the cat (Kety, 1960) or iodinated antipyrin in the rat (Goldman and Sapirstein, 1969; Table I). Wide differences exist between the flow in various parts of the brain. Cerebral white matter has a much lower blood supply than several parts of the cortex. The lateral nuclei of the hypothalamus receive a particularly rich blood supply and here hormones and other substances are known to enter quite rapidly.

In the brain, capillaries are much less permeable to a variety of water-soluble substances than in other parts of the body. Here the glial connective tissue cells are closely applied to the basement membrane of the capillary endothelium and electron micrographs indicate that this glial sheath is about 85% complete (Maynard *et al.,* 1957). Beneath this sheath the basement membrane is homogeneous, relatively dense, and ~ 300-500 A thick. The endothelium appears to be a continuous sheet of cells without visible pores. A substance leaving the capillaries in the CNS has, therefore, to traverse not only the capillary endothelium itself, but also the membranes of glial cells in order to gain access to the interstitial fluid. The composition of this fluid differs strikingly from that of interstitial fluid elsewhere by the nearly complete absence of protein; there are also some differences in the ionic composition. Because of being surrounded by this cellular sheath the permeability characteristics of brain capillaries are rather like those of cell membranes than like capillaries elsewhere in the body. This cellular sheath impedes the passage of ionized or nonionized water-soluble

TABLE I. Regional Cerebral Blood Flow in the Conscious Animal[a]

	Cat^b (n = 6)	Rat^c (n = 15)
Cortex		
Frontal		0.92 ± 0.06
Sensori-motor	1.09 ± 0.04	
Auditory	1.22 ± 0.11	
Parietal		0.89 ± 0.06
Visual	1.17 ± 0.04	
Occipital		0.92 ± 0.05
Misscellaneous-association	0.81 ± 0.05	
Olfactory	0.74 ± 0.05	0.77 ± 0.06
White matter	0.21 ± 0.01	
Deep cerebral structures		
Medial geniculate body	1.43 ± 0.11	
Lateral geniculate body	1.64 ± 0.14	
Basal ganglia		0.79 ± 0.05
Caudate nucleus	1.02 ± 0.07	
Thalamus	1.06 ± 0.07	
Hypothalamus	0.68 ± 0.06	0.78 ± 0.05
Amygdala	0.54 ± 0.03	
Hippocampus	0.62 ± 0.04	0.68 ± 0.04
Optic tract	0.20 ± 0.01	
Midbrain		0.81 ± 0.04
Inferior colliculus	1.74 ± 0.08	
Superior colliculus	1.10 ± 0.16	
Pons and medulla		0.81 ± 0.04
Superior olive	1.08 ± 0.07	
Inferior olive	0.75 ± 0.03	
Reticular formation	0.65 ± 0.03	
Vestibular nuclei	0.92 ± 0.03	
Cochlear nuclei	0.95 ± 0.11	
Pyramid	0.22 ± 0.02	
Cerebellum		0.70 ± 0.04
Nuclei	0.84 ± 0.03	
Cortex	0.83 ± 0.03	
White matter	0.24 ± 0.01	

[a]Values are mean ± S.E. in ml/min/gm.
[b]Reivich *et al.* (1968).
[c]Goldman and Sapirstein (1969).

substances unless they are quite small and accounts for the "blood-brain barrier." Lipid-soluble compounds do, however, enter the brain easily and rapidly. The blood-brain barrier would, therefore, represent a quantitative rather than a qualitative difference in capillary permeability as compared with other tissues. Hormones that act upon the CNS after systemic administration must obviously have a suitable combination of those properties that confer ready penetration, namely, low ionization at plasma pH, low binding to plasma protein, and fairly high lipid/water partition coefficient (Rall and Zubrod, 1962). For example, norepinephrine (NE) is practically unable to enter the brain when administered intravenously; but its precursor, L-dopa, passes readily into brain tissue, where it is converted to NE.

   b. Cerebrospinal Fluid. The CSF which fills the cerebral ventricles and surrounds the CNS in the subarachnoid spaces has aroused the interest of investigators for many years. Yet the functions of this fluid are still unknown. The introduction of various substances into the ventricular lumen has become a popular technique in neuroendocrinology and neuropharmacology, particularly following refinements by Feldberg and his associates (Feldberg and Sherwood, 1953; Carmichael *et al.,* 1964). Not only does this approach provide direct access to the brain of substances otherwise excluded from this tissue when administered via the general circulation, but it has been shown that many compounds, when reaching the brain via the CSF spaces, have powerful actions which often bear no relation to those the same substances produced when reaching the brain via the bloodstream (Feldberg and Fleischauer, 1965). Evidence suggests that the uptake of substances from the CSF by the nervous tissue must be regarded as an active transport across the ependymal borders of the ventricles, possibly mediated by metabolically active glial cells. Feldberg (1963), in fact, proposes that the regional differences in uptake by gray matter may be due to regional differences in distribution of the various types of neuroglia cells.It may be of interest to point out here that, although both the pineal and the pituitary gland can take up substances circulating in the bloodstream, only the pineal body is apparently able to take up substances after intraventricular administration.

   c. Entry of Hormones into the Central Nervous System. Considerable information concerning the site of action of hormones in the CNS is derived from work using hormone implants and is consistent with the notion that these implants act directly upon a discrete neurological mechanism. But for this to have any physiological significance, it is necessary to know that a particular hormone can cross the blood-brain barrier and thereby reach and gain entry to its specific site of action from the general circulation.

   Most of this information has been obtained using measurements of uptake and metabolism of labeled hormones whenever such material with high specific activity has been available. Extensive work on the uptake, distribution and metabolism of radioactive epinephrine after intravenous or intraventricular administration has been reported in the literature and will be dealt with in depth in Chapter 8. Studies on the uptake of ^{3}H-epinephrine and ^{3}H-nonepinephrine have revealed preferential uptake by the pituitary and median eminence regions, decreasing considerably in the remaining hypothalamus (Axelrod *et al.*, 1959; Weil-Malherbe *et al.*, 1961; Samorajski and Marks, 1962). Access to other brain areas is limited by the blood-brain barrier except in the immature animal (Spooner *et al.*, 1968). It appears that the rate of development of the blood-brain barrier differs for different substances.

The administration of radioactive 1-thyroxine results in a higher uptake of radioactivity in the hypothalamus than in the remaining CNS (Jensen and Clark, 1951). Of interest is the observation that, following the administration of radioactive 1-thyroxine the isotope concentration was higher in the neuro-hypophysis than in the adenohypophysis. The pattern of uptake described for nonsteroidal hormones is also followed by most steroids.

Recent studies of uptake and distribution of ^{3}H-testosterone in immature rats showed differential distribution in various areas of the CNS. The order of preference was as follows: olfactory bulbs were the highest, followed by lower spinal cord, posterior hypothalamus, anterior hypothalamus, upper spinal cord, cerebral cortex, and remaining brain (Woolley *et al.*, 1969a). However, Sherratt *et al.* (1969) failed to show any preferential uptake of testosterone by the hypothalamus of 4-day-old female rats.

Similar findings have been reported in studies with ^{3}H-estradiol (Woolley *et al.*, 1969b) in rats, the order of preference being: brain stem, hypothalamus, septum, and cerebral cortex. Using radioautographic techniques, Michael (1962, 1965) reported on the distribution of tritiated hexestrol injected subcutaneously into ovariectomized cats. His data indicate a bilaterally symmetrical, estrogen-sensitive, neurological system involving the lateral spetal area, preoptic region, and hypothalamus (Michael, 1965), accumulating estrogens selectively without prior metabolic modification (Glascock and Michael, 1962), with higher radioactivity than the blood up to 24-26 hours after administration. All other brain areas studied, including thalamus, midbrain, caudate nucleus, and cerebral cortex, showed low uptake within 2 hours of injection and rapidly lost radioactivity thereafter. The radioactivity in the hypothalamic neurons that take it up selectively appears to be associated with both cellular and nuclear membranes. The distribution of estrogens in the brain cannot be accounted for solely on the basis of differential permeability, since there is no evidence of localization in other areas of known high blood-brain permeability, such as the area postrema. Similarly, Waelsch (1955) has shown that the uptake is equally specific and localized in neonatal animals in which the blood-brain barrier is supposedly not fully developed.

As in the case of the uterus, investigations have also suggested that "receptors" exist in the brain which specifically accumulate and bind estradiol (Kato and Villee, 1967; Eisenfeld and Axelrod, 1967). It has also been inferred that these brain hormone receptors have characteristics similar to those found in the uterus. The evidence for such a conclusion, however, is not convincing. Comparisons of the uptake and retention of ^{3}H-estradiol between brain and uterus indicate that these structures respond differently to the hormone. Radioactivity increases or remains stable for at least 1 hour in the uterus, but declines rapidly in brain during that period (Green *et al.*, 1969; Eisenfeld, 1967). Comparing the affinity of uterine and hypothalamic tissue to ^{3}H-estradiol in rats under various conditions, McGuire and Lisk (1968) reported great similarity in the response of brain and uterus to estradiol, whereas Whalen and Maurer (1969) concluded that the two organs behaved quite differently. In the latter study, significant variations in radioactivity level occurring in the uterus as a function of the estrous cycle were not evident in brain, nor did ovariectomy decrease the brain's affinity for estrogen.

Autoradiographic evidence does indicate that estradiol is accumulated and retained by brain (Stumpf, 1968; Pfaff, 1968). Estradiol "receptors" have been described in hypothalamic cytoplasm (Kahwanago *et al.*, 1969) by comparing representative sedimentation patterns of radioactivity. No binding of ^{3}H-progesterone or ^{3}H-testosterone by these receptors was observed nor was there any difference between the sexes in the binding of these steroids. Indications that estradiol receptors were localized in nuclear fractions came from the work of King and Gordon (1967) in which ^{3}H-estradiol bound to a nuclear component of pituitary glands was released by treatment with trypsin. Stumpf's (1968) elegant work has supported this view and McEwen and Zigmond (1969) have recently reported that highly purified cell nuclei isolated from the preoptic area and the hypothalamus retained a great proportion of the radioactive estradiol found in the entire structure.

Controversy about brain corticosteroid receptors also exists: uptake, distribution, and retention varying with different steroids. Eik-Nes and Brizzee (1965) have shown that tritiated cortisol can penetrate into the brain tissue from the bloodstream of normal dogs. The steroid was taken up preferentially by several hypothalamic nuclei rather than the cortex cerebri. Also, the neurohypophysis took up more label than the adenohypophysis. This was true whether the administration was intravenous or intraventricular. Furthermore, the concentration of radioactivity in the hypothalamic nuclei and the blood plasma was high at 15 minutes after intravenous ^{3}H-cortisol administration and remained high for the following 24 hours, suggesting that these nuclei rapidly concentrate cortisol and do not readily exchange this steroid with surrounding fluid. Uptake was not preferential to any particular hypothalamic nucleus suggesting a more diffuse site of action throughout the hypothalamus. Pretreatment of dogs with β-methasone to reduce circulating 17-hydroxycorticosteroids (17-OHCS) resulted in a lower distribution of radioactivity in the supraoptic and ventromedial nuclei and a higher distribution in the lateral hypothalamic nucleus and in the median eminence than found in normal dogs with measurable levels of plasma 17-OHCS. Dogs with elevated circulating 17-OHCS showed no difference in percent distribution of radioactivity, except for a relatively high concentration in the anterior pituitary. In addition, anterior and posterior pituitaries, median eminence and supraoptic nucleus area, and cerebral cortex and mammillary body from adult rat (Grosser and Bliss, 1963; Peterson et al., 1965; Sholiton et al., 1965), dog (Eik-Nes and Brizzee, 1965), and mouse (Grosser, 1966) could convert cortisol to cortisone in vitro. Similarly, conversion of cortisol to cortisone by minces of cerebellum, thalamus-hypothalamus, brain stem, and cortex obtained from fetal, newborn and adult baboons has been reported by Grosser and Axelrod (1968). Highest 11-hydroxysteroid dehydrogenase activity was found in the cerebellum of the third trimester brain. The existence of a cortisol-21-O-acetyltransferase has also been reported with widespread distribution in various areas of primate (Purdy and Axelrod, 1968a,b; Purdy et al., 1968) and neonatal rat brain (Grosser and Axelrod, 1967).

The recent work of McEwen and his associates (McEwen et al., 1968, 1969a) would seem to indicate that the uptake and concentration of corticosterone by rat brain structures differs from that of cortisol. Their findings point to the existence of two simultaneous uptake processes for corticosterone: a nonspecific entry of the steroid into all parts of the brain showing increasing uptake with rising blood levels of the hormone; and, a limited capacity retention of the hormone in the hippocampus and septum of adrenalectomized rats. Radioactive corticosterone uptake and retention by the septum occurs also in normal rats as does estradiol, testosterone, hydrocortisone, and aldosterone (McEwen et al., 1969b). On the other hand, the steroid is not accumulated selectively by the hippocampus of normal rats. Pretreatment of adrenalectomized rats with hydrocortisone or dexamethasone reduced corticosterone uptake in the hippocampus and to a lesser extent in the septum. The onset of the increase in binding capacity in the hippocampus after adrenalectomy is very rapid, being apparent 2 hours after the operation and reaching its maximum about 20 hours after adrenalectomy. This time course is strongly reminiscent of the increased sensitivity to the stress-induced secretion of ACTH that occurs after removal of the adrenals (Hodges and Vernikos, 1959; Hodges et al., 1962). The hippocampus and septum have been postulated to exert an inhibitory influence on pituitary ACTH secretion (Dallman and Yates, 1967; Mangili et al., 1966). It is tempting to suggest that in the absence of the adrenals, pituitary ACTH secretion is enhanced because steroids facilitate the activity of the septum and the hippocampus. McEwen has also provided some evidence for the intracellular site of action of bound corticosterone. They found that highly purified cell nuclei isolated from the hippocampus retain up to 50% of the radioactive material present in the entire structure (McEwen et al., 1969a).

IV. EFFECTS OF HORMONES ON BRAIN FUNCTIONS

A. Taste, Smell, and Hearing

Henkin and his associates (Henkin and Bartter, 1966; Henkin and Solomon, 1962; Henkin *et al.*, 1963, 1967) have reported a considerable number of clinical observations on the effects of changes in adrenocortical and gonadal function on thresholds for taste, smell, and hearing. They report that patients with adrenocortical insufficiency had decreased thresholds for salt, sweet, bitter, and sour, and that their taste perception was approximately 100 times more accurate than that of normal subjects. Treatment with DOC for 2-7 days did not change the taste threshold but prednisolone for 18-36 hours returned this threshold to normal. When prednisolone treatment was stopped, increased taste sensitivity did not return for 3-4 days, hence, the authors point out that changes in extracellular sodium or potassium concentration or in extracellular fluid volume could not account for the prednisolone effect. Prednisolone had no effect on the taste threshold in normal subjects. However, these subjects showed a diurnal variation in taste threshold, with greatest sensitivity in the afternoon and lowest in the early morning hours, when plasma 17-OHCS are highest.

Using galvanic current as well as sodium chloride, Kosowicz and Proszewicz (1967) have reported that patients with adrenocortical insufficiency recognize the taste sensation of galvanic current at lower intensity than the most sensitive of normal subjects. Also, in patients with chromatin-negative gonadal dysgenesis, Henkin (1967) observed that, although the median detection and recognition thresholds for salt and sweet were normal, those for sour and bitter were increased above normal.

Studying olfaction, in these same subjects, he found that the median detection and recognition thresholds for vapors of pyridine, thiophene, and nitrobenzene were all increased above normal. Treatment with gonadal steroids sufficient to induce secondary sexual characteristics did not return either taste or smell sensitivity to normal. Henkin suggested the possibility of a genetic neurophysiological abnormality in the dysfunction of olfaction, since mothers of these patients showed a similar olfactory abnormality. Similarly, in Addison's disease, Henkin and Bartter (1966) have reported the olfactory threshold is approximately 100,000 times more acute than in normal subjects. Administration of DOC had no effect but prednisolone returned the olfactory threshold to normal. As with taste, when prednisolone treatment ceased, the increased olfactory sensitivity did not reappear for 5-7 days. It should be pointed out here that assessment of olfactory thresholds are greatly dependent on the techniques and equipment used and the extent to which the air and control materials are "odorless."

Investigating the hearing disturbance in patients with Addison's disease, Henkin et al. (1967) observed that these patients' auditory sensitivity was more acute than that of normal subjects over most of the frequencies tested and especially in the region of greatest hearing sensitivity of normal subjects, i.e., 1000-3000 Hz. DOC treatment did not alter auditory detection thresholds but prednisolone or other glucocorticoids returned auditory detection thresholds to normal in all patients. The effects of removal and replacement of glucocorticoids on hearing were qualitatively the same irrespective of differences in the auditory system with age (Nixon et al., 1962). Henkin et al. (1966) points out that, although there was an increase in auditory acuity in patients with Addison's disease, they also showed decreased average word discrimination and three times the normal for judgments of equal loudness, while axonal velocity increased by more than 25%. It would appear that when glucocorticoids are absent from the CNS, the normal time pattern of sensory signal transmission is altered, resulting in a loss of information. Thus, although detection thresholds are improved with treatment, integrative functions are worse. In fact, Henkin and Daly (1968) reported recently that increased auditory detection sensitivity and decreased perceptual ability are dependent on the absence of glucocorticoids; replacement therapy with these steroids restores these parameters to normal.

B. Pain

Luft and Olivecrona (1955) noted an incidental and unexpectedly great reduction in or abolition of the pain in 19 of 24 women treated by total hypophysectomy for advanced cancer of the breast. The relief of pain occurred promptly after the operation and was not due to cortisone since it continued when the drug was stopped. It has not been correlated with subsidence of tumor and has occurred both in patients who did and in those who did not show objective evidence of remission. These observations open for consideration the possibility that endocrine potentiation of nervous function is implicated in the full development of pain and open to question the effects of hormones on behavior by assessment of avoidance of pain-involving procedures.

C. Posture and Locomotion

It has been suggested that circulating endocrine secretions affect general motor activity (Beach, 1948) indicating that they may enter into facilitation of postural behavior. Stimulation of the reticular formation through the direct action of epinephrine (E), for example, could provide such an action (Dell et al., 1954). A central action of progesterone has been postulated to explain the decreased tonus and electromyographic activity of abdominal muscles during pregnancy (Kawakami, 1954; Takano, 1956) or following the administration of this hormone (Kawakami, 1954, 1955). This action would favor development of the compensatory lordosis of pregnancy.

D. Body Temperature Regulation

Since changes in body temperature, just as changes in general metabolism may affect behavior, a summary of the known effects of hormones on body temperature is in order at this point. A number of observations indicate that a close relationship exists between the temperature-regulating mechanisms and the endocrine system.

An interesting example of changes in human temperature regulation occurring simultaneously with endocrine changes is the slight but relatively long-standing rise in body temperature which appears in women at the time of ovulation (Bazett, 1959). The 5β-OH steroid hormone metabolites, etiocholanolone, pregnenolone, and 11-ketopregnenolone, raise body temperature in humans. However, the fever-producing action of these steroid metabolites appears to be highly species-specific (Palmer *et al.*, 1961).

When a skin area is cooled, a reflexly induced activation of the adrenal medullae results in increased secretion of catecholamines (CA) (Ekstrom *et al.*, 1943). Intravenously administered E has a significant calorigenic (glycolytic) effect and has, therefore, been suggested to play a role in temperature regulation; its quantitative importance is, however, debatable (Lundholm, 1949). E and NE also constrict skin arterioles, which would be an additional thermoregulatory effect, but the adrenal humoral control of peripheral vessels is quantitatively unimportant in comparison with their nervous vasoconstrictor control (Celander, 1954; Folkow, 1955). The adrenal medullae are under hypothalamic control and Feldberg (1963) has demonstrated the importance of hypothalamic amines in temperature regulation but the possible coordination between adrenomedullary activity and the thermoregulatory effect or systems is not well known (Chatonnet, 1955).

Removal of the thyroid gland (Issekutz, 1937; Pitchotka *et al.*, 1953), the adrenals or the pituitary (Bonvallet and Dell, 1946; Schaeffer and Thibault, 1946) influences temperature regulation, reducing resistance to body cooling and the intensity of the fever response to pyrogens (Gellhorn and Feldman, 1941). This fact does not necessarily imply that these endocrine glands take part in short-term temperature regulation in the intact animal. The endocrine organ ablation effects might be attributed to a gradually altered reactivity of thermoregulatory effect on organs, such as the blood vessels, to their normal mode of control. However, exposure of rabbits to cold is known to evoke within a few hours an increase in thyroxine secretion (Brown-Grant *et al.*, 1954). After a further latency, the metabolic rate of the body responds by an increase. This

thyroid-activating effect of acute cold exposure is mediated by the hypo-
thalamohypophysial system (Von Euler and Holmgren, 1956). Local heating of
the anterior hypothalamus is reported to decrease the blood flow through the
thyroid gland (Söderberg, 1956) and cooling of the preoptic area in the goat
results in activation of the thyroid gland (Anderson et al., 1962).

A relatively immediate effect on temperature regulation seems to be exerted
by ACTH. Douglas and Paton (1952) showed that the intravenous injection of
1 U ACTH/kg in rabbits induced a decrease of approximately 1.4°C in rectal
temperature within 1 hour. The temperature remained depressed for another
hour and gradually returned to normal within 3 hours of injection. ACTH was
also effective in counteracting pyrogen fever. In contrast 0.1 U/kg of posterior
pituitary extract had no effect on body temperature. Is the hypothermic effect
of ACTH mediated by the adrenal cortex? Clinical and laboratory studies have
revealed that corticosteroids, when injected before or together with pyrogen,
prevent or modify the rise in body temperature (Atkins et al., 1955; Spink,
1957). Evidence that this action of corticosteroids is on the CNS came from
experiments that showed that the injection of plasma from pyrogen-cortisone-
treated dogs, in which no rise in body temperature was observed, caused a rise in
body temperature in the recipient dogs (Atkins et al., 1955; Petersdorf et al.,
1957). Furthermore, the direct injection of hydrocortisone into the preoptic
region of rabbits, partially prevented the pyrogen-induced rise in body
temperature (Chowers et al., 1968). Hydrocortisone was much less effective
when injected intravenously or in other loci of the CNS including the corpus
callosum, the caudate nuclei, and the anteriomedian nuclei of the thalamus. In
contrast to the intravenous effect of ACTH, cortisol did not appear to depress
body temperature significantly. Therefore, the hypothermic mechanism of
action of ACTH becomes of interest particularly in view of the extraadrenal
effects of ACTH, including Martini's short-loop theories (Martini et al., 1968;
Mess and Martini, 1968) and the behavioral effects of ACTH, melanocyte-
stimulating hormone (MSH), and short peptide moieties of the ACTH molecule
(De Wied, 1965, 1966; De Wied and Bohus, 1966; Koranyi and Endroczi, 1967).

The effects of peptide hormones in thermoregulation may have been
overlooked as had been their extraendocrine target organ effects. The recent
observation of Thoman et al. (1968) that Nembutal anesthesia did not depress
the body temperature of lactating rats may provide indirect evidence for a role
of prolactin in temperature control. The effects of hormones on body
temperature have been inadequately explored.

E. The Biological Clock

The results of numerous experiments and observations indicate that
important functions of the body are regulated not only by homeostatic

mechanisms, but by even more primitive mechanisms. These regulate with remarkable consistency recurring rhythmic biological and behavioral events of varying periods. Ovulation and the menstrual and estrual cycles are obvious examples. However, only 24-hour, or circadian, rhythms will be briefly mentioned here.

The putative "biological clock" mechanisms are relatively unaffected by most internal and external influences with the exception of light. Richter (1960) postulates a central clock located in the hypothalamus regulating circadian and also indirectly the 48-hour rhythm of mental illnesses. Menninger-Leichental (1960) suggests the diencephalon controls these periodic rhythmic processes. Wurtman and Anton-Tay (1969) have recently proposed that the pineal gland of mammals serves as a transducer receiving light and darkness signals from the environment and delivering time signals to centers in the brain that mediate and synchronize other rhythms. Some evidence does exist that some form of biological clock or pacemaker is inherent to cells controlling the rate of their activities (von Mayersbach, 1967). Hence the function of the central clock would be more consistent with that of an integrator, responsible for the coordination, synchronization, or merely modulation of the multitude of oscillating processes within the body ensuring that their rate of activity will be maintained within limits. Biological clock research in animals and man during the past 40 years has indicated a number of timing devices that exert a definite control over the endocrine glands but which differ from the normal neuro-endocrine regulatory pathways and which, therefore, show differential sensitivity to target organ feedback inhibition. For example, frontal deafferentation of the hypothalamus abolishes pituitary-adrenocortical rhythmicity but does not affect the stress response (Halasz et al., 1967); small doses of dexamethasone that do not block the stress response inhibit the afternoon rise in plasma steroids in rats (Zimmerman and Critchlow, 1967) and the inhibition of this diurnal steroid rhythm following cessation of intake of dexamethasone in drinking water in rats far outlasts that of the stress response (Hodges and Smidgley, 1969). However, malfunction of the endocrine system often coincides with malfunction of the CNS oscillations and therefore may result in mental disorders of various types. Jenner (1968) has admirably reviewed the relevance of biological rhythm research findings on periodic psychoses and the relationship of various endocrine changes to these. It would appear that endocrinopathies cannot be conceived as causative in these cases since the biological clock seems remarkably resistant. To bear this out, the following impressive list of metabolic, neurological, or endocrinological disturbances have been reported to be without effect on the "clock" as measured by the activity rhythm (Richter, 1960).

a. Metabolic. Starvation for 5-7 days; dehydration for 67 hours; restriction of vitamin B_1; total body irradiation.

b. Neurological. Prolonged anoxia; electroshock convulsions; caffeine ad-
minstration in the fourth ventricle; tranquillization with chlorpromazine; LSD or
alcohol intoxication; severe stress, such as forced swimming up to 42 hours.

c. Endocrinological. Gonadectomy, mating, pregnancy and lactation, adrenalectomy, total hypophysectomy, posterior lobectomy, pinealectomy, pan-
createctomy, and hyper- or hypothyroidism.

On the other hand, prolonged hypothermia and the restriction of water
intake (5-10 ml/day) have had some effect on the biological clock, either
resetting it, slowing it down, or stopping it. It is evident, however, that only by
studying the correlation between several parameters as affected by these
treatments can any definite conclusions be drawn about the biological clock.

It may be speculated that hormones may be useful only in restoring an
already disturbed "clock" mechanism or that their role here too is "permissive"
as has been suggested periodically for other processes. Whatever their functions,
more sophisticated neurophysiological, neuroendocrine, and pharmacological
techniques would contribute much to a more accurate description of the
biological clock mechanism which may play a cardinal role in the mechanism by
which hormones affect neural function as a whole.

F. Electrophysiological Effects of Hormones

1. Brain Excitability

Several steroid hormones including DOC, progesterone, and other adrenal
steroids have been demonstrated to have anesthetic effects in a number of
animals (Selye, 1941). Large doses of DOC and progesterone produced deep
anesthesia in rats undergoing prolonged abdominal operations. In man, progesterone has been reported to have a soporific effect in minimal anesthetic doses
(Merryman *et al.*, 1954). Similarly, compound S has been shown to elicit
sedation in moderate doses, with seizure activity following if the dose was
increased further (Heuser *et al.*, 1965).

A recent study by Gyermek *et al.*, (1967) has shown that the CNS
depressant effect of progesterone is greater than that of some short-acting
barbiturates, and that the related 5-β-pregnane derivatives were even more potent
in depressing arousal from reticular formation stimulation than hydroxydione.
However, anesthetic activity of these steroids can be dissociated from hormonal
activity by structural modification of the molecule (Figdor *et al.*, 1957).

On the other hand, an increased incidence of convulsive seizures has been
reported following administration of some hormones, as well as in various
clinical endocrine disorders (Woodbury and Vernadakis, 1967). Convulsions have
been produced in rabbits with high doses of ACTH (Pincus *et al.*, 1951) and
tonic-clonic convulsions in rats and cats have followed injections of high doses of

compound S (Heuser and Eidelberg, 1961). Similarly, in patients treated with ACTH and cortisone for collagen disease, generalized seizures have occurred (Wayne, 1954). In contrast to the seizure-enhancing effects of ACTH and cortisone in adults, these hormones appear to exert an anticonvulsant effect in infants with several types of seizure disorders (Millichap and Bickford, 1962). In peripheral nerves, single doses of DOC and corticosterone increase their excitability whereas large doses diminish it: cortisone, hydrocortisone, and compound S decrease nerve excitability (Chauchard, 1952; Lecor, 1954). All of these hormones increase excitability in both pre- and postganglionic fibers and ACTH diminishes somatic motor nerve excitability. The effect of ACTH on transmission at the neuromuscular junction has been studied in myasthenia (Torda and Wolff, 1949). In these subjects ACTH has been found to prevent the decline in muscle action potential amplitude evoked by repetitive indirect stimulation. However, in normal rats ACTH and cortisone did not alter the amplitude of muscle action potentials, suggesting that the action of these hormones is to improve neuromuscular transmission only when it is abnormal.

In studying the effects of hormones in relation to the changes they induce in the excitability of nervous tissues, the measurement of the minimal strength of electroshock needed to produce convulsions (EST) has provided a useful index. Use of this technique has demonstrated a relationship between excitability and thyroid function consistent with the behavioral manifestations of hyper- and hypofunction of the gland. Thus, in the rat, the threshold and duration of seizures are increased by thyroidectomy and reduced by giving thyroid hormone (Woodbury, 1954), triiodothyronine activity being several times greater than that of thyroxine (Timiras et al., 1955).

Excitability is markedly and differentially influenced by the sex hormones, most workers agreeing that estrogens have an excitatory and androgens an inhibitory effect. Thus, the EST of the female rat is lower than that of the male (Woolley et al., 1961a) and fluctuates with phases of the estrous cycle, reaching its lowest level at the time of ovulation (Woolley et al., 1961b). Moreover, the onset of susceptibility to electroshock is advanced when estradiol is given to newborn rats (Heim and Timiras, 1963). Studies with adrenocortical hormones have led to the conclusion that the effect of these hormones on brain excitability depends on changes in plasma electrolytes. In the adrenalectomized rat both plasma sodium and EST fall abruptly; both changes are reversed by administration of DOC (Davenport, 1949). The mechanisms underlying these effects on brain excitability as measured by EST are discussed more fully in Section V,B.

2. Electrical Activity and Sleep

Clinical and neuroendocrine studies have, for the greater part, provided most of the information and guidelines concerning the effects of hormones on brain electrical activity. Thus, the well-known target organ hormone feedback action is now believed to be exerted on the brain as well as on the pituitary gland (Mangılı *et al.,* 1966). Local stereotaxic implantation experiments have shown that adrenal and gonadal steroid "receptors" may be found in the basal hypothalamus (Barraclough and Cross, 1963; Davidson and Feldman, 1963; Smelik and Sawyer, 1962) and as remotely as the midbrain (Corbin *et al.,* 1965; Endroczi *et al.,* 1961), septum (Davidson and Feldman, 1963), or hippocampus (Slusher, 1966). Evidence for a direct effect of peptide hormones on the CNS has emerged in the past few years following the suggestion by the electrophysiological experiments of Sawyer and Kawakami (1959) that pituitary tropic hormones may exert an "internal" feedback action on the brain, bypassing the target organs. Such "short-loop" adenohypophyseal feedback controls have been described for all pituitary hormones by local implantation techniques (Martini *et al.,* 1968; Motta *et al.,* 1968) or implantation of pituitary tissue into the "hypophysiotropic" area of rat hypothalamus (Halasz and Szentagothai, 1960). With unit recording techniques Ramirez *et al.* (1967) and Kawakami and Saito (1967) found that luteinizing hormone (LH) exerted rather specific effects on discrete hypothalamic units in the rat and cat, respectively. Unfortunately, in animal experiments electrophysiological effects of hormones have generally been described as relating to neuroendocrine-regulating mechanisms and not to behavior, with the exception of the extensive and admirable work of Sawyer and his collaborators and disciples through the years, relating the electrophysiological effects of gonadotropins and gonadal steroids to sex behavior.

On the other hand, clinical observations have also yielded information on the effects of hormones on brain electrical activity that may be indirectly useful to the behavioral psychologist seeking a mechanism or site of action of a hormone that affects a particular form of behavior. Thus, it has long been known that Addisonian patients show seizure phenomena (Klippel, 1899) and a slowing of the frequency of the electroencephalogram (EEG) which can be restored by cortisone (Thorn, 1949; Thorn and Forsham, 1949).

Studying the effects of adrenocortical insufficiency on the EEG, Engel and Margolin (1942) described diffuse slow activity with frequencies of 2-6/sec and voltages higher than those of α waves and up to 75 mV. A rough correlation between changes in the EEG in Addison's disease and the blood sugar level was suggested. In their hands, glucose administration tended to prevent EEG alterations induced by hyperventilation in Addison's disease, although others could not find such a correlation and in some patients replacement therapy did not correct abnormalities in EEG (Hoffman *et al.,* 1942). No changes in cerebral blood flow and oxygen consumption were found in such patients (Woodbury, 1958). In fact, patients with Addison's with adequate blood volume, blood pressure, and electrolyte concentration may show abnormal EEG's (Hoffman *et al.,* 1942) and mental disturbances (Cleghorn, 1951). It would appear that the neurological, electrical, and mental disturbances are not necessarily related to the severity of the metabolic changes observed.

In a study of 14 cases of Klinefelter's syndrome, 12 pathological EEG patterns were found; in 4 of these a typical epileptic pattern with generalized spikes and slow waves or focal sharp waves was recorded (Dumerfurth, 1961). It has also been found that sufficient slowing of the EEG occurs in association with menstruation to convert a normal EEG to an abnormal one (Dusser de Barenne and Gibbs, 1942) and in the final weeks of pregnancy when progesterone levels are high, the EEG is slow compared to postpartum tracings. However, the postmenopausal EEG is not significantly altered by progesterone or stilbestrol (Cress and Greenblatt, 1945).

Insulin-induced hypoglycemia results in progressive decrease in α-wave frequency of the EEG which may be reversed if glucose is supplied (Hill, 1948). Thyrotoxicosis produces an abnormal EEG consisting of increased frequency of α rhythms, and hypothyroidism may show EEG's with an absence of α waves and a decrease in the amplitude of the other brain waves. In addition, Danowski et al. (1960) have observed calcification in the region of the basal ganglia often visible on skull x-rays of hypoparathyroid patients. The reason for these calcifications is not known and they do not regress following successful therapy of the hypoparathyroid condition. They suggest the finding is a reflection of long-standing hypocalcemia. EEG abnormalities may be present in the form of slow waves occurring 2-3 or 5-6/sec either singly or in series (enhanced by hyperventilation but unaffected by the parenteral administration of calcium) and an increase in the amount of fast activity and simple spikes. The correction of the hypoparathyroidal state results in the disappearance of the characteristic waves.

The changes in neurological and psychiatric manifestations in various endocrine diseases have been reviewed by Gabrilove (1966) and Relkin (1969).

Detailed physiological studies in experimental animals have provided a great deal of information for the effects of but a few hormones on brain electrical activity and most have been concerned with the reactions of subcortical structures.

Certain endocrine secretions have been shown to influence directly the activity of specific areas of the CNS. For example, Dell (1958) has shown the facilitatory effects of E upon the ascending reticular activating system. Dell et al. (1954) point out that the excitatory action of E upon the reticulocortical and reticulospinal system heightens considerably the level of activity of the whole somatic system. On the other hand, Sawyer (1958) has shown that the sexual hormones may lower the threshold of a response to electrical stimulation of the reticular formation.

In guinea pigs hormone-induced estrus was shown to be accompanied by a decrease in the amounts of both paradoxical and slow wave sleep (Malven and

Sawyer, 1966), while in the intact cat, large doses of estrogen produced no significant change in cortical electrical activity (Marcus et al., 1966).

Progesterone has been demonstrated to have an inhibitory influence on cerebrocortical electrical activity. Kawakami and Sawyer (1959) have found that a few hours after subcutaneous treatment with progesterone in the estrogen-primed rabbit, its threshold of EEG arousal on direct stimulation of the midbrain reticular formation is much reduced from its preprogesterone threshold. Twenty-four hours after progesterone treatment, when the rabbit is usually anestrus, its threshold of EEG arousal is markedly elevated. In addition, in the rat, pregnanediol has also been observed to cause an inhibitory modulation of the EEG (Arai et al., 1967).

Perhaps some of the most significant of findings in this field are those of Sawyer and Kawakami (1959) who showed that the behavioral "after-reaction" akin to paradoxical sleep, which follows coitus in the female rabbit is associated with changes in electrical activity which can also be elicited by giving LH but not follicle-stimulating hormone (FSH). Since the stimulus of coitus in the female rabbit operating through a neurohumoral pathway originating in the hypo-thalamus is known to induce the release of LH by the pituitary, these findings indicate that LH, in addition to causing ovulation, reacts back upon the CNS to cause behavioral and EEG changes which block further release of "ovulating hormones." Further work along similar lines (Kawakami and Sawyer, 1959) has shown that progesterone markedly elevates the threshold for the EEG manifestations of the after-reaction, is associated with a reluctance to accept the male and causes inhibition of the gonadotropic activity of the pituitary. Similar effects would also be expected during pregnancy when high blood levels of progesterone are maintained by the corpus luteum.

In an attempt to clarify the functional relationship between the anovulatory effect of progesterone and its central depressant action, progesterone was found not only to suppress the activity level of the posterior hypothalamus, but the limbic midbrain area as well (Kobayashi et al., 1962). During the estrous cycle, for instance, the activity of the hippocampus decreases during estrus (when estrogen levels are higher than progesterone) and increases during the postcoital stage and pregnancy (when the reverse hormonal pattern occurs), while the excitability of the amygdala increases at estrus and decreases in postcoital and pregnant stages. The same relationship is reported (Kawakami et al., 1966) in alterations of the amplitude and latency of evoked potentials recorded from the periventricular arcuate nucleus in the hypothalamus of rabbits by stimulation of the hippocampus and amygdala. The authors point out that an inverse relationship of excitability exists between the hippocampus and the amygdala at the estrous and postestrous stages. After injection of progesterone the arcuate nucleus potential evoked by stimulation of the hippocampus was facilitated, whereas the arcuate potential evoked by stimulation of the amygdala was inhibited. LH injection facilitated both negative and positive components of this potential evoked by hippocampal stimulation and inhibited both components evoked by amygdaloid stimulation. Since electrical stimulation of the hippocampus resulted in increased progesterone synthesis and secretion, Kawakami *et al.*, (1967) suggested that the hippocampus is the critical area of positive feedback control and the medial amygdaloid complex of negative feedback control of progesterone.

Considerably less is known about the mechanism of action of androgens on neural tissue. Although it has been generally assumed that gonadal hormones have little direct influence on central neural tissue outside of certain areas of the forebrain, Hart (1967) found that testosterone administration influenced quantitatively the sexual reflexes of castrated spinal male rats. Hart and Haugen (1968) further reported that testosterone implanted into the spinal canal near spinal neurons which mediate sexual reflexes had a facilitatory influence on such reflexes suggesting a direct effect on spinal neural tissue.

On the other hand, it has been suggested that elevated levels of androgens exert a protective effect against increased brain excitability since patients with the adrenogenital syndrome are quite resistant to even large doses of cortisone (Woodbury, 1954).

The relationship between effects of gonadal hormones on the CNS and reproductive behavior have been admirably reviewed by Beyer and Sawyer (1969).

Several other hormones have been shown to cause changes in brain electrical activity. Both in rats and man large doses of insulin are thought to be due to the hypoglycemia since the EEG changes may be reversed if glucose is supplied (Hill, 1948). It may be of interest that, peripherally, insulin has been reported, in the cat, to be involved in the mechanism of normal transmission of the superior cervical ganglion (Minker and Koltai, 1965).

Slowing of the α frequency has been reported in the EEG of hypothyroid subjects. In rats, thyroidectomy was first thought not to affect spontaneous brain electrical activity despite decreased basal metabolic rate (Lee and Van Buskirk, 1928). Later investigations showed that thyroidectomy depressed both spontaneous activity and the metabolic rate; dinitrophenol restored the basal metabolic rate to normal but did not correct the spontaneous activity (Hall and Lindsay, 1938) suggesting that the effects of thyroid hormone on the CNS are independent of its effect on the general metabolism of the animal. In an experiment in which EEG's were taken from animals which had been thyroidectomized neonatally, there was a reduction in frequency and voltage (Bradley *et al.*, 1960) and the capacity of the cortex to "block" in response to auditory stimuli or to "follow" the frequency of photic stimulation was either delayed in appearance or absent. Since axonal and dendritic hypoplasia in the sensorimotor cortex occurs (Eayrs, 1955) under these conditions, the failure of sensory input to synchronize or desynchronize cortical rhythms may be equated with afferent axonal hypoplasia. Other work prompted the suggestion that the prolonged duration of electrocortical potentials was related primarily to metabolic factors and the decreased amplitude primarily to the processes of growth and maturation. This hypothesis was based on the observation that alterations in the former could be rectified by thyroid hormone administration, but the latter could not (Bradley *et al.*, 1964). Since it appears that the origin of the slow potentials associated with electrocortical activity depends on the summation of postsynaptic dendritic potentials (Clare and Bishop, 1955), Eayrs (1964) postulated that the reduced amplitude of recordings in animals having had neonatal thyroidectomy, but not in those having had thyroidectomy when mature, may be attributable to a comparable reduction in the probability of axodendritic interaction as originating and maintaining these potentials. Further evidence of changes in brain electrical activity was obtained in rats in which hypothyroidism was shown to delay the development of the evoked transcallosal response, whereas hyperthyroidism accelerated it (Hatotani and Timiras, 1967).

It may be of interest also that, peripherally, partial or complete absence of thyroid hormone may interfere with transmission of stimuli in the inferior mesenteric ganglion (Babichev, 1964). Actually, it is reported (Babichev, 1965) that, depending on the concentration, circulating thyroxine may either facilitate or inhibit conduction in sympathetic ganglia. As the concentration of thyroxine increases, the primary change was in the properties of presynaptic endings.

Melatonin, the only known principle of the pineal gland, has been reported to have acute effects on sleep mechanisms (Barchas *et al.*, 1967). It increased by 50% the hexobarbital sleeping time in mice and induced sleep for about 45 minutes following intravenous administration in 4-day-old chicks in which the blood-brain barrier is relatively undeveloped. Similarly, Marczynski *et al.* (1964) found that crystalline melatonin injected through steel cannulae implanted directly into areas of the hypothalamus of cats caused sleep lasting about 2 hours.

A recent study (Nir *et al.*, 1969) has also shown that pinealectomy in female rats results in changes in cerebrocortical electrical activity characterized by intermittent general paroxysmal outbursts of slow waves with high amplitudes of centrocephalic origin. These seizurelike discharges occur against a background of basic electrical activity of permanent symmetrical monomorphic and mono-rhythmic waves of 9-12 Hz. The authors suggest that the cortical hyperactivity of the pinealectomized rat may be due to an indirect effect mediated by the gonads (high estrogen levels of permanent estrus) rather than a direct effect of the pineal hormones on the CNS. On the other hand, pineal extract has been found to suppress electrically induced seizures in the cerebral cortex (Roldan and Anton-Tay, 1968). MSH has also been implicated in producing hyper-excitability in mice (Sakamoto, 1966). Kastin *et al.* (1968) have described

similar anxiety, nervousness, and motor restlessness in 3 out of 6 subjects
receiving infusions of MSH, and consider these symptoms to resemble akathisia,
a term used to describe such symptoms in extrapyramidal disease (Ayd, 1961),
while Cotzias *et al.* (1967) found that larger doses of MSH aggravated
Parkinson's disease. Kastin *et al.* pointed out that these investigators implied that
the extrapyramidal symptoms seen in some patients on tranquillizing drugs may
result from an abnormality in the mechanism controlling the release of MSH
from the pituitary gland. This is supported by the observation in animals that
tranquillizers do indeed release pituitary MSH (Kastin and Schally, 1966). It is
also of interest that Kastin *et al.* (1968) found a significant decrease in serum
calcium following MSH infusion. Similar decrease in serum calcium induced by
MSH has also been described in rabbits (Friesen, 1964; Dyster-Aas, 1965).
Patients with hypocalcemia seem to be more sensitive to extrapyramidal
symptoms induced by tranquillizing drugs (Schaaf and Payne, 1966; Lichtigfeld
and Simpson, 1967). Kastin *et al.* (1968) suggest the intriguing concept that the
decline in serum calcium induced by MSH is responsible for the increase in
responsiveness of the CNS to MSH. Hypocalcemia is indeed generally considered
to be responsible for the psychic and neurological alterations in hypoparathy-
roidism, which include emotional lability, anxiety, irritability, and delirium.

Clinical observations on the increased excitability of the CNS during
adrenocortical therapy are corroborated by animal experiments. As discussed
previously, it has been demonstrated by the EST technique in rats, that
cortisone and hydrocortisone markedly increased brain excitability and that the
DOCA-elevated seizure threshold could be lowered by ACTH, cortisone,
hydrocortisone, and adrenocortical extract (Woodbury, 1954). In dogs, cortisone and ACTH decreased the threshold for seizures and increased the incidence
of convulsions produced by electrical stimulation of the cerebral cortex
(Pasolini, 1952), and in rats ACTH and cortisone were found to increase the
sensitivity to Metrazol (Torda and Wolff, 1951). Other work has shown that
glucocorticoids exert marked effects on the brain stem of cats. Feldman *et al.*
(1961) observed an increase in the amplitude of evoked potentials in cats a few
minutes after the injection of ACTH, suggesting that the effect of ACTH may be
attributed to the secondary secretion of hydrocortisone. The effect of
adrenocortical hormones upon evoked potentials is very apparent in the
mesencephalic reticular formation, the hypothalamus, and the intralaminar
nuclei of the thalamus, with much less effect upon the specific sensory
pathways. Feldman *et al.* propose that this effect on "evoked potentials at the
brain stem level suggests that these hormones do not have their primary effect
on conduction of impulses in the laterally placed sensory pathways but rather
upon the multisynaptic systems of neurons extending through the central part of
the midbrain and diencephalon." These areas are known to be involved in
mechanisms of consciousness (Magoun, 1952), mental stability (Adey, 1956),

visceral and endocrine regulation (Harris, 1955; Anderson *et al.*, 1957), as well as regulation of the electrical activity of the brain in the normal state and in centrencephalic epilepsy (Penfield and Jasper, 1954). Increase in the amplitude of the evoked potentials suggests lowering of the threshold for synaptic transmission and consequently involvement of more individual units in the response. Changes in the level of circulating hydrocortisone have been reported to modify spontaneous electrical activity as well as single-cell firing in the hypothalamus (Feldman, 1962; Feldman and Davidson, 1966; Feldman and Dafny, 1966). It is of interest that, although there was a short delay between the administration of hydrocortisone and increase in the amplitude of the evoked potentials (5-15 minutes), the effect persisted for 2-3 hours. The authors (Feldman *et al.*, 1961) attribute this in part to changes in intracellular electrolytes and γ-aminobutyric acid (GABA) concentration in brain as suggested by Woodbury (1958).

The opposite effect on brain electrical activity is seen in the hypoadrenal state. This is characterized by a generalized slowing in electrical activity in the cortex as well as in subcortical structures (Bergen, 1951). The conduction time of somatosensory impulses and neuronal recovery are prolonged in the polysynaptic pathways of the midbrain reticular formation and the anterior hypothalamus, but not in the medial lemniscus (Feldman and Robinson, 1968). The involvement of polysynaptic pathways in hypoadrenalism is also indicated by the experiments of Cook *et al.* (1960) and Chambers *et al.* (1963) studying blockage of the EEG arousal response and the conduction from the midbrain to the cortex in adrenalectomized cats. Furthermore, adrenalectomized rats are particularly sensitive to anesthetics and smaller amounts of pentobarbital are required to abolish the evoked potentials in the reticular formation and anterior hypothalamus of these animals as compared to intact rats. It is of interest that in a study of the changes in the electrical activity of the brain of rats implanted chronically with cortical and subcortical electrodes decrease in wave frequency with time after adrenalectomy reached its lowest at about 7 days. Since the hypothalamus is considered the site of action through which corticosteroids inhibit ACTH secretion (Davidson and Feldman, 1963; Vernikos-Danellis, 1964), it is of interest that the slowing in wave frequency corresponds to the changes in circulating ACTH and the increase corticotropin-releasing factor (CRF) content of the ME following adrenalectomy (Vernikos-Danellis, 1965). The electrophysiological effects of hypo- and hyperadrenal corticism on the brain have been admirably reviewed by Feldman (1968).

Although it would appear from the above discussion that the effects of ACTH on brain electrical activity are mediated entirely by adrenocortical secretions, there is increasing evidence that certain polypeptide hormones including ACTH, α-MSH, and β-MSH play a role in the nervous system as "modulators of nervous activity" (Krivoy *et al.*, 1963). Reviewing and studying the effects of these and related peptides on the spinal cord, Krivoy (1969) has collected evidence indicating a stimulant action that is independent of the adrenal. It appears that these three peptides act on spinal cord to alter synaptic transmission by a facilitation of normally active pathways so that transmission through these pathways occurs more readily. This action is antagonized by anticholinergic drugs such as atropine and by chlorpromazine and phenobarbital. A long latent period (about 1 hour) precedes the action of these peptides following intracisternal administration whether the action recorded is facilitation of the ventral root response to dorsal root stimulation (Nicolov, 1967; Guillemin and Krivoy, 1960; Krivoy and Guillemin, 1961) or the characteristic "stretching crisis" described by Ferrari *et al.* (1955, 1963). In an attempt to explain the long latency to maximal action, Krivoy (1969) presents evidence that β-MSH, for instance, alters the recovery period of nerve cells causing these cells to remain in a hyperexcitable state for a longer period of time. With continuous input these phenomena will summate with time (Krivoy *et al.*, 1963) and the latent period may represent that amount of time required for sufficient summation to take place so that this hyperexcitability becomes manifest. A similar response was elicited following the injection of synthetic ACTH into the brain of cats using chronically implanted cannulae. The hypothalamic areas lining the third ventricle were reported to be the most sensitive parts of the brain to ACTH as defined by production of the "stretching crisis" (Gessa *et al.*, 1967). Whatever the mechanism or site of action of this effect, it appears to be specific since STH, TSH, oxytocin, LH, FSH, or insulin have no such action.

The occurrence of rapid-eye movement (REM) sleep episodes at the time of the diurnal rise in plasma steroids has prompted the suggestion that the two events are associated (Weitzman *et al.*, 1966). Indirect evidence obtained from sleep deprivation or reversal studies would not support this view (Nichols and Tyler, 1967). Similarly, the diurnal rise in plasma growth hormone in man that occurs during the slow wave sleep period following the onset of sleep may or may not indicate some association between the two events (Takahashi *et al.*, 1968; Parker *et al.*, 1969). Direct evidence appears to be lacking, particularly with respect to the effects of this hormone on sleep mechanisms. However, the rhythmic release of growth hormone in early sleep would be expected to enhance amino acid incorporation and diminish their diversion to gluco-neogenesis through release of free fatty acids, thus exerting an anabolic function during sleep.

3. Electrical Activity—Single Neurons

Work with single unit recording has added support to the hypotheses regarding the site of action of hormones in the CNS, particularly that for steroid hormones. A great deal of this work is attributable to Cross and his co-workers.

Using the technique developed by Cross and Green (1959), Barraclough and Cross (1963), in a study of unit activity in the lateral hypothalamic area in relation to the estrous cycle in the rat, found that the percentage of units inhibited by pain, cold, or cervical stimulation was higher in estrus than diestrus. These observations were confirmed and extended by Lincoln and Cross (1967). They recorded a progressive alteration in the response pattern from units in the lateral hypothalamus, through the anterior hypothalamus and preoptic area to the septum. The lateral hypothalamus contained primarily units giving excitatory responses, the anterior hypothalamus and preoptic area showed approximately equal numbers of units giving excitatory and inhibitory responses, and in the septum there was a large number of units giving inhibitory responses. The effects of endogenous or exogenous estrogen also varied through the same anatomical sequence. In the lateral and anterior hypothalamic areas estrogen enhanced the inhibitory responsiveness to pain, cold, and cervical stimuli, whereas in the septum it decreased the number of inhibitory responses. In the preoptic area estrogen had an effect intermediate between that of the anterior hypothalamus and the septum, since the responsiveness of units to cervical stimuli was enhanced while that to pain and cold was depressed. Exogenous or endogenous progesterone selectively depressed the excitation of hypothalamic neurons by stimuli from the genital tract (Cross and Silver, 1965). The effect of exogenous progesterone was transient being maximally effective 30 minutes to 1 hour after the iv injection of 400 μg progesterone. Progesterone was not found to alter the number of inhibitory responses in lateral hypothalamic neurons.

Prolactin-responsive neurons have recently been described in the rabbit hypothalamus (Clemens et al., 1969). Intravenous prolactin (50 μg) predominantly inhibited the firing rates of single neurons in several sites in the hypothalamus.

Oxytocin has also been reported to influence the firing rate of hypothalamic neurons (Kawakami and Saito, 1967). However, more recent evidence in unanesthetized rats with diencephalic island preparations (Cross and Kitay, 1967), which exclude indirect influences through afferent nervous excitation, contradicts this finding (Cross and Dyer, 1969).

Study of spontaneous unit activity in the posterior diencephalon and midbrain of cats showed an increase in the discharge frequency following both intravenous and intracerebral administration. Neurons in the posterior diencephalon appeared to be more sensitive to local application of the steroid than neurons in the midbrain (Slusher et al., 1966). The technique of microelectrophoresis developed by Ruf and Steiner (1967) has added a new dimension to the study of the site and mechanism of action of hormones and other drugs on the CNS. Its main advantage is the possibility of delivering from multibarreled micropipets minute amounts of material into the immediate extracellular environment of single neurons and observing the response of these cells directly and immediately in terms of changes in the discharge rate of action potentials.

Using this technique it was found that, whereas dexamethasone applied to neurons in the cortex, hippocampus, and thalamus never influenced neuronal activity, the discharge rate of hypothalamic units concentrated in specific areas of the periventricular gray of the third ventricle and aqueduct were markedly depressed (Ruf and Steiner, 1967). The depression of these units was almost instantaneous and complete; the depression of mesencephalic units was somewhat more delayed and progressive. Steroid-sensitive neurons thus identified were then found to be activated by ACTH and by acetylcholine but inhibited by NE and dopamine (DA) (Steiner *et al.*, 1968). The authors suggest that specific nerve cells in the hypothalamus and midbrain are sensitive to both hormonal and humoral factors and involved in negative and positive feedback actions of the hormones.

V. EFFECTS OF HORMONES ON BRAIN MECHANISMS

A. Respiration and Metabolism of Brain Tissue

1. *Adrenal Medullary*

The first chemical agent found to accelerate the cerebral metabolic rate in normal man was E. When administered by continuous intravenous infusion in sufficient amounts to raise the arterial pressure, it was found to produce consistent and significant increases in the rate of cerebral oxygen consumption (King *et al.*, 1952). Because of the relationship of this substance to the phenomenon of "anxiety," it has been suggested that it is the mediator of the stimulation of cerebral metabolic rate in that emotional state (Sokoloff, 1956). Sensenbach and his associates (1953) have failed to find any effect of E on human cerebral metabolic rate, after intramuscular administration in doses that did not alter arterial blood pressure. NE does not appear to have any obvious effect on cerebral metabolism (King *et al.*, 1952; Sensenbach *et al.*, 1953).

2. *Thyroid Hormones*

The accelerative effect which the thyroid hormone has been found to have on the metabolic processes of almost all body tissues does not seem to occur in the brain. In human adults suffering from hyperthyroidism, no alteration in cerebral oxygen consumption has been observed despite marked increases in the total body metabolic rate (Scheinberg, 1950; Sensenbach *et al.*, 1954; Sokoloff *et al.*, 1953). In adult hypothyroidism one study found a reduction in cerebral metabolic rate (Scheinberg *et al.*, 1950); another found no difference from normal during disease and no change following thyroid hormone. In juvenile hypothyroidism, Himwich *et al.* (1942) using cerebral arteriovenous oxygen differences and the thermoelectric flow recorder found qualitative evidence of an increase in cerebral metabolic rate following thyroid administration. In studies in rats, Fazekas *et al.* (1951) found in artificially induced hyperthyroidism that the cortical oxygen consumption rose more rapidly from its postnatal low level to the normal adult level. Once the level of the mature state was reached, there was no difference in the cortical oxygen consumption between hyperthyroid and normal rats. No differences from normal were observed in hypothyroidism. Cohen and Gerard (1937) found that the rate of oxygen consumption by minced brain from hyperthyroid rats was initially about 30% higher than normal without added substrate and that the effects of added glucose or other substrate were increased. On the other hand, Brophy and McEachern (1949) found no increases using slices. Peters and Rossiter (1939) found that thiamine appreciably increased pyruvate oxidation by minced brain from hyperthyroid rats. From all this evidence, it appears that thyroid hormone exerts its effects on the brain chiefly during its period of growth and development. Once maturation has been achieved, the brain appears to be little affected, if at all, by the level of circulating thyroid hormone. Sokoloff and his associates (1953) have suggested that this lack of effect does not appear to be the result of the inability of thyroxine to pass the blood-brain barrier. The difference in the effects of thyroxine on cerebral metabolic rate in mature and immature brain is probably secondary to the effects of the hormone on protein biosynthesis since puromycin blocks the effect of thyroxine on oxygen consumption, at least peripherally (Sokoloff and Klee, 1966).

3. Insulin

Insulin does not appear to exert any direct action on brain tissue metabolism. Insulin added *in vitro,* or administered to the animal, does not obviously affect the respiration rate of brain suspensions (Elliott *et al.,* 1942; Elliott and Libet, 1942). Although the respiration rate of brain tissue removed from an insulinized animal falls off more rapidly than normally in the absence of added substrate, this is due to the tissue containing less glucose and lactate than normal (Kerr and Ghantus, 1936; Elliott, 1946). Rafaelsen (1958, 1961a,b), using isolated pieces of rat spinal cord, has reported that insulin in the incubation medium increased the aerobic glucose uptake and that in alloxan-diabetic rats the glucose uptake was decreased but addition of insulin to the medium increased it.

4. Pituitary, Adrenal Cortex, and Sex Hormones

The relatively few reported studies, particularly in man, on the effects of the pituitary, adrenocortical, and sex hormones on the metabolism of the CNS *in vivo,* with a few exceptions, indicate very little effect of these hormones, at least in the mature individual. Reiss and Rees (1947) observed no changes in the respiration rate of cortex slices from hypophysectomized rats but a 25% increase in average rate of anaerobic glycolysis. Administration of ACTH brought the anaerobic glycolysis back to normal (MacLeod and Reiss, 1940). TSH in hypophysectomized animals caused some increase in respiration but this fell off later and no obvious effect was observed in normal animals (Reiss and Rees, 1947). No change in the respiration of brain slices was observed by Crismon and Field (1940) in adrenalectomized rats. It is generally agreed that adrenalectomy does not appear to alter the oxygen consumption of rat median eminence or hypothalamus (Roberts and Keller, 1955; Levey and Roberts, 1957; Jacobowitz, 1962). But Bergen and co-workers (1953) have observed a fall in cerebral metabolic rate following adrenalectomy which was restored to normal by adrenocortical extract and cortisone but not by DOC. In man neither ACTH (Alman and Fazekas, 1951; Schieve et al., 1951; Sensenbach et al., 1953) nor cortisone (Sensenbach et al., 1953) have been found to have any significant effect on cerebral metabolic rate. In rats, however, several reports concur that addition of corticoids to hypothalamic or other brain tissue in vitro depresses oxygen consumption (Tipton, 1939; Roberts and Keller, 1955; Jacobowtiz, 1962). In addition, Jacobowitz (1962) showed that the increase in oxygen consumption produced by a stress-blocking dose of hydrocortisone was limited to the anterior pituitary and median eminence but was not evident in the remaining hypothalamus.

The anesthetizing actions of large doses of steroids first reported by Selye in 1941 may be traced to their direct effects on cerebral metabolism. The anesthetic 21-hydroxypregnane-3,20-dione (sodium hydroxydione) produces in man a profound reduction in cerebral blood flow, oxygen, and glucose consumption comparable to that of barbiturate anesthesia (Gordan, 1956; Gordan et al., 1955).

Elliott et al. (1957) have studied the in vitro effects of this steroid on rat and guinea pig brain using manometric techniques and measurements of glucose uptake and/or lactic acid production. Their evidence indicates that sodium hydroxydione acts on oxidative reactions to inhibit the entrance of glucose into the tricarboxylic acid cycle. Gordan and Elliott (1947) have demonstrated direct parallels between the anesthetic action of steroids and their ability to inhibit glucose oxidation of rat brain homogenates. This was true for DOC, progesterone, testosterone, and α-estradiol but not for stilbestrol, which is less anesthetic than the first three steroids but the most potent brain respiration inhibitor. The experiments indicated an action of the steroids on the dehydrogenases of the cellular respiratory system and Hoagland (1957) proposed that stilbestrol may exert its effect by competing with cytochrome c as a hydrogen acceptor for lactic dehydrogenase. Bourne and Malatoy (1953) using a histochemical reaction for succinic dehydrogenase have found it to increase in cerebellum of intact rats following cortisone injection. Adrenalectomy caused a marked reduction of succinic dehydrogenase which was restored completely to normal by cortisone but only partially by DOCA. Testosterone was without effect and progesterone had some restorative action on succinic dehydrogenase.

In castrated prepubertal rats there is an elevated cerebral oxygen consumption (Denison et al., 1955; Eisenberg et al., 1949; Gordan, 1956), which is restored to normal by the administration in vivo of any one of a number of steroids such as testosterone, methyltestosterone, epitestosterone, progesterone, anhydrohydroxyprogesterone, DOCA, and ACTH, but not by estradiol-17β (Eisenberg et al., 1950; Gordan, 1956). On the other hand, in postpubertal human males, castration has been reported to cause a fall in cerebral oxygen consumption; and the postoperative administration of the steroids, DOC glucoside or testosterone, cause, if anything, a rise in the cerebral metabolic rate back toward precastration levels (Gordan, 1956). Gordan has suggested that the androgenic and adrenal cortical steroids normally maintain a "braking" action on cerebral metabolic rate and when deficient as in preadolescent testicular eunuchoidism or preadolescent hypopituitarism, there is a release and elevation of the cerebral metabolic rate. He further suggests that the steep fall in cerebral metabolic rate at puberty (Kennedy and Sokoloff, 1957) is the result of the increased production of these steroid hormones at that time (Gordan and Adams, 1956; Gordan, 1956).

B. Water and Electrolytes

One of the primary and possibly the most important effect of most, if not all, of the hormones is directly concerned with the regulation of water and electrolyte metabolism. These range from the well-known role of antidiuretic hormone and adrenal and gonadal steroids on sodium, potassium, and water balance, to those of the thyroid and parathyroid glands on calcium metabolism.

Hodgkin and Katz (1949) have demonstrated that the resting membrane of nerve is more permeable to potassium than it is to sodium. However, the active membrane, in the process of conducting the nerve impulse, becomes more permeable to sodium than to potassium. They presented significant evidence for the view that this reversal of permeability is brought about by a large increase in sodium permeability, while the potassium permeability remained unchanged. This view is in accord with the reversal of the action potential, with respect to the resting potential of the nerve, when the nerve becomes active in conduction. Thus, while the resting potential and excitability are largely dependent upon potassium gradients, the action potential is mainly due to movements of sodium. The nerve impulse itself is thus subject to modification both by sodium and potassium gradients across the nerve membrane suggesting the importance of homeostatic regulation of these cations for normal function of the nervous system and for synaptic conduction.

More recently evidence suggests that calcium ions have a vital role, not only in "stimulus-secretion coupling" events in the neuroendocrine system (Douglas, 1966; Douglas and Rubin, 1963; Milligan and Kraicer, 1969), but also in electrically activated synapses (Penn and Loewenstein, 1966) depressing the discharge of neurons in the cerebral cortex (Krnjevic, 1965), caudate nucleus, and hippocampus (Wang et al., 1966) and elevating EST in rats (Woodbury and Davenport, 1949). The depressant action of calcium in the CNS conforms to its known effect on the excitability of nerve membranes (Cerf, 1963) but is in contrast to its effect on junctional transmission where excess Ca^{2+} enhances the release of transmitter substances from presynaptic endings (Desmedt, 1963). Based on experiments using iontophoretic application to cells in the cerebral cortex, cuneate nucleus, and spinal cord of cats, Somjen and Kato (1968) conclude that calcium blocks synaptic transmission in the CNS predominantly by a postsynaptic action since it did not elevate electrical threshold and produced little or no change of spontaneous and evoked synaptic potentials, membrane potentials, or membrane resistance (Kelly et al., 1968).

Calcium appears to exchange readily between neural and nonneural tissue. The healthy adult rat brain appears to take up about 0.1% of an injected dose of ^{45}Ca without evidence of selective localization within brain stem, cerebellum, and cerebrum (Daniels et al., 1967). Most, if not all, hormones appear to affect, directly or indirectly calcium metabolism and may therefore be expected to exert profound effects on brain maturation and excitability and hence behavior. For example, apart from the well-known regulatory effects of the thyroid and parathyroid glands on calcium metabolism, corticosteroids (Clark and Geoffroy, 1957; Fischer and Hastrup, 1954), estrogens (Schjeide and Urist, 1956), and testosterone (Mandel et al., 1954; Rigamonti, 1957) have all been shown to affect calcium metabolism in a variety of species. The injection of ACTH in rabbits is reported to produce within 2 hours a 20% decrease in serum calcium levels (Natelson et al., 1966) and pinealectomy is thought to decrease calcium turnover in lymphatic organs (Csaba et al., 1967).

The more recent observations on the central effects of angiotensin may be relevant as an example. Intraventricular administration of angiotensin II results in a marked pressor response, an increase in plasma corticosteroids, and increased drinking behavior (Daniels, 1968; Epstein et al., 1969; Booth, 1968; Daniels et al., 1969). A calcium requirement has been demonstrated for the peripheral actions of angiotensin (Khairallah et al., 1965; Benelli et al., 1964) including its ability to release catecholamines by the adrenal medulla (Poisner and Douglas, 1965). Daniels and Buckley (1968) using calcium-free CSF or EDTA-containing medium have shown that the centrally evoked pressor response to angiotensin is also calcium- and NE-dependent and propose that calcium is required for the central adrenergic pressor mechanism by the peptide. Whether the characteristic drinking behavior exhibited by rats following central administration of angiotensin is also calcium-dependent is not yet known and would be interesting to determine. On the other hand, it has been demonstrated that this drinking behavior is neither pituitary- nor adrenal-dependent.

In sharp contrast to the relative absence of information on the effects of hormones on brain calcium, there is an abundance of information on the effects of hormones on brain sodium and potassium metabolism. This is grossly due to the very extensive and thorough works of Woodbury, Timiras, Vernadakis, and Woolley, which have been admirably reviewed in recent years (Woodbury, 1954; Woodbury *et al.*, 1957; Woodbury and Karler, 1960; Woodbury, 1958) and will therefore not be discussed in depth here. Using concurrent measurements of EST and brain and plasma Na and K concentrations, they have provided evidence that ACTH and adrenocortical steroids exert a regulatory influence on brain excitability. "This regulatory function is operative only when changes in excitability occur; the adrenocortical hormones then act to restore normal brain excitability, regardless of the direction in which the deviation tends" (Woodbury *et al.*, 1957). Chronic administration of large doses of DOCA and to a lesser extent, aldosterone decreased excitability, whereas cortisone and hydrocortisone increased brain excitability; corticosterone had little effect. They postulate that DOCA and hydrocortisone affect the active transport of Na across brain cells in opposite manner and thereby modify brain excitability.

The role of the adrenal cortex in the regulation of the metabolism of sodium and potassium and its possible effects on permeability of the blood-brain barrier to potassium is well known, as is the importance of potassium in relation to nerve function. Hoagland and Stone (1948) determined the content of potassium in brains of normal and adrenalectomized rats before and after stress and after the administration of steroids. Adrenalectomy did not significantly affect the rate of exchange of brain potassium, but it decreased plasma sodium concentration, increased intracellular brain sodium concentration, and decreased the ratio of the two (Woodbury and Davenport, 1952). However, the authors point out that the effects of hormones on brain excitability are not invariably accompanied by changes in brain electrolytes.

A relation between ovarian hormones and brain excitability has been known for many years (Gowers, 1885) when it was noted that the incidence of seizures in female epileptics varied with the phases of the menstrual cycle. In 1956, Laidlaw tabulated observations indicating that there was a decrease in seizures in epileptic females during the luteal phase of the menstrual cycle, with an irregular increase immediately before, during, and after menstruation. Experiments in rats have essentially substantiated these observations. Woolley *et al.* (1960) have shown that administration of estradiol has a stimulatory effect on brain excitability as opposed to the depressant action of progesterone. They also refer to a sex influence as shown by the greater depressant effect of progesterone in the female than in male rats. Their data also indicate that estradiol affects brain excitability by mechanisms other than electrolyte changes since the EST was lowered in spite of elevated plasma sodium concentration and an increased extracellular/intracellular cortex sodium ratio.

The thyroid gland has also been shown to affect brain electrolytes and brain excitability by a mechanism distinct from its general stimulatory action on general metabolism. Both thyroidectomy and treatment with propylthiouracil decrease brain excitability and treatment with thyroxine and triiodothyronine increase it (Woodbury *et al.*, 1952; Woodbury, 1954). Triiodothyronine is five times more potent in this respect than thyroxine, although its action is faster and more transient. The effects of thyroxine are still evident after 24 hours. The effects of the thyroid appear to bear a direct relationship to brain sodium concentrations (Lundbaek, 1947; Timiras and Woodbury, 1956). The observation that thyroid hormones increase brain excitability and brain sodium concentration less in adrenalectomized than in intact rats suggests that a dual mechanism may be involved for the action of these hormones on the brain; a direct stimulation of the CNS and an indirect stimulation mediated by increased secretion of adrenocortical (Eartley and Leblond, 1954) or adrenomedullary hormones (Minz and Domino, 1953).

C. Protein Metabolism

The rapid growth that characterizes nervous tissue from the start of its embryonic origin implies rapid synthesis of new protein. The deoxyribonucleic acid (DNA) and ribonucleic acid (RNA) required for protein synthesis are contained within the primitive nerve cells themselves but the rate of growth and differentiation of the nerve cells is determined by humoral controlling influences coming from other tissues external to the nervous system. It is no wonder therefore that hormones would be expected to exert their maximal influence during this period of rapid growth and affect only minimally the protein metabolism of the adult brain.

In the rat brain a number of enzymes normally increase very considerably in activity at about the tenth day after birth, but destruction of the thyroid with ^{131}I leads to a decrease in activity of the succinate dehydrogenase and acetylcholinesterase (AChE) and cholinesterase (Hamburgh and Flexner, 1957; Geel and Timiras, 1967a). Treatment with thyroid hormones restores the enzymic activities to normal if started before the tenth day but not if treatment is delayed beyond the fifteenth day. Similarly, the cerebral hypoplasia and hypofucntion described in hypothyroid, cretinoid animals can be ascribed, in part, to impaired protein synthesis. Studies *in vivo* and *in vitro* have shown a reduction in cerebral RNA concentration per cell (Geel and Timiras, 1967b) and a depressed cerebral protein turnover (Geel *et al.*, 1967), which reflect a reduced rate of protein synthesis and, consequently, a lower functional activity of the cells. Protein synthesis can be restored, however, if thyroxine is administered within the first 12 days after birth. In the foregoing study, changes in the ionic distribution also were observed in the cerebral cortex of thyroid-deficient rats (Geel *et al.,* 1967). A deficiency in the Na-K pump would result in a depressed uptake of labeled amino acid because of the characteristic sensitivity of the brain protein-synthesizing system to ionic environment. On the other hand, the administration of growth hormone, known to enhance cortical growth when given *in vitro* (Zemenhof, 1942; Clendinnen and Eayrs, 1961), has only a slight ameliorating effect upon the cretinoid rat (Eayrs, 1961a).

Experiments with tissue slices and cell-free systems *in vitro* have shown that thyroidectomy decreases the rate of incorporation of labeled amino acids into proteins, while small amounts of thyroid hormones increase it (DuToit, 1952; Sokoloff and Kaufman, 1961; Tata *et al.*, 1963). The stimulant effect of thyroid hormones is specific for the L-isomer of thyroxine and triiodothyronine. Sokoloff and his colleagues have provided some evidence that a component of the mitochondrial system is responsible for the difference in response of young and of adult brain. They have shown that, in the course of cerebral maturation, the mitochondria of the brain lose their capacity to interact with thyroxine during the process of protein biosynthesis (Klee *et al.,* 1963; Gelber *et al.,* 1964; Klee and Sokoloff, 1964). Campbell and Eayrs (1965) propose that this finding may help to explain not only the specificity of the stimulant effect of thyroid hormone on protein synthesis in the nervous system, but also the "irreversibility of behavioral deficits in terms of an inability later in life to develop appropriate synaptic affinities" (Hyden, 1961).

It is generally agreed that the stimulant action of the thyroid hormones is not concerned with the amino acid-activating enzymes. Klee and Sokoloff (1964) conclude that thyroxine stimulates the rate of uptake by the ribosomes of bound amino acids attached to transfer RNA. Tata and Widnell (1964) report evidence that the point of action of the thyroid hormones is the DNA-dependent RNA polymerase, since stimulation of this system by thyroid hormones can be shown to precede the increased incorporation of amino acids into protein: they conclude that the thyroid hormones act primarily on the genetically linked regulatory mechanisms of protein synthesis. It would therefore be expected that the central effects of drugs such as methylthiouracil, which reduce the level of thyroid hormones, are also due to their influence on protein metabolism.

The influence of ACTH and adrenocortical steroids on protein and amino acid metabolism of brain has not been adequately studied, although their effects on other tissues, particularly the liver, have received considerable attention (Tomkins and Maxwell, 1963).

The observations of Loeb *et al.* (1953) that ACTH increased the turnover of ^{32}P in the pentosenucleic acid fraction of the monkey hypothalamus (an effect presumably mediated by the adrenal cortex) might indicate an increase in the rate of synthesis of cellular protein. On the other hand, Goldman (1957) found that the adenine content of the hypothalamus was decreased significantly in both sham and bilaterally adrenalectomized rats indicative of a rapid turnover of adenosine triphosphate (ATP). The low adenine in the sham-operated animals returned to control levels in about 11 days, whereas it remained depressed for as long as 22 days in the adrenalectomized animal. Whether this increase in hypothalamic ATP turnover is directly related to the absence of circulating corticoids has not been ascertained. Application to the brain of data obtained on the action of corticoids on other tissues would be speculative at this time. It would be highly desirable that studies on the action of corticosteroids on brain metabolism be carried out analogous to the extensive investigations carried out on their peripheral effects.

However, there is no doubt that some of the steroids have marked effects on protein metabolism. Thus methyltestosterone has been demonstrated to have specific protein anabolic action. In contrast to this, the 11-oxysteroids of the adrenal cortex normally exert pronounced protein catabolic action as evidenced by a rapid disappearance of lymphocytes and a shift in nitrogen balance with corresponding deposition of liver glycogen. These far-reaching repercussions of the steroids on protein metabolism include a wide variety of tissues and since enzymes are proteins, it is tempting to consider the possible action of adrenal steroids on protein metabolism of the brain. Hyden (1947) and Hyden and Hartelius (1948), using ultraviolet microspectroscopy, found an increase in protein catabolism in single cells of the CNS in connection with increased functional demands when the cells conduct nerve impulses over periods of time. In both motor activity and sensory stimulation a rapid breakdown of nucleoproteins is reported to take place in the cell bodies of central nervous units of the conducting apparatus, and the restitution of the nucleoprotein content of the cells can be demonstrated after the period of action. Hyden's work indicates a surprisingly rapid turnover of nucleoprotein in cells of the CNS, and it is interesting to consider the possibility that this turnover may be modified by steroid hormones just as they regulate protein metabolism in other tissues. Nurnberger (1953a) has investigated the concentrations of nucleic acids and proteins in the cytoplasm, nucleus, and nucleolus of cells of the liver and of the supraoptic neurons in the rat's hypothalamus. Changes of these cellular constituents following fasting and exposures to cold stress were found and correlated with changes in adrenal ascorbic acid. In subsequent studies he (Nurnberger, 1953b), examined cytoplasmic protein and RNA concentrations in liver and in the supraoptic nucleus cells of the hypothalamus from normal and adrenalectomized rats. He found that adrenalectomy approximately doubled the protein concentration of both types of cells. For example, liver cell protein increased from 26 to 51% and that of the supraoptic nucleus from 14 to 32%. Changes in RNA concentration were not significant following adrenalectomy. When intact rats were exposed to 1 hour of cold, cellular protein content was increased from 26 to 40% in liver and RNA fell from 1.8 to 1% with comparable changes occurring in the supraoptic nucleus cells. The most pronounced changes, however, were found in adrenalectomized rats exposed to cold where liver protein fell from 51 to 17% and supraoptic nucleus protein fell from 32 to 11%. These changes in protein concentrations were not accompanied by changes in RNA.

Nurnberger has pointed out that in acute experiments, adrenalectomy produces alterations in the activity of cellular proteins and that these changes represent alterations in cellular gluconeogenesis. It is suggested that the small changes in nucleic acids in the intact animal may serve in the storage and liberation of labile phosphate. It is evident that cell protein changes seem to be very sensitive to the level of adrenocortical function and it is interesting to note that the effect of the adrenal on brain protein metabolism is similar to that on liver cells.

The evidence indicates that a hormone can influence the protein metabolism of nervous tissues in a number of different ways. It may act on the enzymes directly concerned in protein synthesis; it may act indirectly on RNA metabolism; it may act by affecting the transport or metabolism of amino acids, or it may act by influencing the energy metabolism of the cell.

D. Neurohumors and Neurotransmitters

The elementary criteria of a transmitter substance are that, in the relevant tissue at appropriate times, it must be produced, stored, released, exert an appropriate action, and be removed. There is ample evidence for the production, storage, and physiological or pharmacological activity of a number of substances. However, there has been limited evidence that such material is released under physiological conditions in the mammal *in vivo* (Feldberg and Fleischauer, 1965) but substantiated by the CSF cross-circulation experiments of Myers and his associates (Myers and Sharpe, 1968; Myers and Yaksh, 1969).

The presence, in discrete areas of the brain, of acetylcholine, histamine, and compounds containing an indole or a catechol nucleus, and of the enzymes which metabolize them, has provided presumptive evidence that the metabolism of these substances is involved in the function of the CNS. The conclusion that any one of these compounds serves as a synaptic transmitter of neuronal activity, or of the modification of such activity, should be approached with some caution. Studies of the qualitative and quantitative aspects of the metabolic pathways of these compounds and the administration of drugs inhibiting specific metabolic steps has helped to define their relationships to the function of the brain [for extensive discussion see Barchas *et al.*, Chapter 8, this volume, and Green, (1970)]. Several other substances are found in the brain and thought to be of high significance in nervous function (Krnjevic, 1965). For example, evidence that GABA may be an inhibitory transmitter substance is accumulating (Elliott, 1965); glutamate and aspartate are excitatory agents (Curtis and Koizumi, 1961), and a variety of amino acids exert varied effects (Krnjevic, 1965).

In discussing the effects of hormones on brain amines, it becomes evident that the methodological sources of error are monumental (Barchas *et al.*, Chapter 8, this volume; Dewhurst, 1968; Wurtman *et al.*, 1969). Techniques used to estimate brain amine content or turnover include fluorescence microscopy, chemical assay of content in whole brain, synthesis from radioactive precursor, disappearance of unlabeled amine from brain following pharmacological inhibition of enzymes which normally metabolize it, etc. Estimation of brain amine turnover is believed to provide an index of the physiological activity of the neurons which contain the amine and it has been generally assumed that when endocrine manipulations modify brain amine levels by affecting their synthesis, storage, release, or metabolism, they are altering the physiological activity of the neurons involved. Apart from the effects of circulating hormones on those hypothalamic amines representing a component of the feedback system controlling the secretion of the pituitary, hormones may affect neurons with unrelated functions depending on the degree of localization specificity within the CNS.

As in other aspects of the study of the influence of hormones on neural tissue emphasis has been placed on the effects of sex and adrenal steroids.

The CA content of the anterior and middle hypothalamus has been reported to vary during the estrous cycle (Stefano and Donoso, 1967). Using an adaptation for microfluorometry of the histochemical fluorescence method of Falck and Owman (1965), Lichtensteiger (1969) measured the CA fluorescence in the predominantly DA-containing nerve cells of the tuberal region and of the substantia nigra. He found that in the tuberal nerve cells the mean relative fluorescence intensity showed a steady increase from diestrous day 1 to estrous day, while only a slight change with a different rhythm occurred in the substantia nigra. This would indicate that under these conditions the variations in CA are restricted to certain special adrenergic groups in the CNS and caused by a functional involvement of these specific neurons. A similar increase of fluorescence intensity in the tuberoinfundibular dopamine neurons has been described for pregnancy (Fuxe *et al.*, 1967). Ovariectomy on diestrous day 1 interrupted these changes (Lichtensteiger *et al.*, 1969) but 3-7 weeks later evidence of slightly increased amine activity was again evident. Measuring NE turnover in the rat brain, Anton-Tay and Wurtman (1968) found that it increased after gonadectomy. The hypothalamus and midbrain showed the greatest change. Since the rate at which ^{3}H-NE disappeared 6 days after gonadectomy increased, but the content of endogenous brain NE did not change, the authors suggested that synthesis of the amine was probably stimulated. More recent evidence supports this view (Donoso *et al.*, 1969).

Hypophysectomy unlike gonadectomy, had no such effect (Anton-Tay and Wurtman, 1968). This was the first indication that the change in brain amine was possibly due to pituitary gonadotropins rather than gonadal secretions. Subsequent experiments substantiated this view when it was shown that treatment of intact rats with FSH, but not LH, also raised brain NE turnover (Anton-Tay et al., 1969). Since castration in experimental animals is known to result in increased secretion of FSH (Greep and Chester-Jones, 1950), it may therefore follow that the changes in brain NE metabolism which follow castration are mediated by an increase in the secretion of FSH. Donoso and Cukier (1968), however, have reported that estrogen treatment can block the increase in hypothalamic NE content observed in castrated rats and Lichtensteiger et al. (1969) found that a dose of estradiol that reduced serum FSH and LH in ovariectomized rats also reduced the fluorescence intensity of tuberal neurons. Progesterone had no effect on FSH levels nor on the fluorescence, although Coppola (1969) reports decreased turnover rates of CA following 2-day treatment with either estrone or progesterone. It would therefore appear that if the effect of estrogens on brain NE is an indirect one by inhibition of FSH secretion, then adrenergic neurons are not involved in this feedback system. The ability of FSH then to stimulate brain CA turnover is either unrelated to the regulation of pituitary FSH secretion or adrenergic neurons are *only* involved in the "short feedback loop" (Corbin and Story, 1963; Fraschini et al., 1968).

Using the microfluorometric method, Lichtensteiger et al. (1969) also examined the effects of thyroid hormone on tuberal nerve cell CA content. Exposure of female rats on diestrous day 1 to $4°C$ resulted in a marked increase in fluorescence. This change was prevented by thyroxine administered 3 hours before. This provides only indirect evidence for a correlation between this change and TSH secretion. However, LH concentrations did not increase in these animals under these conditions. Hence, it does not appear that these tuberoinfundibular CA-containing neurons are exclusively concerned with the control of gonadotropins or any one particular pituitary hormone. Thyroid also appears to affect brain cholinergic activity. In neonatally hypothyroid rats, there is a decrease in AChE and cholinesterase activity (Geel and Timiras, 1967a). AChE has been used as evidence for the presence of ACh; therefore, a reduction of AChE implies alteration of synaptic transmission. Since cholinesterase activity is predominately present in glial cells, a reduction of this enzyme suggests that the function of glial cells may be altered in the hypothyroid state.

Brain GABA activity is reported to decrease following insulin administration (Lovell and Elliott, 1963). This is presumably because in the absence of glucose, glutamate is oxidatively used up and its concentration and therefore the rate of GABA formation are decreased.

Melatonin has also been described to affect brain GABA concentrations. Two hours after the administration of a small dose (5 μg/100gm ip) of melatonin to rabbits the concentration of aspartic acid, glutamine, and GABA in the hypothalamus are significantly elevated. Larger doses of melatonin depress the levels of these amino acids as well as glutamic acid (Anton-Tay et al., 1966). It has also been shown that the intraperitoneal administration of melatonin to rats caused an increase in brain serotonin (5-hydroxytryptamine,5-HT) concentration especially in the midbrain and hypothalamus. These are also the sites at which circulating ^{3}H-melatonin is most highly concentrated in the brain (Noble et al., 1967). Concentration of 5-HT in the cerebral cortex and the olfactory bulb and tubercle remained essentially unchanged. The effect appears to be primarily on the 5-HT-containing neurons (Dahlstrom and Fuxe, 1964) since the midbrain appeared to be most affected. It is of interest that the increase in brain 5-HT was not associated with changes in NE concentration (Anton-Tay et al., 1968).

That hormones can affect the activity of the brain neurotransmitters by peripheral mechanisms has been demonstrated by the interesting work of Curzon and Green (1968a,b). Tryptophan, primarily oxidized by liver tryptophan pyrrolase to formylkynurenine, is also metabolized by a minor route to 5-HT. Since pituitary-adrenal activation results in increased pyrrolase synthesis (Knox and Auerbach, 1955) they worked on the premise that this might result in decreased 5-HT synthesis. Indeed injection of hydrocortisone decreased brain 5-HT significantly. Brain 5-hydroxyindolylacetic acid (5-HIAA) also fell suggesting decreased brain 5-HT synthesis. Injection of the pyrrolase inhibitors allopurinol (Becking and Johnson, 1967) or yohimbine (Madras and Sourkes, 1966) with the steroid blocked the fall in brain 5-HT. Similar findings were reported following the stress of immobilization for 5 hours. Like Corrodi et al. (1968), Curzon and Green (1969) observed a 20-45% fall of brain 5-HT while liver tryptophan pyrrolase rose considerably. Pretreatment of the animals with allopurinol lessened the decrease in brain 5-HT, indicating that at least part of the mechanism by which it occurred involved pyrrolase increase.

Adrenocortical hormones have been shown to affect E synthesis in the adrenal medulla (Wurtman and Axelrod, 1965; Wurtman, 1966). They do this by induction of the enzyme phenylethanolamine-N-methyltransferase (PNMT) that converts NE to E. Small amounts of E have been identified in mammalian brain (Vogt, 1954) and more recently PNMT activity was demonstrated in various regions of brain (Pohorecky et al., 1969) with the greatest activity in the olfactory tubercle. In contrast to PNMT in the adrenal medulla, hypophysectomy had no effect on the brain enzyme activity, whereas pretreatment with dexamethasone for 7 days elevated olfactory tubercle PNMT activity in the rat. It may be of interest to determine if the preferential uptake of ^{3}H-testosterone in olfactory bulbs of immature rats (Woolley et al., 1969a) bears any relationship to E synthesis in that tissue.

Acute or chronic treatment of rats with hydrocortisone did not affect NE content of the whole brain (Jacobowitz et al., 1963). However, Gorny (1968) reports that 12-day treatment with small doses (0.1 mg/100 gm body weight) of hydrocortisone decreased brain E, DOC had no effect but hydrocortisone plus DOC caused an increase in brain E. Javoy *et al.* (1968) measuring central turnover of NE after adrenalectomy in the rat found no effect immediately after the operation but an accelerated turnover 6 days after adrenalectomy.

Interpretation of these results may be complicated by the fact that CA may have in the CNS as they do in the periphery both excitatory and inhibitory effects (Vogt, 1965) and that hormones by acting simultaneously at many sites, may produce effects which cancel each other.

VI. CONCLUDING REMARKS

It is quite clear from this survey that information concerning the effects of hormones on the CNS is limited, scattered, and for the greater part, indirect. Most of what is known is derived from and relates to neuroendocrine feedback studies. This is evidenced by the remarkable absence of information on the central effects of those hormones that are not presently known to be regulated by target organ feedback, e.g., growth hormone, prolactin, thyrocalcitonin, oxytocin, etc. Similarly, the field is permeated by the persistent notion that any effects of pituitary peptide hormones on brain mechanisms are mediated by the secretion of their target organs. This is in spite of excellent indications to the contrary. The work of De Wied (1966), Koranyi and Endroczi (1967), and others draw attention to the fact that biologically active polypeptides acting specifically on one or more target organs can influence neural processes through direct action or by altering the biochemical and vascular environment of neural elements.

It is evident that totally contradictory conclusions may be drawn about the site and action of a hormone depending on methodology used, e.g., labeled hormone uptake and distribution vs electrical activity vs effect on brain electrolyte or protein metabolism.

It is also evident that gross errors of judgment may result concerning the site, mechanism of action, and functional implication of some hormonal-neural relationships unless caution is exercised concerning the limitations of the conclusions that may be drawn from the findings described here. For instance, does a gross change in the CNS recorded simultaneously with some endocrine or behavioral parameter imply a cause and effect relationship? Does the peripheral administration of a hormone and a change in brain activity imply a direct effect? Is endocrine organ ablation the opposite of hormone administration? Is there respect for the lack of specificity of pharmacological tools and surgical techniques, for the existence of biological rhythms and for the fact that the bulk of neuroendocrine and behavioral information is obtained from the nocturnal rat during its quiescent hours? Do acute, delayed, and chronic effects of hormones involve the same site, act in the same sequence, and by the same mechanism of action?

On the other hand, it is encouraging that in recent years attempts have been made to narrow the radius of action of various hormones to more discrete loci and mechanisms.

Recording of single unit activity, autoradiography, microfluorometry, and microelectrophoresis have contributed greatly to knowledge regarding the specificity of hormonal effects on neurons. Application of these techniques to other hormones and other brain functions, as has been done to some extent for drugs, amino acids, and amines (Krnjevic, 1965), could result in an invaluable mapping of the selective sensitivity of neuronal activity. For instance, are light-sensitive neurons adrenergic or serotoninergic? By what hormones are they affected and how? How do osmosensitive neurons believed to be involved in the regulation of drinking (Cross and Green, 1959) respond to angiotensin? Are they adrenergic as the indirect evidence might suggest? How do other hormones that affect electrolyte metabolism alter the activity of these neurons? Are glucose-sensitive neurons (Oomura et al., 1969) also sensitive to insulin and growth hormone? The possibilities of this approach are obviously infinite.

Hormones are a structurally diverse group of compounds ranging from polypeptides to steroids to monoamines. Hence, describing a universal mechanism of hormone action on neural tissue would be premature based on the limited information available. Certain general concepts, however, emerge: Neurons sensitive to one hormone respond to other hormones as well as to neurohumors in a manner characteristic for that neuron. The initial effect of the hormone is transient, coincides with the time of rising at that site, and can be reproduced by raising peripheral levels of that hormone (Jones, 1970). A secondary or delayed and long-lasting action of the hormone when site-concentration may be low (McEwen et al., 1969a) probably involves effects on protein metabolism. A hormone may influence the protein metabolism of nervous tissues in a number of different ways. It may act by affecting the transport or metabolism of amino acids or by influencing the energy metabolism of the cell; it may act indirectly on the RNA metabolism or on the enzymes directly concerned with protein synthesis. A hormone may thus also influence the metabolism of brain neurohumors that may be involved in neural transmission. It has been suggested that the mode of action of these neurotransmitters on nervous tissue is mediated by adenosine $3'5'$-monophosphate (cyclic AMP) as are the actions of numerous hormones on peripheral tissues (Sutherland et al., 1968). Various nerve tissue preparations respond to CA, indolalkylamines, and histamine by increasing levels of cyclic AMP (Kakiuchi and Rall, 1968a,b; Klainer et al., 1962; Weiss and Costa, 1968), which has also been implicated in the release of ACh at motor nerve endings under certain conditions (Breckenridge *et al.*, 1967). It may therefore be feasible to propose that the cyclic nucleotide may be involved in the regulation of a variety of homeostatic mechanisms integrated at the level of the hypothalamus (Breckenridge and Lisk, 1969).

Acknowledgments

My most sincere thanks are due to Professor B. H. Marks and Dr. H. Goldman for critically reviewing the manuscript, and to Dr. C. M. Winget for his advice, constructive criticism, and encouragement throughout the writing of this chapter. I also wish to thank all those investigators who so generously supplied me with reprints, manuscripts, and unpublished information of their work related to this subject.

References

Adey, W. R. (1956). *Australas. Ann. Med.* **5**, 153.

Allen, B. M. (1938) *Biol Rev. Cambridge Phil. Soc.* **13**, 1.

Alman, R. W., and Fazekas, J. F. (1951). *AMA Arch. Neurol. Psychiat.* **65**, 680.

Anderson, B., Ekman, L., Gale, C. C., and Sundsten, J. W. (1962). *Acta Physiol. Scand.* **54**, 191.

Anderson, E., Bates, R. W., Hawthorne, E., Haymaker, W., Knowlton, K., Rioch, D. M., Spence, W. T., and Wilson, H. (1957). *Recent Progr. Horm. Res.* **13**, 21.

Anton-Tay, F., and Wurtman, R. J. (1968). *Science* **159**, 1245.

Anton-Tay, F., Ortega, B., and Cruz, R. M. (1966). Unpublished observations quoted in Wurtman and Anton-Tay, *Recent Progr. Horm. Res.* **25**, 493.

Anton-Tay, F., Chou, C., Anton, S., and Wurtman, R. J. (1968). *Science* **162**, 277.

Anton-Tay, F., Pelham, R. W., and Wurtman, R. J. (1969). *Endocrinology* **84**, 1489.

Arai, Y., Hiroi, M., Mitra, J., and Gorski, R. A. (1967). *Neuroendocrinology* **2**, 275.

Atkins, E., Allison, F., Smith, M. R., and Wood, W. B. (1955). *J. Exp. Med.* **101**, 353.

Axelrod, J., Weil-Malherbe, H., and Tomchick, R. (1959). *J. Pharmacol. Exp. Ther.* **127**, 251.

Ayd, F. J. (1961). *J. Amer. Med. Ass.* **175**, 1054.

Babichev, V. N. (1964). *Biull. Eksp. Biol. Med.* **58**, 1029.

Babichev, V. N. (1965). *Fed. Proc. Fed. Amer. Soc. Exp. Biol.* **24**, 1777.

Barchas, J., DaCosta, F., and Spector, S. (1967). *Nature (London)* **214**, 919.

Barraclough, C. A. (1961). *Endocrinology* **68**, 62.

Barraclough, C. A., and Cross, B. A. (1963). *J. Endocrinol.* **26**, 339.

Barraclough, C. A., and Gorski, R. A. (1961). *Endocrinology* **68**, 68.

Barraclough, C. A., and Gorski, R. A. (1962). *J. Endocrinol.* **25**, 175.

Bazett, H. C. (1949). *In* "Physiology of Heat Regulation and the Science of Clothing" (L. H. Newburgh, ed.), p. 109. Saunders, Philadelphia, Pennsylvania.

Beach, F. A. (1948). "Hormones and Behavior." Harper (Hoeber), New York.

Becking, G. C., and Johnson, W. J. (1967). *Can. J. Biochem.* **45**, 1667.

Benelli, G., Della Bella, D., and Gandini, A. (1964). *Brit. J. Pharmacol.* **22**, 211.

Bergen, J. R. (1951). *Amer. J. Physiol.* **164**, 16.

Bergen, J. R., Hunt, C. A., and Hoagland, H. (1953). *Amer. J. Physiol.* **175**, 327.

Beyer, C., and Sawyer, C. H. (1969). *In* "Frontiers in Neuroendocrinology" (W. F. Ganong and L. Martini, eds.), pp. 255-287. Oxford Univ. Press, London and New York.

Bonvallet, M., and Dell, P. (1946). *C. R. Soc. Biol.* **140**, 942.

Booth, D. A. (1968). *J. Pharmacol. Exp. Ther.* **160**, 336.

Bourne, G. H., and Malatoy, H. A. (1953). *J. Physiol. (London)* **122**, 178.

Bradley, P. B., Eayrs, J. T., and Schmalbach, K. (1960). *Electroencephalogr. Clin. Neurophysiol.* **12**, 467.

Bradley, P. B., Eayrs, J. T., and Richards, N. M. (1964). *Electroencephalogr. Clin. Neurophysiol.* **17**, 308.

Breckenridge, B. McL., and Lisk, R. D. (1969). *Proc. Soc. Exp. Biol. Med.* **131**, 934.

Breckenridge, B. McL., Burn, J. H., and Matschinsky, F. M. (1967). *Proc. Nat. Acad. Sci. U.S.* **57**, 1893.

Brophy, D., and McEachern, D. (1949). *Proc. Soc. Exp. Biol. Med.* **70**, 120.

Brown-Grant, K., von Euler, C., Harris, G. W., and Reichlin, S. (1954). *J. Physiol. (London)* **126**, 1.

Campbell, H. J., and Eayrs, J. T. (1965). *Brit. Med. Bull.* **21**, 81.

Carmichael, E. A., Feldberg, W., and Fleischauer, K. (1964). *J. Physiol. (London)* **173**, 354.

Celander, O. (1954). *Acta Physiol. Scand. Suppl.* **32**, 116,1.

Cerf, J. A. (1963). *In* "Ions Alcalino Terreux" (Z. M. Bacq, ed.). Suppl. 17, Vol. 1, pp. 164-285. Springer-Verlag, Berlin and New York.

Chambers, W. F., Freeman, S. L., and Sawyer, C. H. (1963). *Exp. Neurol.* **8**, 458.

Chatonnet, J. (1955). *Arch. Scand. Physiol.* **9**, C103.

Chauchard, P. (1952). *Rev. Sci. Med.* **90**, 120.

Chowers, I., Conforti, N., and Feldman, S. (1968). *Amer. J. Physiol.* **214**, 538.

Clare, M. C., and Bishop, G. H. (1955). *Amer. J. Psychiat.* **111**, 818.

Clark, I., and Geoffroy, R. F. (1957). *Fed. Proc. Fed. Amer. Soc. Exp. Biol.* **16**, 165.

Cleghorn, R. A. (1951). *Can. Med. Ass. J.* **65**, 449.

Clemens, J. A., Gallo, R. V., Whitmoyer, D. I., and Sawyer, C. H. (1969). *The Physiologist* **12**, 199 (abstract).

Clendinnen, B. G., and Eayrs, J. T. (1961). *J. Endocrinol.* **22**, 183.

Cohen, R. A., and Gerard, R. W. (1937). *J. Cell. Comp. Physiol.* **10**, 223.

Cook, S., Mavor, H., and Chambers, W. F. (1960). *Elecgroencephalogr. Clin. Neurophysiol.* **12**, 601.

Coppola, J. A. (1969). *Neuroendocrinology* **5**, 75.

Corbin, A., and Story, J.C. (1963). *Endocrinology* **73**, 696.

Corbin, A., Mangili, G., Motta, M., and Martini, L. (1965). *Endocrinology* **76**, 811.

Corrodi, H., Fuxe, K., and Hokfelt, T. (1968). *Life Sci.* **7**, 107.

Cotzias, G. C., Van Woert, M. H., and Schiffer, L. M. (1967). *New Engl. J. Med.* **276**, 374.

Cress, C. H., Jr., and Greenblatt, M. (1945). *Proc. Soc. Exp. Biol. Med.* **60**, 139.

Crimson, J. M., and Field, J. (1940). *Amer. J. Physiol.* **130**, 231.

Cross, B. A., and Dyer, R. G. (1969). *J. Physiol. (London)* **203**, 70P.

Cross, B. A., and Green, J. D. (1959). *J. Physiol. (London)* **148**, 554.

Cross, B. A., and Kitay, J. I. (1967). *Exp. Neurol.* **19**, 316.

Cross, B. A., and Silver, I. A. (1965). *J. Endocrinol.* **31**, 251.

Csaba, G., Kiss, J., and Bodoky, M. (1967). *Experientia* **23**, 148.

Curry, J. J., and Heim, L. M. (1966). *Nature (London)* **209**, 915.

Curtis, D. R., and Koizumi, K. (1961).*J. Neurophysiol.* **24**, 80.

Curzon, G., and Green, A. R., (1968a). *Nature (London)* **220**, 1095.

Curzon, G., and Green, A. R., (1968b). *Life Sci.* **7**, 657

Curzon, G., and Green, A. R. (1969). *Biochem. J.* **111**, 15P.

Dahlstrom, A., and Fuxe, K. (1964). *Acta Physiol. Scand. Suppl.* **62**, 232, 1.

Dallman, M. F., and Yates, F. E. (1967). *Proc. Roy. Soc. Med.* **60**, 904.

Daniels, A. E. (1968). Ph.D. Thesis, Univ. of Pittsburgh, Pittsburgh, Pennsylvania.

Daniels, A. E., and Buckley, J. P. (1968). *Eur. J. Pharmacol.* 4, 152.

Daniels, A. E., Severs, W. B., and Buckley, J. P. (1967). *Life Sci.* 6, 545.

Daniels, A. E., Ogden, E., and Vernikos-Danellis, J. (1969). *The Physiologist* 12,205.

Danowski, T. S., Lasser, E. C., and Wechsler, R. (1960). *Metabolism* 9, 1064.

Davenport, V. D. (1949). *Amer. J. Physiol.* 156, 322.

Davidson, J. M., (1969). *In* "Frontiers in Neuroendocrinology" (W. F. Ganong and L. Martini, eds.). pp. 343-388. Oxford Univ. Press, London and New York.

Davidson, J. M., Feldman. S., (1963). *Endocrinology* 72, 936.

Davidson, J. M., Feldman, S., Jones, L. E., and Levine, S. (1967). *Rass. Neurolog. Vegetativa* 21, 9.

Dell, P. (1958). *In* "The Reticular Formation of the Brain" (H. H. Jasper, ed.), Chapter 18, pp. 365-379. Little, Brown, Boston, Massachusetts.

Dell, P., Bonvallet, M., and Hugelin, A. (1954). *Electroencephalogr. Clin. Neurophysiol.* 6, 599.

Denison, M. E., Jasper, R. L., Hiestand, W. A., and Zarrow, M. X. (1955). *Fed. Proc. Fed. Amer. Soc. Exp. Biol.* 14, 37.

Desmedt, J. E. (1963). *In* "Ions Alcalino Terreux" (Z. M. Bacq, ed.). Suppl. 17, Vol. 1, pp. 295-336. Springer-Verlag, Berlin and New York.

Dewhurst, W. G. (1968). *In* "Studies in Psychiatry" (M. Shepherd and D. L. Davies, eds.), pp. 289-317. Oxford Univ. Press, London and New York.

De Wied, D. (1965). *Int. J. Neuropharmacol.* 4, 157.

De Wied, D. (1966). *Proc. Soc. Exp. Biol. Med.* 122, 28.

De Wied, D., and Bohus, B. (1966). *Nature (London)* 213, 1484.

Donoso, A. O., and Cukier, J. O. (1968). *Nature (London)* 218, 969.

Donoso, A. O., De Gutierrez Moyano, M. B., and Santolaya, R. C. (1969). *Neuroendocrinology* 4, 12.

Douglas, W. W. (1966). *Pharamacol. Rev.* 18, 471.

Douglas, W. W., and Paton, W. O. M. (1952). *Lancet* 1, 342.

Douglas, W. W., and Rubin, R. P. (1963). *J. Physiol. (London)* 167, 288.

Dumerfurth, G. (1961). *Helv. Paediat. Acta* 16, 102.

Dusser de Barenne, D., and Gibbs, F. A. (1942). *Amer. J. Obstet. Gynecol.* 44, 687.

Du Toit, C. H. (1952). *In* "Phosphorous Metabolism" (W. D. McElroy and B. Glass, eds.), Vol. 2, p. 597. Johns Hopkins Press, Baltimore, Maryland.

Dyster-Aas, K. (1965). *Acta Univ. Lund. Sect. 2*, 12, 1.

Eartley, H., and Leblond, C. P. (1954). *Endocrinology* 54, 249.

Eayrs, J. T. (1954). *J. Anat.* 88, 164.

Eayrs, J. T. (1955). Acta Anat. 25, 160.

Eayrs, J. T. (1960). *Brit. Med. Bull.* 16, 122.

Eayrs, J. T. (1961a). *Reg. Neurochem. Reg. Chem. Physiol. Pharmacol. Nerv. Syst., Proc. Int. Neurochem. Symp., 4th, 1960* (S. S. Kety and J. Elkes, eds.).

Eayrs, J. T. (1961b). *Growth* 25, 175.

Eayrs, J. T. (1964). Brain-thyroid relationships. *Ciba Found. Study Group* [Pap.] No. 18, 60.

Eayrs, J. T. (1967). *Rev. Neuropsiquiatria (Lima)* 30, 117.

Eayrs, J. T., and Horn, G. (1955). *Anat. Rec.* 121, 53.

Eayrs, J. T., and Taylor, S. H. (1951). *J. Anat.* 85, 350.

Eik-Nes, K. B., and Brizzee, K. R. (1965). *Biochem. Biophys, Acta* 97, 320.

Eisenberg, E., Gordan, G. S., and Elliott, H. W. (1949). *Science* 109, 337.

Eisenberg, E., Gordan, G. S., and Elliott, H. W. (1950). *Fed. Proc. Fed. Amer. Soc. Exp. Biol.* 9, 269.

Eisenfeld, A. J. (1967). *Biochim. Biophys. Acta* 136, 498.

Eisenfeld, A. J. and Axelrod, J. (1967). *Biochem. Pharmacol.* 16, 1781.

Ekstrom, T., Lundgren, N., and Schmiterlow, C. G. (1943). *Acta Physiol. Scand.* 6, 52.

Elliott, K. A. C. (1946). *Proc. Soc. Exp. Biol. Med.* 63, 234.

Elliott, K. A. C. (1965). *Brit. Med. Bull.* 21, 70.

Elliott, K. A. C., and Libet, B. (1942). *J. Biol. Chem.* 143, 227.

Elliott, K. A. C., Scott, D. B. M., and Libet, B. (1942). *J. Biol. Chem.* 146, 251.

Elliott, K. A. C., Krueckel, K., and Sutherland, R. E. (1957). Unpublished observations quoted in "Hormones, Brain Function and Behavior" (H. Hoagland, ed.). Academic Press, New York.

Endroczi, E., Lissak, K., and Tekeres, M. (1961). *Acta Physiol.* 18, 291.

Engel, G. L., and Margolin, S. G. (1942). *Arch. Intern. Med.* 70, 236.

Epstein, A. N., Fitzsimons, J. T., and Simons, B. J. (1969). *J. Physiol. (London)* 200, 98P.

Etkin, W. (1955). *In* "Analysis of Development.' (B. H. Willier, P. A. Weiss, and V. Hamburger, eds.), p. 631. Saunders, Philadelphia, Pennsylvania.

Falck. B., and Owman, C. (1965). *Acta Univ. Lund. Sect.* 2 7, 5.

Fazekas, J. F., Graves, F. B., and Alman, R. W. (1951). *Endocrinology* 48, 169.

Feldberg, W. (1963). "A Pharmacological Approach to the Brain, from its Inner and Outer Surface." Williams & Wilkins, Baltimore, Maryland.

Feldberg, W., and Fleischauer, K. (1965). *Brit. Med. Bull.* 21, 36.

Feldberg, W., and Sherwood, S. L. (1953). *J. Physiol. (London)* 120, 3P.

Feldman, S. (1962). *Arch. Neurol. (Chicago)* 7, 460.

Feldman, S. (1968). *Actual. Neurophysiol.* 8, 293.

Feldman, S., and Dafny, N. (1966). *Isr. J. Med. Sci.* 2, 621.

Feldman, S., and Davidson, J. M. (1966). *J. Neurol. Sci.* 3, 462.

Feldman, S., and Robinson, S. (1968). *J. Neurol. Sci.* 6, 1.

Feldman, S., Todt, J. C., and Porter, R. W. (1961). *Neurology* 11, 109.

Ferrari, W., Floris, E., and Paulesu, F. (1955). *Boll. Soc. Ital. Biol. Sper.* 31, 862.

Ferrari, W., Gessa, G. L., and Vargiu, L. (1963). *Ann. N. Y. Acad. Sci.* 104, 330.

Figdor, S. K., Kodet, M. J., Bloom, B. M., Agnello, E. J., P'an, S. Y., and Laubach, G. D. (1957). *J. Pharmacol. Exp. Ther.* 119, 299.

Fischer, F., and Hastrup, B. (1954). *Acta Endocrinol. (Copenhagen)* 16, 141.

Folkow, B. (1955). *Physiol. Rev.* 35, 629.

Fraschini, F., Motta, M., and Martini, L. (1968). *Neuroendocrinology* 24, 270.

Friesen, H. (1964). *Endocrinology* 75, 692.

Fuxe, K., Hokfelt, T., and Nilsson, O. (1967). *Life Sci.* 6, 2057.

Gabrilove, J. L. (1966). *In* "Endocrines and the CNS" (R. Levine, ed.), p. 419. Williams & Wilkins, Baltimore, Maryland.

Geel, S., and Timiras, P. S. (1967a). *Endocrinology* 80, 1069.

Geel, S., and Timiras, P. S. (1967b). *Brain Res.* 4, 135.

Geel, S., Valcana, T., and Timiras, P. S. (1967). *Brain Res.* 4, 143.

Gelber, S., Campbell, P. L., Deibler, G. E., and Sokoloff, L. (1964). *J. Neurochem.* 11, 221.

Gellhorn, E., and Feldman, J. (1941). *Endocrinology* 29, 467.

Gessa, G. L., Pisano, M., Vargiu, L., and Ferrari, W. (1967). *Rev. Can. Biol.* 26, 229.

Glascock, R. F., and Michael, R. P. (1962). *J. Physiol. (London)* 163, 38P.

Goldman, H. (1957). Ph.D. Thesis, Univ. of Chicago, Chicago, Illinois.

Goldman, H. and Sapirstein, L. (1969). Unpublished observations.

Gordan, G. S. (1956). *Recent Progr. Horm. Res.* 12, 153.

Gordan, G. S., and Adams, J. F. (1956). *In* "Hormones and the Aging Process" (E. T. Engle and G. Pincus, eds.), p. 299. Academic Press, New York.

Gordan, G. S., and Elliott, H. W. (1947). *Endocrinology* 11, 517.

Gordan, G. S., Gaudagni, N., Picchi, J., and Adams, J. E. (1955). *Presse Med.* 63, 1483.

Gorny, D. (1968). *Acta Physiol. Pol.* 19, 722.

Gowers, W. R. (1885). "Epilepsy and Other Chronic Convulsive Diseases." Wood, New York.

Granich, M., and Timiras, P. S. (1967). *Fed. Proc. Fed. Amer. Soc. Exp. Biol.* 26, 709.

Green, J. P. (1970). *In* "Handbook of Neurochemistry" (A. Lajtha, ed.), Vol. 3, pp. 221-250. Plenum, New York.

Green, R., Luttge, W. G., and Whalen, R. E. (1969). *Endocrinology* 85, 1969.

Greep, P. O., and Chester-Jones, I. (1950). *Recent Progr. Horm. Res.* 5, 197.

Gregory, K. M., and Diamond, M. C. (1968). *Exp. Neurol.* 20, 394.

Grosser, B. I. (1966). *J. Neurochem.* 13, 475.

Grosser, B. I., and Axelrod, L. R. (1967). *Steroids* 9, 229.

Grosser, B. I., and Axelrod, L. R. (1968). *Steroids* 11, 827.

Grosser, B. I., and Bliss, E. L. (1963). *Fed. Proc. Fed. Amer. Soc. Exp. Biol.* 22, 271.

Guillemin, R., and Krivoy, W. A. (1960). *C. R. Acad. Sci.* 25, 1117.

Gyermek, L., Genther, G., and Fleming, N. (1967). *Int. J. Neuropharmacol.* 6, 191.

Halasz, B., and Szentagothai, J. (1960). *Acta Morphol.* 9, 251.

Halasz, B., Vernikos-Danellis, J., and Gorski, R. (1967). *Endocrinology* 81, 921.

Hall, V. E., and Lindsay, M. (1938). *Endocrinology* 22, 66.

Hamburgh, M., and Flexner, L. B. (1957). *J. Neurochem.* 1, 279.

Hamburgh, M., Lynn, E., and Weiss, E. P. (1964). *Anat. Rec.* 150, 147.

Harris, G. W. (1955). "Monographs of Physiological Society," No. 3, pp. 103-129. Williams & Wilkins, Baltimore, Maryland.

Harris, G. W., and Levine, S. (1962). *J. Physiol. (London)* 163, 42P.

Hart, B. L. (1967). *Science* 155, 1283.

Hart, B. L., and Haugen, C. M. (1968). *Physiol. Behav.* 3, 735.

Hatotani, N., and Timiras, P. S. (1967). *Neuroendocrinology* 2, 147.

Heim, L. M. (1966). *Endocrinology* 78, 1130.

Heim, L. M., and Timiras, P. S. (1963). *Endocrinology* 72, 598.

Held, R. (1965). *Sci. Amer.* 213, 89.

Henkin, R. I. (1967). *J. Clin. Endocrinol. Metab.* 27, 1436.

Henkin, R. I., and Bartter, F. C. (1966). *J. Clin. Invest.* 45, 1631.

Henkin, R. I., and Daly, R. L. (1968). *J. Clin. Invest.* 47, 1269.

Henkin, R. I., and Solomon, D. H. (1962). *J. Clin. Endocrinol. Metab.* 22, 856.

Henkin, R. I., Gill, J. R., Jr., and Bartter, F. C. (1963). *J. Clin. Invest.* 42, 727.

Henkin, R. I., Daly, R. L., and Ojemann, G. E. (1966). *J. Clin. Invest.* 45, 1021.

Henkin, R. I., McGlone, R. E., Daly, R. L., and Bartter, F. C. (1967). *J. Clin. Invest.* 46, 429.

Heuser, G., and Eidelberg, E. (1961). *Endocrinology* 69, 915.

Heuser, G., Ling, G. M., and Buchwald, N. A. (1965). *Arch. Neurol.* (Chicago). 13, 195.

Hill, D. (1948). *Folia Psychiat. Neerl.* 51, 95.

Himwich, H. E., Daly, C., Fazekas, J. F., and Herrlich, H. C. (1942). *Amer. J. Psychiat.* 98, 489.

Hoagland, H., ed. (1957). "Hormones, Brain Function and Behavior." Academic Press, New York.

Hoagland, H., and Stone, D. (1948). *Amer. J. Physiol.* 152, 423.

Hodges, J. R., and Smidgley, S. (1969). Unpublished observations.

Hodges, J. R., and Vernikos, J. (1959). *Acta Endocrinol. (Copenhagen)* 30, 188.

Hodges, J. R., Jones, M., and Vernikos-Danellis, J. (1962). *J. Physiol. (London)* **162**, 19.
Hodgkin, A. L., and Katz, B. T. (1949). *J. Physiol. (London)* **108**, 37.
Hoffman, W. C., Lewis, R. A., and Thorn, G. W. (1942). *Bull. Johns Hopkins Hosp.* **70**, 335.
Hyden, H. (1947). *Symp. Soc. Exp. Biol.* **1**, 152.
Hyden, H. (1961). *Sci. Amer.* **205**, 62.
Hyden, H., and Hartelius, H. (1948). *Acta Psychiat. Scand. Suppl.* **48**, p. 1-117.
Ifft, J. D. (1966). *Neuroendocrinology* **1**, 350.
Issekutz, B. V., Jr. (1937). *Pfluegers Arch. Gesamte Physiol. Menschen Tiere* **238**, 787.
Jacobowitz, D. M. (1962). Ph.D. Thesis, Ohio State Univ., Columbus, Ohio.
Jacobowitz, D. H., Marks, B. H., and Vernikos-Danellis, J. (1963) Unpublished observations.
Javoy, F., Glowinski, J., and Kordon, C. (1968). *Eur. J. Pharmacol.* **4**, 103.
Jenner, F. A. (1968). *Int. Rev. Neurobiol.* **11**, 129.
Jensen, J. M., and Clark, D. E. (1951). *J. Lab. Clin. Med.* **38**, 663.
Jones, M. T. (1970). Personal communication.
Kahwanago, I., Heinrichs, W. L., and Herrmann, W. L. (1969). *Nature (London)* **223**, 313.
Kakiuchi, S., and Rall, T. W. (1968a). *Mol. Pharmacol.* **4**, 367.
Kakiuchi, S., and Rall, T. W. (1968b). *Mol. Pharmacol.* **4**, 379.
Kastin, A. J., and Schally, A. V. (1966). *Endocrinology* **79**, 1018.
Kastin, A. J. Kullander, S., Borglin, N. E., Dahlberg, B., Dyster-Aas, K., Krakau, C. E. T., Ingvar, D. H., Miller, M. C., Bowers, C. Y., and Schally, A. V. (1968). *Lancet* **1**. 1107.
Kato, J., and Villee, C. A. (1967). *Endocrinology* **80**, 1133.
Kawakami, M. (1954). *Jap. J. Physiol.* **4**, 274.
Kawakami, M. (1955). *Jap. J. Physiol.* **5**, 251.
Kawakami, M., and Saito, H. (1967). *Jap. J. Physiol.* **17**, 466.
Kawakami, M., and Sawyer, C. H. (1959). *Endocrinology* **65**, 631.
Kawakami, M., Koshino, T., and Hattori, Y. (1966). *Jap. J. Physiol.* **16**, 551.
Kawakami, M., Seto, K., Terasawa, E., and Yoshida, K. (1967). *Progr. Brain Res.* **27**, 69.
Kelly, J. S., Krnjevic, K., and Somjen, G. (1968). *Int. Congr. Physiol. Sci., Proc., 24th, 1968.* Washington, D.C. Federation of Amer. Soc. Biol., Abstract.
Kennedy, C., and Sokoloff, L. (1957). *J. Clin. Invest.* **36**, 1130.
Kerr, S. E., and Ghantus, M. (1936). *J. Biol. Chem.* **116**, 9.
Kety, S. S. (1960). *In* "Handbook of Physiology" (J. Field, H. W. Magoun, and V. E. Hall, eds.), Vol. III, pp. 1751-1760. Amer. Physiol. Soc., Washington, D.C.
Khairallah, P. A., Vadaparampil, G. J., and Page, I. H. (1965). *Arch. Int. Pharmacodyn. Ther.* **158**, 155.
King, B. D., Sokoloff, L., and Wechsler, R. L. (1952). *J. Clin. Invest.* **31**, 273.
King, R. J., and Gordon, J. (1967). *J. Endocrinol.* **39**, 533.
Klainer, L. M., Chi, Y. M., Freidberg, S. L., Rall, T. W., and Sutherland, E. W. (1962). *J. Biol. Chem.* **237**, 1239.
Klee, C. B., and Sokoloff, L. (1964). *J. Neurochem.* **11**, 709.
Klee, C. B., Cason, J., and Sokoloff, L. (1963). *Fed. Proc. Fed. Amer. Soc. Exp. Biol.* **22**, 580.
Klippel, M. (1899). *Rev. Neurol.* **7**, 898.
Knox, W. E., and Auerbach, V. H. (1955). *J. Biol. Chem.* **214**, 307.
Kobayashi, T., Takeyawa, S., Oshima, K., and Kawamura, H. (1962). *Endocrinol. Jap.* **9**, 302.
Kollros, J. J. (1943). *Physiol. Zool.* **16**, 269.
Koranyi, L., and Endroczi, E. (1967). *Neuroendocrinology* **2**, 65.
Kosowicz, J., and Proszewicz, A. (1967). *J. Clin. Endocrinol. Metab.* **27**, 214.

Krivoy, W. A. (1969). *Psychopharmacol. Bull.* **5**, 29.

Krivoy, W. A., and Guillemin, R. (1961). *Endocrinology* **69**, 170.

Krivoy, W. A., Lane, M., and Kroeger, D. C. (1963). *Ann. N. Y. Acad. Sci.* **104**, 312.

Krnjevic, K. (1965). *Brit. Med. Bull.* **21**, 10.

Laidlaw, J. (1956). *Lancet* **271**, 1235.

Lecor, R. (1954). *Rev. Pathol. Comp.* **54**, 529.

Lee, M. D., and Van Buskirk, E. F. (1928). *Amer. J. Physiol.* **84**, 321.

Levey, H. A., and Roberts, S. (1957). *Amer. J. Physiol.* **189**, 86.

Levine, S., and Mullins, R. F., Jr. (1966). *Science* **152**, 1585.

Lichtensteiger, W. (1969). *J. Physiol. (London)* **203**, 675.

Lichtensteiger, W., Korpela, K., Langeimann, H., and Keller, P. J. (1969). *Brain Res.* **16**, 199.

Lichtigfeld, F. J., and Simpson, G. M. (1967). *New Engl. J. Med.* **276**, 874.

Lincoln, D. W., and Cross, B. A. (1967). *J. Endocrinol.* **37**, 191.

Loeb, G., Cleland, R. S., and Anderson, A. J. (1953). *Stanford Med. Bull.* **11**, 106.

Lovell, R. A., and Elliott, K. A. C. (1963). *J. Neurochem.* **10**, 479.

Luft, R., and Olivecrona, H. (1955). *Cancer (Philadelphia)* **8**, 261.

Lundbaek, K. (1947). *Acta Med. Scand.* **127**, 193.

Lundholm, I. (1949). *Acta Physiol. Scand. Suppl.* **19**, 67.

McEwen, B. S., and Zigmond, R. (1969). Unpublished observations quoted in McEwen, B. S., Weiss, J. M., and Schwartz, L. S. (1969a).

McEwen, B. S., Weiss, J. M., and Schwartz, L. S. (1968). *Nature (London)* **220**, 911.

McEwen, B. S., Weiss, J. M., and Schwartz, L. S. (1969a). *Brain Res.* **16**, 227.

McEwen, B. S., Pfaff, D. W., and Zigmond, R. (1969b). Unpublished observations quoted in McEwen, B. S., Weiss, J. M., and Schwartz, L. S. (1969a).

McGuire, J. L., and Lisk, R. D. (1968). *Proc. Nat. Acad. Sci. U.S.* **61**, 497.

MacLeod, L. D., and Reiss, M. (1940). *Biochem. J.* **34**, 820.

Madras, B. K., and Sourkes, T. L. (1966). *Fed. Proc. Fed. Amer. Soc. Exp. Biol.* **25**, 195.

Magoun, H. W. (1952). *AMA Arch. Neurol. Psychiat.* **67**, 145.

Malven, P. V., and Sawyer, C. H. (1966). *Exp. Neurol.* **15**, 229.

Mandel, P., Ebel-Gries, A., and Fontaine, R. (1954). *C. R. Soc. Biol.* **148**, 713.

Mangili, G., Motta, M., and Martini, L. (1966). *In* "Neuroendocrinology" (L. Martini and W. F. Ganong, eds.), Vol. I, pp. 297-370. Academic Press, New York.

Marcus, E. M., Watson, C. W., and Goldman, P. L. (1966). *Arch. Neurol. (Chicago)* **15**, 521.

Marczynski, T. I., Yamaguchi, N., Ling, G. M., and Grodzinska, L. (1964). *Experientia* **20**, 435.

Martini, L., Fraschini, F., and Motta, M. (1968). *In "Endocrinology and Human Behaviour"* (R. P. Michael, ed.), pp. 175-187. Oxford Univ. Press, London and New York.

Maynard, E. A., Schultz, R. L., and Pease, D. C. (1957). *Amer. J. Anat.* **100**, 409.

Menninger-Leichenthal, E. (1960). "Periodizitat in der Psychopathologie (Neuro-und allgemeinpathologie)." Maudrich Verlag, Wien, Bonn, and Bern.

Merryman, W., Boiman, R., Barnes, L., and Rothchild, I. (1954). *J. Clin. Endocrinol. Metab.* **14**, 1567.

Mess, B., and Martini, L. (1968). *In* "Recent Advances in Endocrinology" (V. H. T. James, ed.), pp. 1-49. Churchill, London.

Michael, R. P. (1962). *Int. Congr. Physiol. Sci., Symp. Spec. Lect., 21st, 1959,* Excerpta Medica Int. Congr. Ser. No. 47, p. 650.

Michael, R. P. (1965). *Brit. Med. Bull.* **21**, 87.

Miller, N. E. (1968). *Unesco/IBRO Symp. Brain Res. Human Behaviour, Unesco House, Paris, March, 1968.*

Millichap, J. G., and Bickford, R. G. (1962). *J. Amer. Med. Ass.* **182**, 523.

Milligan, J. V., and Kraicer, J. (1969). *The Physiologist* **12**, 303.

Minker, E., and Koltai, M. (1965). *Naturwissenschaften* **52**, 189.

Minz, B., and Domino, E. F. (1953). *J. Pharmacol. Exp. Ther.* **107**, 204.

Motta, M., Fraschini, F., Piva, F., and Martini, L. (1968). *Mem. Soc. Endocrinol.* **17**.

Myers, R. D., and Sharpe, L. G. (1968). *Science* **161**, 572.

Myers, R. D., and Yaksh, T. L. (1969). *J. Physiol. (London)* **202**, 483.

Natelson, S., Walker, A. A., and Pincus, J. B. (1966). *Proc. Soc. Exp. Biol. Med.* **122**, 689.

Nichols, C. T., and Tyler, F. H. (1967). *Annu. Rev. Med.* **18**, 313.

Nicolov, N. (1967). *Folia Med. (Plovdiv)* **9**, 249.

Nir, I., Behroozi, K., Assael, M., Ivriani, I., and Sulman, F. G. (1969). *Neuroendocrinology* **4**, 122.

Nixon, J. C., Glorig, A., and High, W. S. (1962). *J. Laryngol. Otol.* **76**, 288.

Noble, E. P., Wurtman, R. J., and Axelrod, J. (1967). *Life Sci.* **6**, 281.

Nurnberger, J. I. (1953a). *Res. Publ. Ass. Res. Nerv. Ment. Dis.* **32**, 132.

Nurnberger, J. I. (1953b). *Neurology Symp., 25th Anniversary Program, Columbia Presbyterian Med. Ctr., October 12, 1953.*

Oomura, Y., Ono, T., Ooyama, H., and Wayner, M. J. (1969). *Nature (London)* **222**, 282.

Palmer, R. H., Ratkovits, B., and Kappas, A. (1961). *J. Appl. Physiol.* **16**, 345.

Parker, D. C., Sassin, J. F., Mace, J. W., Gotlin, R. W., and Rossman, L. G. (1969). *J. Clin. Endocrinol. Metab.* **29**, 871.

Pasolini, F. (1952). *Boll. Soc. Ital. Biol. Sper.* **28**, 298.

Peczely, P. (1966). *Acta Biol. (Budapest)* **16**, 291.

Penfield, W., and Jasper, H. (1954). "Epilepsy and the Functional Anatomy of the Human Brain," pp. 195–238. Little, Brown, Boston, Massachusetts.

Penn, R. D., and Loewenstein, W. R. (1966). *Science* **151**, 88.

Peters, R. A., and Rossiter, R. J. (1939). *Biochem. J.* **33**, 1140.

Petersdorf, R. G., Keene, W. R., and Bennett, I. L. (1957). *J. Exp. Med.* **106**, 787.

Peterson, N. A., Chaikoff, I. L., and Jones, C. (1965). *J. Neurochem.* **12**, 273.

Pfaff, D. W. (1968). *Science* **161**, 1355.

Pfeiffer, C. A. (1936). *Amer. J. Anat.* **58**, 195.

Phoenix, C. H., Goy, R. W., Gerall, A. A., and Young, W. C. (1959). *Endocrinology* **65**, 369.

Pincus, J. B., Natelson, S., and Lugovoy, J. K. (1951). *Proc. Soc. Exp. Biol. Med.* **78**, 24.

Pitchotka, J., von Kugelgen, B., and Damann, R. (1953). *Naunyn-Schmiedebergs Arch. Pharmakol. Exp. Pathol.* **220**, 398.

Pohorecky, L. A., Zigmond, M., Karten, H., and Wurtman, R. J. (1969). *J. Pharmacol. Exp. Ther.* **165**, 190.

Poisner, A. M., and Douglas, W. W. (1965). *Fed. Proc. Fed. Amer. Soc. Exp. Biol.* **24**, 488.

Purdy, R. H., and Axelrod, L. R. (1968a). *Int. Congr. Endocrinol. 3rd, Mexico City, 1968,* Excerpta Medica Foundation, Abstract, p. 170.

Purdy, R. H., and Axelrod, L. R. (1968b). *Steroids* **11**, 851.

Purdy, R. H., Grosser, B. I., and Axelrod, L. R. (1968). *Steroids* **11**, 837.

Rafaelsen, O. J. (1958). *Lancet* **2**, 941.

Rafaelsen, O. J. (1961a). *J. Neurochem.* **7**, 33.

Rafaelsen, O. J. (1961b). *J. Neurochem.* **7**, 45.

Rall, D. P., and Zubrod, C. G. (1962). *Annu. Rev. Pharmacol.* **2**, 109.

Ramirez, V. D., Komisaruk, B. R., Whitmoyer, D. I., and Sawyer, C. H. (1967). *Amer. J. Physiol.* **212**, 1376.

Reiss, M., and Rees, D. S. (1947). *Endocrinology* **41**, 437.

Reivich, T., Isaacs, G., Evarts, E., and Kety, S. (1968). *J. Neurochem.* **15**, 301.

Relkin, R. (1969). *N. Y. State J. Med.* **69**, 2133.

Richter, C. P. (1960). *Proc. Nat. Acad. Sci.* **46**, 1506.

Rigamonti, J. (1957). *Arch. Sci. Med.* **104**, 317.

Roberts, S., and Keller, M. R. (1955). *Endocrinology* **57**, 64.

Roldan, E., and Anton-Tay, F. (1968). *Brain Res.* **11**, 238.

Ruf, K., and Steiner, F. A. (1967). *Science* **156**, 667.

Sakamoto, A. (1966). *Nature (London)* **211**, 1370.

Salas, M., and Schapiro, S. (1969). *The Physiologist* **12**, 346.

Samorajski, T., and Marks, B. H. (1962). *J. Histochem. Cytochem.* **10**, 392.

Sawyer, C. H. (1958). *In* "The Reticular Formation of the Brain" (H. H. Jasper, L. D. Proctor, R. S. Knighton, W. C. Noshay, and R. T. Costello, eds.), pp. 223-230. Little, Brown, Boston, Massachusetts.

Sawyer, C. H., and Kawakami, M. (1959). *Endocrinology* **65**, 622.

Schaaf, M., and Payne, C. A. (1966). *New Engl. J. Med.* **275**, 991.

Schaeffer, G., and Thibault, O. (1946). *C.R. Soc. Biol.* **140**, 765.

Scheinberg, P. (1950). *J. Clin. Invest.* **29**, 1010.

Scheinberg, P., Stead, E. A., Brannon, E. S., and Warren, J. V. (1950). *J. Clin. Invest.* **29**, 1139.

Schieve, J. F., Scheinberg, P., and Wilson, W. P. (1951). *J. Clin. Invest.* **30**, 1527.

Schjeide, O. A., and Urist, M. R. (1956). *Science* **124**, 1242.

Selye, H. (1941). *J. Pharmacol. Exp. Ther.* **73**, 127.

Sensenbach, W., Madison, L., and Ochs, L. (1953). *J. Clin. Invest.* **32**, 226.

Sensenbach, W., Madison, L., Eisenberg, S., and Ochs, L. (1954). *J. Clin. Invest.* **33**, 1434.

Sherratt, M., Exley, D., and Rogers, A. W. (1969). *Neuroendocrinology* **4**, 374.

Sholiton, L. J., Werk, E. E., Jr., and MacGee, J. (1965). *Metabolism* **14**, 1122.

Slusher, M. A. (1966). *Exp. Brain Res. (Berlin)* **1**, 184.

Slusher, M. A., Hyde, J. E., and Laufer, M. (1966). *J. Neurophysiol.* **29**, 157.

Smelik, P. G., and Sawyer, C. H. (1962). *Acta Endocrinol. (Copenhagen)* **41**, 561.

Söderberg, U. (1956). *Int. Congr. Physiol. Sci., 20th, 1956, Brussels, Excerpta Medica Foundation*, Abstracts, p. 839.

Sokoloff, L. (1956). *Progr. Neurobiol.* **1**, 216.

Sokoloff, L., and Kaufman, S. (1961). *J. Biol. Chem.* **236**, 795.

Sokoloff, L., and Klee, C. B. (1966). *In* "Endocrines and the CNS" (R. Levine, ed.), pp. 371-385. Williams & Wilkins, Baltimore, Maryland.

Sokoloff, L., Wechsler, R. L., Mangold, R., Balls, K., and Kety, S. S. (1953). *J. Clin. Invest.* **32**, 202.

Somjen, G. G., and Kato, G. (1968). *Brain Res.* **9**, 161.

Spink, W. W. (1957). *New Engl. J. Med.* **257**, 579.

Spooner, C. E., Mandell, A. J., Winters, W. D., Sabbot, I. M., and Cruikshank, M. K. (1968). *Proc. West. Pharmacol. Soc.* **11**, 98.

Stefano, F. J. E., and Donoso, A. O. (1967). *Endocrinology* **81**, 1405.

Steiner, F. A., Pieri, L., and Kaufmann, L. (1968). *Experientia* **24**, 1133.

Steiner, F. A., Ruf, K., and Akert, K. (1969). *Brain Res.* **12**, 74.

Stumpf, W. E. (1968). *Science* **162**, 1001.

Sutherland, E. W., Robison, G. A., and Butcher, R. W. (1968). *Circulation* **37**, 279.

Takahashi, Y., Kipnis, D. M., and Daughaday, W. H. (1968). *J. Clin. Invest.* **47**, 2079.

Takano, H. (1956). *Jap. J. Physiol.* **6**, 22.

Tata, J. R., and Widnell, C. C. (1964). *Biochem. J.* **92**, 26P.

Tata, J. R., Ernster, L., Lindbergh, O., Arrhenius, E., Pedersen, S., and Hedman, R. (1963). *Biochem. J.* **86**, 408.

Taurog, A., Tong, W., and Chaikoff, I. L. (1958). *Endocrinology* **62**, 646.

Thoman, E. B., Wetzel, A., and Levine, S. (1968). *Commun. Behav. Biol.* **2**, 165.

Thorn, G. W. (1949). "Adrenal Cortex." *Trans. Macy Conf. 1st, 1949,* p. 189. Josiah Macy, Jr. Found., New York.

Thorn, G. W., and Forsham, P. H. (1949). *Recent Progr. Horm. Res.* **4**, 243.

Timiras, P. S., and Vernadakis, A. (1967). *In* "Endocrine Aspects of Disease Processes" (G. Jasmin, ed.), pp. 151-159. Green, St. Louis, Missouri.

Timiras, P. S., and Woodbury, D. M. (1956). *Endocrinology* **58**, 181.

Timiras, P. S., Woodbury, D. M., and Agarwal, S. L. (1955). *J. Pharmacol. Exp. Ther.* **115**, 154.

Tipton, S. R. (1939). *Amer. J. Physiol.* **127**, 710.

Tomkins, G. M., and Maxwell, E. S. (1963). *Annu. Rev. Biochem.* **32**, 677.

Torda, C., and Wolff, H. G. (1949). *J. Clin. Invest.* **28**, 1228.

Torda, C., and Wolff, H. G. (1951). *Fed. Proc. Fed. Amer. Soc. Exp. Biol.* **10**, 137.

Trojanova, M., and Mourek, J. (1966). *Physiol. Bohemoslov.* **5**, 231.

Tusques, J. (1956). *Biol. Med. (Paris)* **45**, 395.

Vernadakis, A., and Timiras, P. S. (1967). *Experientia* **23**, 467.

Vernadakis, A., and Woodbury, D. M. (1960). *Fed. Proc. Fed. Amer. Soc. Exp. Biol.* **19**, 153.

Vernadakis, A., and Woodbury, D. M. (1963). *J. Pharmacol. Exp. Ther.* **139**, 110.

Vernikos-Danellis, J. (1964). *Proc. Int. Congr. Endocrinol. 2nd, 1964, London, Excerpta Medica Foundation,* pp. 549-555.

Vernikos-Danellis, J. (1965). *Endocrinology* **76**, 122.

Vogt, M. (1954). *J. Physiol. (London)* **123**, 451.

Vogt, M. (1965). *Brit. Med. Bull.* **21**, 57.

Von Euler, C., and Holmgren, B. (1956). *J. Physiol. (London)* **131**, 137.

von Mayersbach, H., ed. (1967). "The Cellular Aspects of Biorhythms." Springer-Verlag, Berlin and New York.

Waelsch, H. (1955). *In* "Biochemistry of the Developing Nervous System" (H. Waelsch, ed.), pp. 187-201. Academic Press, New York.

Walker, D. G., Simpson, M. E., Asling, C. W., and Evans, H. M. (1950). *Anat. Rec.* **106**, 539.

Walker, D. G., Asling, C. W., Simpson, M. E., Li, C. H., and Evans, H. M. (1952). *Anat. Rec.* **114**, 19.

Wang, H. H., Tarby, T. J., Kado, R. T., and Adey, W. R. (1966). *Science* **154**, 1183.

Wayne, H. L. (1954). *J. Clin. Endocrinol. Metab.* **14**, 1039.

Weil-Malherbe, H., Whitby, L. G., and Axelrod, J. (1961). *J. Neurochem.* **8**, 55.

Weiss, B., and Costa, E. (1968). *J. Pharmacol. Exp. Ther.* **161**, 310.

Weiss, P., and Rossetti, F. (1951). *Proc. Nat. Acad. Sci. U.S.* **37**, 540.

Weitzman, E. D., Schaumburg, H., and Fishbein, W. (1966). *J. Clin. Endocrinol. Metab.* **26**, 121.

Whalen, R. E., and Maurer, R. A. (1969). *Proc. Nat. Acad. Sci. U.S.* **63**, 681.

Wilkins, L. (1957). "The Diagnosis and Treatment of Endocrine Disorders in Childhood and Adolescence," 2nd ed., p. 99. Blackwell, Oxford.

Woodbury, D. M. (1954). *Recent Progr. Horm. Res.* **10**, 65.

Woodbury, D. M. (1958). *Pharmacol. Rev.* **10**, 275.

Woodbury, D. M., and Davenport, V. D. (1949). *Amer. J. Physiol.* **157**, 234.

Woodbury, D. M., and Davenport, V. D. (1952). *Arch. Int. Pharmacodyn. Ther.* **92**, 97.

Woodbury, D. M., and Karler, R. (1960). *Anesthesiology* **21**, 686.

Woodbury, D. M., and Vernadakis, A. (1967). *In* "Neuroendocrinology" (L. Martini and W. F. Ganong, eds.), Vol. II, pp. 335-375. Academic Press, New York.

Woodbury, D. M., Hurley, R. E., Lewis, N. G., McArthur, M. W., Copeland, W. W., Kirschvink, J. F., and Goodman, L. S. (1952). *J. Pharmacol. Exp. Ther.* **106**, 331.

Woodbury, D. M., Timiras, P. S., and Vernadakis, A. (1957). *In* "Hormones, Brain Function and Behavior" (H. Hoagland, ed.), pp. 27-54. Academic Press, New York.

Woolley, D. E., Timiras, P. S., and Woodbury, D. M. (1960). *Proc. West. Pharmacol. Soc.* **3**, 11.

Woolley, D. E., Timiras, P. S., Rosenzweig, M. R., Krech, D., and Bennett, E. L. (1961a). *Nature (London)* **190**, 515.

Woolley, D. E., Timiras, P. S., Srebnik, H. H., and Silva, A. (1961b). *Fed. Proc. Fed. Amer. Soc. Exp. Biol.* **20**, 198.

Woolley, D., Talens, G., and Saari, M. (1969a). *The Physiologist* **12**, 400.

Woolley, D. E., Holinka, C. F., and Timiras, P. S. (1969b). *Endocrinology* **84**, 157.

Wurtman, R. J. (1966). *Endocrinology* **79**, 608.

Wurtman, R. J., and Anton-Tay, F. (1969). *Recent Progr. Horm. Res.* **25**, 493.

Wurtman, R. J., and Axelrod, J. (1965). *Science* **150**, 1464.

Wurtman, R. J., Anton-Tay, F., and Anton, S. (1969). *Life Sci.* **8**, 1015.

Zamenhof, S. (1942). *Physiol. Zool.* **15**, 281.

Zamenhof, S., Mosley, J., and Schuller, E. (1966). *Science* **152**, 1396.

Zimmerman, E., and Critchlow, V. (1967). *Proc. Soc. Exp. Biol. Med.* **125**, 658.

3

*Hormones and Reproductive Behavior**

Julian M. Davidson

That the reproductive process depends upon the appropriate functioning of certain behavioral responses seems patently obvious. Yet the reproductive biologist too often assumes that, given only the appropriate physiological conditions for gametogenesis, fertilization, and subsequent events, the essential behavioral events will occur as a matter of course. The main purpose of this chapter is to examine the relationship between hormones, sexual behavior, and the reproductive process.

Our relative ignorance of the physiological basis of sexual behavior in humans can be understood in part as the outcome of historical stigmata associated with such behavior; gradual breakdown of taboos is resulting in the blossoming of research in this field. Widely divergent views are expressed on the relative importance of "physiological" and "psychological" factors in the control of human sexual behavior (Kinsey *et al.,* 1953; Money, 1961). Clarification of this issue would be of great significance.

The study of the relationship between hormones and sexual behavior has implications for the physiological control of a broad spectrum of behavior.

*Portions of this chapter will also appear in *Reproductive Biology*, to be published by Excerpta Medica Foundation.

Whether or not sexual behavior is more dependent on variables of blood chemistry than nonreproductive behavior, in no other field have hormonal relationships been so thoroughly identified and investigated. Much information is also available on the neural factors involved in sexual behavior.

Without slighting the large body of interesting information available on sexual behavior of submammalian forms, the discussions of this chapter are limited to mammals. Within Mammalia much of the research on hormones and behavior has been carried out with laboratory rodents. Where striking interspecific differences are known they will be discussed, and in a final section we will consider the degree to which some of the principles derived from rodents and other mammals can be applied to the human species.

I. COPULATORY PATTERNS

Although physiologists use indirect indices of copulatory behavior, such as searching for sperm in the vaginal smear or other indirect indices of mating, systematic investigations of its physiological control must be based on a sound knowledge of the behavioral patterns themselves (cf. Beach, 1966). To treat mating behavior as an all-or-none event is to ignore the intricacies of the qualitative and quantitative influences of experimental variables and to lose crucial information.

Walton (1952) has discussed the extent to which interspecific differences in copulatory behavior are reflected in differences of genital morphology. Thus, in the nonerect state, the "vascular-type" penis of the horse is completely flaccid and withdrawn into the prepuce. Tumescence of the erectile tissue and protrusion of the organ take place slowly, an occurrence which appears to be dependent on continual reception of stimuli during courting behavior. In this species, therefore, foreplay appears to be an essential part of the mating pattern. The fibroelastic penis of the bull, on the other hand, is "relatively rigid even in the nonerect condition" and, while undergoing little enlargement on erection, increases in rigidity. Erection and protrusion usually occur rapidly during the first mount, a factor which is apparently related to the relative absence of foreplay in this species (Walton, 1952).

The specific mating pattern observed in a given species may be correlated with its socioecological circumstances. Thus, the rapid copulation observed in cattle may be seen as adaptive behavior in animals which are typically preyed upon in the wild, since copulating animals are particularly vulnerable to predators (Walton, 1952). An extreme example of this kind of adaptation is seen in the gerenuk antelope (*Litocranius walleri*) in which coitus lasts only a few seconds. The male runs after the female and copulates rapidly while both male and female continue to run, the male on his hind legs with his forelegs in the air

(Backhaus, 1958). Predominantly predatory animals such as bears, lions, ferrets, wolves, and dogs have, on the other hand, relatively lengthy copulation. The complex pattern of multiple intromissions leading to ejaculation found in such rodent species as rats,* mice and hamsters, represents an adaptation of a different sort. Multiple stimulation of the female tract is necessary to activate endocrine mechanisms essential for the attainment of normal pregnancy (see IIIB).

Beach *et al.* (1966) have compared several aspects of the ejaculatory response in a number of mammalian species, including man. One phenomenon found to be rather widespread in species which show multiple serial ejaculations was a progressive increase in the postejaculatory refractory period with successive ejaculations. This phenomenon has been observed in rats, hamsters, deer mice, mice, cats, sheep, swine, and cattle. This change in the refractory period is therefore observed both in species showing multiple intromissions and in those which show only one intromission with ejaculation. It should be noted that similarity in patterns of copulatory behavior is not a necessary correlate of phylogenetic proximity. The multiple-intromission type of copulation is not limited to rodents, being present in species as distant, from an evolutionary viewpoint, as *Macaca mulatta*. Furthermore, multiple intromissions are not universal in rodents; the guinea pig has but one intromission with ejaculation, and copulation is not repeated for some time.

Any consideration of the evolution of human coital patterns is necessarily extremely speculative. Obviously, specific adaptation as a result of vulnerability is no longer of much significance, although the extension of this concept to psychological vulnerability of people engaging in "illegitimate intercourse" has been interestingly alluded to by Bermant (1967). Coitus in humans is often very prolonged, though not as lengthy as the coitus of the mink and sable, where a single intromission may last as long as 8 hours (Ford and Beach, 1951, p. 48). Unique features of copulation in humans are utilization of the face-to-face position and the phenomenon of female orgasm.

Face-to-face copulation facilitates more intense stimulation of the female genitalia, particularly the clitoris. Apparently the animal kingdom offers no real analogy to the phenomenon of the human female's orgasm, with the possible exception of the violent postcopulatory "after-reaction" in the domestic cat (Ford and Beach, 1952). Morris (1969) has offered the interesting speculation

---

*Male copulatory behavior in the rat is characterized by a series of mounts, most of which result in intromission with pelvic thrusting, and which are separated by periods of 0.5-1.0 minutes of grooming. A series of intromissions is terminated with an ejaculatory mount. After a postejaculatory period of approximately 5 minutes a new series commences. Intromissions and ejaculations can be clearly distinguished from mounts and from each other by the accompanying behavioral patterns, and the latencies and frequencies of these acts are found to be reproducible and predictable to an extent.

that female orgasm evolved in order to provide rewards to the female which would facilitate permanent pair formation necessary for nurture of the slowly developing offspring. Zumpe and Michael (1968) have suggested that the "clutching reaction" of the female rhesus monkey which occurs during the ejaculatory mount (Carpenter, 1942) is a form of female orgasm. Similar clutching is found throughout copulation in pigtailed macaques.

The possible uniqueness of female orgasm in humans is commonly discussed in terms of "climactic" events corresponding to the human experience. However, as described by Masters and Johnson (1966), orgasm involves a set of specific physiological events involving the skeletal musculature, the cardiovascular, and other systems. These systemic changes, which largely correspond to similar events in the male, have not been studied to any extent in subhuman species. Conclusions about orgasm in these species cannot be drawn until both physiological and behavioral studies investigating the "consummatory" properties of possible orgasmic events are performed. Since failure of female orgasm is a major psychosexual problem in man, identifying an animal model of this phenomenon would certainly be valuable. Both in lower animals and in humans the possible relationship of coitus-induced hormone secretion to female orgasm (see III) could then be evaluated.

II. HORMONAL DETERMINATION OF SEXUAL BEHAVIOR

If a normal, adult, sexually experienced laboratory rat is placed with a normal female on the evening before her ovulation, there is a high degree of probability that mating will commence within a matter of minutes or seconds. If, however, either partner has been gonadectomized some time before the encounter, mating will not occur. This simple observation raises the main question with which this chapter will deal; however, the problems to be illuminated are exceedingly complex. In the discussions that follow we will first consider the nature of the relationships between the gonads and behavior and then consider the mechanism of action of these gonadal influences on behavior.

A. Males

There is little doubt that the principal, if not the only, means whereby the testes influence behavior is via testosterone secretion. Despite suspicions about the possible role of the small amounts of testicular estrogen and other unknown hormones produced by the male (see Davidson, 1966a, p. 598), no evidence implicates such factors in the control of mating behavior.

Table I shows the amounts of testosterone required to maintain a normal level for two androgen-dependent organs, sexual behavior, and plasma luteinizing hormone (LH) level in castrates. The daily dose of testosterone required to maintain complete and normal mating patterns in 100% of treated animals is only 50% of that estimated to be the physiological replacement dose, based on accessory sex gland and pituitary weights.* This evidence suggests that a wide safety margin exists in the hormonal control of behavior in the male rat. The indication that the testosterone level is not a limiting factor in sex behavior under normal conditions is supported also by other lines of evidence. In castrated rats (Beach and Fowler, 1959; Whalen et al., 1961) and guinea pigs (Grunt and Young, 1952, 1953; Riss and Young, 1954) testosterone does not restore performance markedly beyond the precastration level, even when high doses are used. The implication of Young's work, based on the guinea pig, was that no amount of testosterone could "improve" behavioral performance above the normal level (Young, 1961, p. 1185). However, such increases can be obtained in intact rats (Kagan and Beach, 1953; Beach and Holz-Tucker, 1949) and rabbits (Cheng and Casida, 1949; Cheng et al., 1950). More study would clarify whether or not there are species differences involved. The development of simplified and highly sensitive methods for analysis of blood steroids is facilitating the probing of this question by allowing correlation of inter- and intraindividual differences with circulating levels of testosterone.

Consideration of the dose-response relationship between testosterone and male sex behavior reveals several anomalies. One such anomaly is the rather long latency to restoration of mating following initiation of testosterone therapy in castrates. This restoration latency may be analogous to other physiological mechanisms. After removal of an endocrine gland there is commonly a decrease in sensitivity of the target tissues' responses to the hormones of that gland, such that prolonged treatment with the hormone is necessary before full responsiveness can be reestablished. It seems reasonable to assume that the tissues underlying the behavioral response to testosterone show a similar decrease in sensitivity after withdrawal of the hormone, and that this desensitization is responsible for the slow recovery of these responses on replacement therapy in castrates. Following several weeks' administration of testosterone to long-term castrate rats, considerably more hormone must be administered to maintain sexual behavior than when androgen treatment commences immediately following castration (Fig. 1). In fact, the discrepancy between "maintenance" and "restoration" treatments is greater for behavioral responses than for accessory sex gland growth. Unlike the latter, the sensitivity of the behavioral

*It may be seen from Table I that the amount of hormone required to reverse the castration-induced increase in plasma LH is significantly higher than this amount. This has been used as evidence that some testicular hormone other than testosterone participates in the negative feedback regulation of LH secretion (Ramirez and McCann, 1965; Davidson and Bloch, 1969).

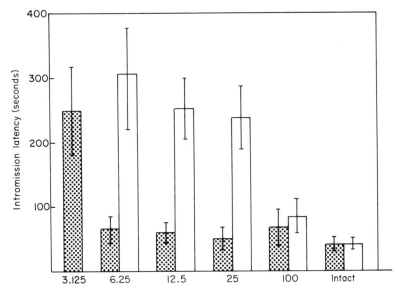

Fig. 1. Effects of testosterone on intromission latency under "maintenance" (dark bars) and "restoration" (white bars) conditions. See Table I for explanations [From data of Smith *et al.* (1971).] Means and standard errors are shown in this figure and Figs. 2 and 3.

"substrate" is not restored in long term castrates with "maintenance" doses even after prolonged (2 months) treatment with testosterone (Table I).

In males of various species studied a major discrepancy between the behavioral and physiological effects of androgens is the frequently prolonged lag

TABLE I. Minimum Approximate Doses of Testosterone Propionate[a] Required to Maintain or Restore Various Androgen-Dependent Parameters to the Level Found in Normal Intact Rats[b]

	Sex behavior[c]	Seminal vesicle weight[d]	Pituitary weight[d]	Plasma LH level[d] (OAAD assay)
Maintenance[e]	12.5	25.0[f]	25.0	25.0–100.0
Restoration[g]	100.0	25.0[f]	100.0	25.0–100.0

[a] μg/(day–100 gm body wt.) administered for 2 months.
[b] From data of Smith *et al.* (1971).
[c] Dose required for 100% normal behavior.
[d] Dose required to reach level not significantly different from that in normal intact rats.
[e] Administration from the day of castration. For dose levels used, see Fig. 1.
[f] At doses lower than this, seminal vesicle stimulation is significantly lower under restoration than under maintenance condition.
[g] Administration commencing 2 months after castration. For dose levels used, see Fig. 1.

between castration and complete loss of mating behavior. Since castrates may be very slow to respond in the testing situation, the retention of postcastration behavior may be underestimated if the animals are tested for several minutes only (Bloch and Davidson, 1968). Complete ejaculatory patterns may in fact be observed in rats for as long as 5 months after castration (Davidson, 1966b), which, it may be noted, is a considerable portion of the organism's life span. How does this apparently androgen-dependent behavior persist so long after complete disappearance of the testicular hormone from the circulation? One suggested possibility is that sexual behavior is maintained by adrenal androgen after castration [refs. in Young (1961), p. 1184]. This is clearly not so in the rat (Bloch and Davidson, 1968) and hamster (Warren and Aronson, 1956), in which no effect of adrenalectomy on sexual behavior before or after castration and testosterone replacement therapy could be demonstrated. Neither the frequency of successful matings nor any other measure of sex behavior was affected by absence of the adrenals (Bloch and Davidson, 1968).

Does the actual experience of the behavioral act "fix" the mechanism, permanently, in the central nervous system (CNS)? Rosenblatt and Aronson (1958) demonstrated a more prolonged postcastration retention of mating behavior in cats which had had precastration mating experience than in those which had had no experience. This was not, however, the case in rats (Bloch and Davidson, 1968) or dogs (Hart, 1968a). For these species, at least, it seems most logical to postulate a mechanism, set in motion by, and initially dependent upon androgen which, without androgen, continues to function for a period of time.

Implicit in the above discussions on the involvement of testosterone in male sexual behavior is the rather simplistic assumption of a 1:1 relationship between the hormone and the behavior studied, analogous to the effect of this hormone on seminal vesicle growth. This relationship becomes somewhat more sophisticated if we consider a motivational component separate from the actual neuromuscular execution of the behavior. Several such "dualistic" notions of mating behavior have been described (cf. Young, 1961, p. 1177 ff.), but perhaps most notably by Beach (1958), who distinguishes an "arousal mechanism" (AM) and a "consummatory mechanism" (CM).

In the immediate postcastration period, during which mating continues in the absence of circulating testosterone, the AM and CM appear to be differentially changed. Rats which continue to copulate following orchidectomy show an immediate and continuing increase in intromission latency and postejaculatory interval* indicating a decrease in "motivation" or "arousal" within the mating situation. On the other hand, measures denoting consum-

---

*Intromission and ejaculation latencies are the times from the onset of a test to the first intromission and from the first intromission to ejaculation, respectively. Intromission frequency is the number of intromissions before ejaculation, and postejaculatory interval is the time from ejaculation to the first intromission of the next series (Beach and Fowler, 1969).

mation, i.e., intromission frequency and ejaculation latency* show decreases, suggesting an increased "efficiency" of mating during these weeks (Davidson, 1966b). Therefore, testosterone might actually prolong the mating patterns in male rats by increasing the numbers of intromissions and the amount of time elapsed between onset and termination of mating. Subsequent investigation showed, however, that these changes could not be reversed with testosterone (Davidson, 1969b; Fig. 2) and that, in fact, the trauma accompanying surgery might have been responsible for these effects. However, it should be emphasized that these behavioral trends are eventually reversed; in long-term castrates ejaculation latency and intromission frequency are elevated (Davidson, 1966b). It is of parenthetical interest that a single exposure to an environmental stimulus, such as excessive noise, surgical trauma, or anesthetization, can have relatively lasting effects on behavioral patterns (Davidson, 1969b), and the possible relevance of this to human sexual behavior deserves consideration.

Meaningful statements about the possible differential dependence of the AM and the CM on androgen cannot presently be made. Beach (1958, 1967) has pointed out the maintenance, in castrated dogs and cats, of certain clearly consummatory responses, e.g., penile stimulation-induced erectile, ejaculatory, and postural reflexes in dogs. Although there is often a prolonged postcastration maintenance of these responses, both Beach (1967) and Hart (1968b), who has

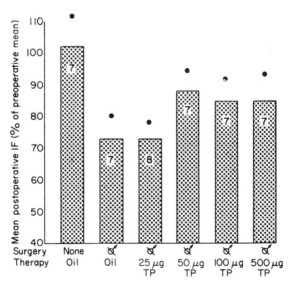

Fig. 2. Effects of castration and replacement therapy with testosterone propionate (TP) on intromission frequency (IF). Postoperative scores were averaged over tests performed twice during the 3 weeks following castration, during which time testosterone was injected sc daily in the doses shown.

performed the most complete studies on spinal sexual reflexes, found definite decrements in measures such as duration of the genital lock in dogs. In fact, the persistence of mounting in the absence or decline of ejaculatory responses in rats (Beach and Holz-Tucker, 1949; Davidson, 1966b), guinea pigs (Grunt and Young, 1953), cats (Rosenblatt and Aronson, 1958), and dogs (Hart, 1968a; LeBoeuf, 1970) suggests that the CM is more dependent on androgen than the AM. However, a fair percentage of subjects show rather rapid disappearance of attempts to mount, and in these cases we can infer nothing about CM. Indeed, the inter- and intraindividual variability in postcastration behavior is so great as to make it difficult to draw conclusions on the basis of existing data. Studies correlating the behavior of individual castrates in the normal mating situation with their responses to artificial penile stimulation would certainly advance our understanding of this problem. The future investigator would be well advised, however, to maintain a healthy skepticism toward existing concepts of dualistic nature of sexual behavior.

B. Females

A striking difference between the male and the female in the hormonal control of reproductive behavior is the general absence in the female of the period of behavioral persistence following gonadectomy. The disappearance of sexual behavior in female rats and guinea pigs after gonadectomy is rapid and complete (see Beach, 1947, p. 300). The apparently simpler behavior patterns associated with sexual receptivity in the female* seem to have more of a one-to-one relationship to gonadal hormones than in the male, whose behavioral patterns appear more complex and less "reflex." In addition to the rapid disappearance of sexual behavior following gonadectomy, the more direct relationship between dose and response is illustrated by the more rapid restoration of behavior following the onset of replacement therapy with ovarian hormones. A dose-responsive curve relating the amount of administered estrogen to the degree of receptivity ("lordosis quotient" or "lordosis-to-mount ratio") can be demonstrated (Fig. 3). The amount of estrogenic hormone required to restore sexual behavior (0.8-1.6 μg/day estradiol benzoate for lordosis and uterine and pituitary weights) seems to be close to the amount needed to establish "physiological" levels of circulating hormone, which is not true, as we have seen, for testosterone in the male (Davidson *et al.,* 1968a).

*Most of the experimental work on female sexual behavior in subprimate laboratory animals is based on a single index: lordosis in response to mounting or simulated mounting (by manual stimulation). The courtship and mating patterns in females of different species obviously include a variety of other behavioral responses, e.g., ear wiggling and hopping in rats. Nevertheless, measurement of the incidence, and possibly the intensity of the lordosis response is a generally quite adequate way to study female sexual behavior in laboratory rodents.

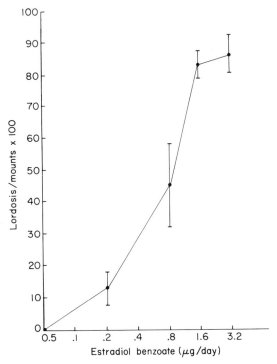

Fig. 3. Effects of estradiol benzoate administered sc daily commencing 3 weeks postoperatively, on sexual behavior (lordosis quotient) in spayed adult rats.

1. Estrogen vs Progesterone: Facilitation

The respective roles of estrogenic and progestational hormones in the control of female sexual behavior is a question of considerable interest. In reproductive physiology, various interactions between estrogen and progesterone can be found, from frank antagonism to marked synergism. How do these interactions affect reproductive behavior? The experimental facts in rodents are relatively straightforward (if not universally recognized), but their interpretation is not so clear. Estradiol can restore apparently normal female sex behavior in spayed rats, if it is given acutely in high doses (Boling and Blandau, 1939) or if it is administered chronically in approximate physiological doses for about 1 week (Fig. 3). In the guinea pig, too, estrogen alone can restore lordosis behavior, although the quality of the behavioral response may be inferior to that obtained with combined estrogen-progesterone treatment (Boling et al., 1938). This apparent nonessentiality of progesterone for estrous behavior in estrogen-treated castrates is not due to secretion of progesterone from the adrenal, since adrenalectomy has no effect on this behavior (Davidson et al., 1968b).

Despite the above considerations, progesterone administered to an animal previously "primed" with one or two doses of estrogen results in a definite facilitation of receptive behavior. How do these experimental observations illuminate the control of sexual behavior during the normal estrous cycle? One might argue that the acute-dose experiments are more relevant, since rats have short physiological and behavioral cycles of 4-5 days, and the waxing and waning of receptivity in these animals must be the result of fairly rapid changes in hormone titers. On the other hand, the fact that prolonged administration of estrogen is necessary to induce normal receptivity with physiological doses of estrogen in spayed rats may be the result of insensitivity caused by prior absence of hormone. Thus, the amount of time required to restore sex behavior with chronic daily administration of estrogen may merely be an index of the time required to restore the sensitivity of the "substrate" tissues.

Circumstantial evidence does, however, indicate that progesterone secretion does have a role in the rapid onset of receptivity which occurs in the rat shortly before ovulation. The results of studies in which plasma progesterone levels were sampled frequently in relation to cyclic changes in behavior, have shown both for the rat (Feder et al., 1967) and the guinea pig (Feder et al., 1966) that a sharp rise in plasma progesterone coincides with, or slightly precedes the appearance of lordosis behavior. Following subcutaneous administration of progesterone to estrogen-primed rodents, it takes some 4 hours for lordosis to appear. Lisk (1960) has reported, however, that intravenous progesterone administration leads to an almost immediate appearance of receptivity in rats, although this finding was not confirmed by others (e.g., Hamburg, 1966).

Does mating occur in rats if they are deprived of the progesterone secreted on the day of proestrous? Schwartz and Talley (1965) found that ovariectomy on the day before proestrus prevented mating (as detected by presence of sperm in the vaginal contents), and presumed that this decrement was due to the removal of estrogen secretion. No significant behavioral decrements resulted from ovariectomy on the morning of proestrus, suggesting the nonessentiality of ovarian progesterone. Recently, however, Powers (1970), using the more appropriate procedure of direct observation of lordoses in response to a male, found that marked inhibition followed ovariectomy on proestrus just prior to the period of progesterone secretion. Further work by Nequin and Schwartz (1971) resulted in a reinterpretation of the role of progesterone. They found that adrenalectomy combined with ovariectomy on the morning of proestrus would prevent mating, and the suggestion was that a factor from the adrenal, presumably progesterone, could substitute for or augment ovarian progesterone in the activation of mating behavior (Schwartz, 1969). That conclusion is consistent with the finding of Feder and Ruf (1969) that ACTH-induced progesterone secretion from the adrenal gland could facilitate estrogen-induced lordosis behavior.

Thus the evidence seems to indicate an acute facilitation of mating behavior by progesterone in the proestrous rat following the burst of estrogen secretion which commences the previous day (Hori *et al.*, 1968). In line with this conclusion are the results of Zucker (1967a), who found that the schedules of progesterone treatment effective in advancing or retarding ovulation in 4- or 5-day cycling rats (Everett, 1948; Zeilmaker, 1966) had essentially parallel effects on the time of onset of estrous behavior. In these experiments, it may be assumed that the administered progesterone was mediating behavior via its influence on the time of ovulatory LH secretion and therefore of LH-induced progesterone secretion. This would imply that the occurrence of behavioral estrus is a function of the timing of endogenous progesterone secretion.

The situation in the ewe, in which the appropriate sequence of hormonal secretion for production of estrous behavior is progesterone followed by estrogen, has long puzzled investigators. However, this "reversed" sequence does make sense in terms of the cyclic pattern of secretion of the two steroids. Moore *et al.* (1969) have recently shown that ovarian secretion of progesterone remains high until shortly before estrus, when a rapid fall occurs, immediately preceding an abrupt rise in estrogen production.

In reflex ovulators, in which appreciable progesterone secretion would not be expected until after LH release, i.e., after mating had occurred, the relative roles of estrogen and progesterone need further definition. Estrous behavior may be produced with ease with estrogen alone in cats (Bard, 1939; Michael and Scott, 1964) and rabbits (Sawyer and Everett, 1959). Although the latter investigators showed that progesterone has some facilitatory effect on receptivity in estrogen-primed rabbits, single or multiple injections of rather low doses of estrogen alone are effective in this species (McDonald *et al.*, 1970; Palka and Sawyer, 1966).

2. Progesterone: Inhibition

Though estrogen and progesterone may have complementary actions in many physiological systems, progesterone may also be shown to have inhibitory effects on the induction of lordosis behavior.

This apparent contradiction between facilitation and inhibition may be resolved, in rabbits (Sawyer and Everett, 1959) and guinea pigs (Zucker, 1966a), by postulating a biphasic sequence of effects—initial facilitation in the estrogen-primed animal, followed by secondary inhibition. In fact, Zucker and Goy (1967) showed that in guinea pigs any progesterone dose capable of facilitating sexual behavior was also able to induce a refractory state at a later time period. Zucker (1968) has been able to relate this dual action of progesterone to the pattern of receptivity during the normal estrous cycle of the guinea pig which is behaviorally refractory during the late luteal phase.

Ovariectomy at this time rapidly restores behavioral responsiveness (Zucker, 1968). Similar biphasic effects of progesterone on ovulatory thresholds have been described by Sawyer and Everett (1959) in the rabbit and by Zeilmaker (1966) in the rat.

It is apparently more difficult to demonstrate inhibitory effects of progesterone on female sex behavior in the rat than in the guinea pig. Although some investigators have found mild inhibitory effects of progesterone under certain carefully specified conditions (Whalen and Nakayama, 1965; Lisk, 1969), Zucker (1967b) was unable to demonstrate such an inhibitory effect in ovariectomized rats. While rats are clearly refractory during pregnancy and pseudopregnancy (Powers and Zucker, 1969), presumably this refractory period results in part from prolonged very high levels of progesterone. The difficulty of demonstrating inhibitory effects of progesterone in the rat may be related to the absence of a prolonged phase of luteal activity following ovulation. Since it is present only relatively briefly, progesterone does not appear to play a role in preventing mating during "inappropriate" stages of the cycle. Consistent with this view is the finding of Kuehn and Zucker (1968) that the Mongolian gerbil, another short-cycling animal, exhibits the same apparent lack of responsiveness to the inhibitory effect of progesterone on estrous behavior. However, progesterone inhibition of estrous behavior is easily demonstrable in the reflex-ovulating rabbit (Sawyer and Everett, 1959; Beyer et al., 1969).*

In contrast to the variable but predominantly facilitatory effects of progesterone in infraprimate species, it is reported that progesterone is predominantly inhibitory in monkeys. Thus Michael et al. (1967) have presented preliminary evidence that progesterone inhibits sexual receptivity in macaques by activating a "refusal" mechanism toward the males' advances. Other evidence suggesting inhibitory effects of progesterone comes from the laboratory of Goy (1968) and the early work of Ball (1941). Since there has been but little systematic work on primates, however, future investigations might reveal conditions under which progesterone is facilitatory.

The several interspecific roles of progesterone provide a striking model for the aphorism ascribed to Medawar and Hisaw that it is not the hormones which have evolved so much as the uses to which they are put.

III. BEHAVIOR AS STIMULUS

The great preponderance of studies on psychosexual endocrinology have been concerned with the effects of hormones on various aspects of reproductive

---

*Recently, Nadler (1970) has suggested that the difficulties in demonstrating inhibitory effects of progesterone are due to the use of superthreshold "priming" doses of estrogen.

behavior, i.e., with hormones as the independent variable and behavior as the dependent variable. However, this approach toward such complex relationships does not suffice to describe the gamut of endocrine-behavior interactions in the area of sex. Situations are now coming to light in which behavioral stimuli precipitate changes in endocrine function as well as other physiological and behavior events. As reproductive behavior is a form of social behavior, the effects of stimuli derived from social interaction, per se, on endocrine systems are relevant to this discussion.

Social and behavior-derived stimuli can affect endocrine function in several ways. First, behavioral stimuli originating in individual A may affect hormone secretion in the same individual. Second, stimuli emanating from individual A may affect endocrine function in individual B. In either case, the changed levels of hormones may affect further behavioral events in either individual A or B. In some cases the communication between individuals A and B is effected by secretion of chemical agents known as pheromones, which are disseminated into the environment and act, presumably, through olfactory receptors, on endocrine and/or behavioral function in individual B. The extent to which conditioning is involved in these interactions in unknown. However, since the secretions of the posterior pituitary are believed to be prone to conditioning of the Pavlovian type (Corson and Corson, 1968) and a variety of visceral responses are subject to operant conditioning (Miller, 1969), this conditioning might well be a factor of importance. The potential medical importance of the conditioning of endocrine secretion may be tremendous, and phenomena of this type present significant questions to potential investigators in this virtually unexplored area.

A. Reflex Ovulation

The fact that ovulation in a number of species (e.g., cats, rabbits, ferrets, minks, ground squirrels, and many avian species) occurs as a result of sexual stimuli—usually copulation itself—is well known. Stimuli derived from the act of mating activate a neuroendocrine reflex resulting in the release of pituitary LH leading to ovulation. The effect is apparently mediated via neural activation of the secretion of LH releasing factor from the basomedial hypothalamus. Thus, copulation-induced ovulation can be prevented in rabbits either by discrete lesions in this area (Sawyer, 1959) or by implantation therein of small amounts of crystalline estrogen (Davidson and Sawyer, 1961a). In birds, at least, reflex ovulation may be prone to conditioning; ovulation in pigeons can result from the mere presence of another male or even female pigeon. Interestingly, ovulation can also be induced merely by placing a mirror in the cage of the female pigeon (Matthews, 1939), a phenomenon which may be the only case of narcissism in endocrinology.

It is now becoming increasingly clear that the LH releasing action of sexual stimuli is not limited to the classic "reflex ovulators," making it necessary to reconsider the traditional distinction between those species and the "spontaneous ovulators." Thus, if ovulation is blocked in rats by various drugs (Everett, 1952; Harrington et al., 1966), or if receptivity is induced prematurely by estrogen treatment (Aron et al., 1965, 1966), copulation may induce ovulation. A similar phenomenon may be demonstrated in immature rats in which ovulation evoked by pregnant mare serum (PMS) is blocked by chlorpromazine (Zarrow and Clark, 1968). The existence of an inherent mechanism for copulation-induced ovulation in "spontaneous ovulators" might either be simply a vestigial function or may serve as a safety factor in cases where the ovulatory mechanism is inadequately functioning. Claims that similar effects occur in humans under certain conditions (cf. Hartman, 1962) have not been adequately substantiated.

The nature of the adequate stimulus for reflex LH release (as reflected in ovulation or luteinization) has been studied. Artificial mechanical stimulation of the vagina and cervix was shown by Aron et al., (1968) and Zarrow and Clark (1968) to be sufficient for ovulation in the rat. The latter investigators found that such stimulation produced a greater response than electrical stimulation of the cervix, suggesting that vaginal receptors are important as well as uterine ones. However, Aron et al. (1968) claim that intromission is not a necessary part of the stimulus pattern in mating-induced ovulation, i.e., either genital stimulation or other unspecified stimuli resulting from mounting by the male are each effective in the absence of the other. This apparent nonspecificity is reminiscent of earlier findings in the reflex-ovulating rabbit that genital deafferentation did not block copulation-induced ovulation (e.g., Brooks, 1935). However, following daily single mounts with lordosis, rabbits of the Dutch belted breed did not ovulate if intromission was prevented (Staples, 1967). Ovulation did occur in submissive does if they were *repeatedly* mounted by other does, but not in females who assumed the dominant role. The conclusion arrived at by Staples (1967) was that the "degree of excitement attained by the submissive female" was the factor necessary to produce ovulation. Clearly, more work is required to identify precisely the appropriate afferent stimuli.

Interestingly enough, it has been reported that LH is released following coitus in male rats (Taleisnik et al., 1966) and also in rabbits, in which increases in testosterone secretion have been demonstrated, presumably secondary to LH release (Endroczi and Lissak, 1962; Saginor and Horton, 1968).* This phenomenon may have physiological significance, since aging male rats show a decrease in incidence of spontaneous reproductive system atrophy when given

---

*Recently in our laboratory (Davidson et al., 1970) and in others (Spies and Niswender, 1971), the findings of Taleisnik et al. (1966) could not be repeated using the more reliable method of LH radioimmunoassay.

the opportunity to copulate (Drori and Folman, 1964). Further, Thomas and Neiman (1968) found, interestingly, that reproductive system atrophy in male rats was not prevented by mounts alone and that ejaculations were more effective than intromissions in this regard. The implication here that "sex is good for you" should come as no surprise.

B. Behavioral Influences on Prolactin Secretion

A whole series of "social" and behavioral effects on the reproductive system of rodents appear to be mediated via changes in the secretion of pituitary prolactin-luteotropin.* These include both effects of coital stimuli on prolactin secretion, as well as responses to noncoital stimuli deriving from other animals.

1. Copulatory Stimuli

As mentioned above, the ovulation-inducing (LH-releasing) effect of stimuli resulting from mating behavior is at best only of subsidiary importance in "spontaneously ovulating" species. Another effect of copulation is, however, overwhelmingly important—the induction of luteal activity in short-cycled animals such as the rat, mouse, and hamster. This phenomenon is easiest to demonstrate by sterile mating, when a period of "pseudopregnancy" ensues, though this mechanism apparently operates in the case of fertile matings, and seems to play an important role in ensuring the successful outcome of pregnancy.

For the purpose of this discussion, the oversimplification is made that prolonged periods of active luteal function in rodents results from prolactin secretion. However, LH has been shown to stimulate progesterone secretion in rodents as well as in other species (Armstrong, 1968) so that the ovarian changes to be discussed may derive both from LH and from prolactin secretion. Nevertheless, the luteotropic effect of mating is clearly distinguishable from the ovulatory release of gonadotropin, and the two can be experimentally dissociated, as demonstrated by Everett (1961, p. 532). In reflex ovulators, mating induces ovulation, and luteal activation either follows automatically (cat, rabbit, ferret) or may require additional environmental stimuli (mink) (Everett, 1961, p. 533). Of parenthetical interest is the finding of postcopulatory release of prolactin and ACTH in the rabbit (Desjardins, et al., 1967), although neither of these hormones is apparently luteotropic in this species. Coital release of oxytocin has been reported both in lower animals and in women and may be involved in sperm transport (Cross, 1966).

---

*The name luteotropin is hardly justifiable as an alternative for prolactin, since only in rodents has it been shown unequivocally to have luteotropic effects.

In the induction of pseudopregnancy, sterile mating may be replaced by mechanical (Long and Evans, 1922) or electric (Shelesnyak, 1931) stimulation of the cervix. However, cervical stimulation is apparently not the only mediator of pseudopregnancy; Ball (1934) found that, although cervicotomy diminished the responses to single matings, pseudopregnancy still invariably resulted when multiple vaginal plugs were deposited. A more recent analysis of the adequate stimulus for behavioral induction of luteal activity in the mouse (Land and McGill, 1967) indicated that intromissions alone were not sufficient for the effect. Furthermore, repeated mating with animals which had had their seminal vesicles surgically removed was effective in inducing pseudopregnancy. Since vaginal plugs could not be deposited by these males, the authors concluded that some event resulting from the ejaculatory process other than plug deposition provides the stimulus for luteal activation in mice (McGill et al., 1968; McGill, 1970).

That the successful outcome of pregnancy in rats is dependent on stimuli derived from mating is suggested by the finding of Wilson et al. (1965): a high frequency rate of pregnancy seemed to depend on the female rat receiving multiple intromissions. Early work by Blandau (1945) indicated that the presence of a vaginal plug was necessary to facilitate sperm passage through the cervix. Adler recently provided evidence (1969) that the low rate of successful fetal implantation found in rats given only few intromissions before ejaculation was due both to failure of sperm transport through the cervix and to the secretion of insufficient progesterone to ensure normal implantation and gestation. The adequate stimuli in the rat may thus differ from those in the mouse where high intromission rates were not found to be necessary for pseudopregnancy (Land and McGill, 1967). It should be noted, however, that there are many more pelvic thrusts per intromission in the mouse than in the rat. Further research is required in order to elucidate the possible significance for reproduction of various elements of the diverse mating patterns in different species.

Although maternal behavior is not one of the areas with which this review is primarily concerned, certain phenomena relating to mother-infant interactions should be mentioned because of their relevance in the present context. It is well known that suckling by the young provides a stimulus for milk ejection in the lactating mother, and that this reflex is mediated by the secretion of oxytocin from the posterior pituitary (Denamur, 1965). Less well known is the fact that suckling induces the release of other hormones, particularly prolactin (Meites and Turner, 1942). Furthermore, self-licking of the nipple lines by the pregnant rat facilitates mammary development (Roth and Rosenblatt, 1968). Grosvenor and co-workers (1969) have provided evidence that, in multiparous animals, prolactin release becomes conditioned to the exteroceptive stimulus of the presence of the young, obviating the need for either suckling or self-licking. The importance of such conditioning of endocrine secretions has previously been mentioned.

2. Pheromones.

A considerable body of evidence now exists indicating that regulation of the estrous cycle in mice is dependent upon "social" stimuli. The mechanism of this endocrine effect of behavioral phenomena is quite different from those discussed above; it results from the chemoreception or ingestion of pheromones, which are chemical agents excreted into the atmosphere by the "stimulus" animal. Much is known about pheromones in insects, including, in some cases, their chemical structure. Wilson and Bossert (1963) classify pheromones as either "primer"— acting on a series of physiological events, such as changes in the endocrine system, or "releaser"—acting directly to change the recipient animal's behavior. There is evidence for both these types of phenomena in mammals. Among the primer pheromone effects well established in mice is the Lee-Boot effect (Van der Lee and Boot, 1956)—suppression of estrous cycles when all-female groups are housed together. Another primer action is the Whitten effect, whereby introduction of males into the cages of female mice accelerates the appearance of estrus and synchronizes estrous cycles (Whitten, 1956a). The latter phenomenon may be duplicated by exposure to male urine (Whitten, 1956a,b) and both effects are suppressed by removal of the females' olfactory bulbs. It is presumed that the Lee-Boot effect results from a stimulation of prolactin secretion, while the Whitten effect is the result of inhibition of prolactin secretion. Although most of the work has been done on mice, these phenomena are present in other mammalian species, indicated by the variety of reports on acceleration of estrus in ewes by the presence of rams [see Anderson (1969) for review].

The well-known Bruce effect, whereby exposure to the presence or the odor of an alien male prevents implantation in a recently fertilized mouse (Bruce, 1959) is apparently also due to inhibition of prolactin secretion, and the effect can be abolished by exogenous prolactin (Parkes and Bruce, 1961) or progesterone (Dominic, 1966). Whitten (1966) has suggested that the same pheromone is involved in the Whitten and Bruce effects. The possibility that male odors have stimulatory effects on gonadotropin secretion is suggested by the finding of Vandenbergh (1969) that males or their urine accelerate sexual maturation in female mice. Since prolactin secretion is often inversely related to FSH and LH secretion, the same pheromone could be operating again in this case. However, Clemens et al. (1969a) reported precocious puberty in female rats with prolactin administration, a finding possibly, but not necessarily, relevant to this discussion.

As yet, there appears to be no evidence for primer pheromone effects in *male* mammals. The pituitary-gonadal response to mating in male rats and rabbits is probably not triggered by female odors, since Thomas and Neiman (1968) failed to duplicate the accessory sex gland-stimulating effect of cohabitation by exposure to urine from estrous females.

Little information is available on signaling or "releaser" pheromones in mammals. However, LeMagnen (1952) demonstrated the ability of male rats to distinguish the odors of estrous from anestrous females. This capacity is androgen-dependent (Carr and Caul, 1962; Carr *et al.,* 1965). A similar olfactory discriminative ability is possessed by rams (Lindsay, 1965) and probably other mammalian species. The olfactory "preference" of male dogs for females in induced estrus was dramatically demonstrated by Beach and Merari (1968). When confronted with cotton balls soaked in vaginal secretions, the males spent considerably longer time sniffing and licking the balls with vaginal discharge from spayed females injected with estrogen. Interest on the part of the male was further increased when the donor female had also received progesterone. Michael and co-workers have recently obtained evidence for estrogen facilitation of pheromone-like activity of vaginal secretions having marked influence on the behavior of the male rhesus monkey (Michael and Keverne, 1968).

The possible biological significance of presumed signaling and primer mammalian pheromones is discussed in the excellent review by Bronson (1968). The utility of signaling pheromones in facilitating mating is obvious, although the sex attractant effect is probably not as important in this class as it is in insects. Among the examples of "primer" pheromone phenomena, the Whitten effect seems to promote fertility while the Lee-Boot effect may be advantageous in seasonally breeding animals to synchronize births (see Bronson, 1968).

IV. MECHANISM OF ACTION
OF HORMONES ON SEX BEHAVIOR

Elucidation of the mechanism whereby gonadal hormones influence sexual behavior presents a challenge of great importance to behavioral physiologists because of the far-reaching implications of such information for our understanding of the physiological basis of behavior in general. Since little is known about the action of gonadal hormones on the cellular and subcellular levels, this discussion will be almost entirely limited to consideration of the locus of this action. Even on this level, the search for answers is difficult and complex. However, such answers become the necessary precursors of future investigations into the cellular and molecular events underlying hormonal influences on behavior.

Assuming, as we must, that CNS events are crucial to the manifestation of sexual behavior, there are three possible loci for the action of gonadal hormones.

They may act peripherally, on genital or other tissues, to influence afferent nervous input to the CNS. Secondly, they may act on regions widespread throughout the CNS. Finally, their action may be specifically to effect changes in discrete neural regions. The CNS-gonadal hormone relationship is further complicated by the fact that these three possibilities are not mutually exclusive.

A. Females

A variety of attempts to eliminate various sensory modalities (vision, olfaction, audition) by surgical or pharmacological interventions has led to the conclusion that no one specific modality is essential for sexual receptivity in female animals (Beach, 1947; Fletcher and Lindsay, 1968). Deafferentation of the genital region likewise has remarkably little effect on female sexual behavior in a variety of species [refs. in Beach (1947) and Sawyer (1960)], and sexual reflexes may be found in spinally sectioned cats (Maes, 1939; Bard, 1940) and guinea pigs (Dempsey and Rioch, 1939). Unlike Maes (1939), Bard (1940) found that the postural responses which resemble those of the intact copulating cat were not estrogen-dependent. Recently, Hart (1969) was unable to influence with estrogen the weak lordosis responses which could be evoked in spinal rats. The hormone was only partially effective in facilitating other sexual reflexes which could be elicited by mechanical stimulation in the spinal bitch (Hart, 1970).

These findings suggest that the locus of action of the ovarian hormones in influencing female sexual behavior is primarily central rather than peripheral. Further evidence of this central locus of action comes from reports that hypothalamic lesions of various types prevent the occurrence of female responses even after administration of ovarian hormones [refs. in Lisk (1967a)]. Although these findings are suggestive of the locus of hormonal action, it remains possible that the lesions were removing structures essential for sex behavior which are not themselves sensitive to the hormones.

In 1958 Harris et al. reported the results of an important investigation in which, for the first time, intracerebral implantation of crystalline steroid was used to study sexual behavior. Receptivity was induced in spayed cats following hypothalamic implantation of crystalline estrogen (stilbestrol) in the absence of vaginal cornification or uterine stimulation. When estrogen was administered subcutaneously, a lower dose was required to produce vaginal and uterine changes than the dose needed to induce behavioral receptivity. Thus the effects of the brain implants were presumably not due to release of steroid into the circulation. Later reports (Harris and Michael, 1964; Michael, 1965) indicated that estrogen implants were effective when located in a rather wide region of the hypothalamus, from the medial preoptic to the posterior hypothalamus. Although an abstract by Sawyer (1963) indicated that the anterior hypothalamus was the more effective region in this regard, Palka and Sawyer (1966) found that in spayed female rabbits estrogen implants in the ventromedial-premammillary hypothalamus precipitated estrous behavior. Lisk (1962) reported that implants in the preoptic-anterior hypothalamic region elicited lordosis behavior in the ovariectomized rat and that implants elsewhere in the hypothalamus were ineffective.

In the above-mentioned studies, behavioral data were not analyzed quantitatively (except for latencies) but rather were reported as presence or absence of receptivity. Experiments on rats in our laboratory, utilizing implants similar to Lisk's, suggest that this procedure might obscure relevant information (Davidson, 1966d, 1969b, p. 136). Implantation of estradiol in various areas both in and outside of the hypothalamus resulted in some degree of lordosis, but in no case were the levels of responding similar to those of naturally estrous females (Table II). Furthermore, even implants which had only a slight effect on behavior resulted in the release of sufficient estrogen into the circulation to induce vaginal cornification. Since higher doses of estradiol are required to precipitate normal behavior than those required to induce cornification, the finding that anterior hypothalamic estrogen implants result in low grade behavior *and* cornification illustrates the difficulty of demonstrating a clearly hypothalamic effect of estrogen on behavior, at least in these (Long-Evans) rats. Whalen (1969) has also found that small intrahypothalamic estrogen implants outside the circumscribed anterior region stimulated lordosis behavior in female rats. Thus, before the precise extent of the estrogen-sensitive region can be mapped, the estrogen implant experiment needs to be further refined. The array of evidence, however, still suggests that in a variety of species the action of estrogenic hormones on the hypothalamic region does activate a certain degree of female sex behavior in response to the adequate stimuli. The complex questions raised by this statement may be better understood after analysis of the neuroendocrine basis of male behavior patterns.

B. Males

Where does androgen act in conditioning the male organism to respond with copulatory behavior to the appropriate sexual stimuli? The complexity of the behavioral patterns involved in the male might lead us to expect fairly widespread CNS action. On the other hand, the male genitalia are to a greater or lesser degree dependent on androgen for their structural maintenance. We must question the extent to which erection requires androgenic stimulation, as well as the possible importance of androgen for normal sensory feedback from the genitalia during mating behavior. While it would be presumptuous at this time to eliminate from consideration any of the possible targets of androgen—penis, afferent nerves, spinal cord, or brain—experiments on intracerebral implantation

TABLE II. Effects of Intracerebral Implantation of Estradiol on Lordosis Behavior in Females Ovariectomized Three Weeks Prior to Implantation[a]

Area	N	Lordoses/mounts × 100						Vaginal smears (% cornified)
		Day after implantation						
		1	4	5	7	8	11	
Cortex	7	10 ± 1	17 ± 9	19 ± 9	42 ± 16	32 ± 11	31 ± 11	98
Anterior hypothalamus	8	8 ± 4	36 ± 13	33 ± 14	50 ± 11	57 ± 9	49 ± 11	84
Posterior hypothalamus	8	4 ± 2	29 ± 9	14 ± 6	38 ± 11	47 ± 12	40 ± 13	89

[a]Estradiol fused inside the tip of 27–gauge tubes. Each group includes 1 or 2 animals in which the implants were located just outside the areas cited. There was no correlation within the groups between precise location of implant and behavior.

TABLE III. Activiation of Male Sexual Behavior in Long-Term Male Castrates by intracerebral Testosterone Propionate Implants[a]

Area	No. rats	Tests positive %[b]	Intromission latency (sec)	
			Before castration	After implantation
Hypothalamus[c]	16	44	37 ± 8	136 ± 42
Medial preoptic	8	57	17 ± 8	141 ± 43
Other regions	22	13	24 ± 4	336 ± 67
Cholesterol controls	15	0		

[a]From data of Davidson (1966).
[b]Ejaculatory pattern present.
[c]Excluding supraoptic, including area anterior to habenulointerpeduncular tract.

of crystalline androgen (Davidson, 1965, 1966c) seem to indicate the hypothalamus as (see below) the primary site of action of the hormone in adult male rats.

Adult castrate rats which had ceased to manifest mating behavior were given single 200 μg implants of testosterone propionate in various cerebral locations and received five mating tests in the next 3 weeks. Animals with implants in the hypothalamus showed complete restoration of mating patterns on approximately half of these tests in the absence of histologically detectable stimulation of the sexual accessory glands (Table III). Copulation culminated in normal ejaculatory behavior, although intromission latency was markedly increased. Since it was also shown that more systemically administered testosterone was required to restore ejaculatory behavior than to effect minimal histological changes in the seminal vesicles and prostates, the androgen was apparently acting locally rather than via absorption into the circulation. Although the area from which behavior was most consistently obtained was the anterior hypothalamic-medial preoptic "continuum," responses were also obtained from other parts of the hypothalamus, and there were insufficient data to establish clearly whether or not the anterior region was the most effective site. Evidence was adduced that the effects of posterior hypothalamic implants were not due to diffusion to an active site in the anterior region. It was therefore concluded that a relatively widespread testosterone-sensitive system was present throughout the hypothalamus, and that activation of any one portion of this system was sufficient to activate mating, in the absence of effective amounts of androgen elsewhere in the organism (Davidson, 1966c).*

*Recent unpublished experiments of P. J. Johnston and J. M. Davidson have shown, however, that implants in the anterior region are clearly more effective than those in the posterior hypothalamus.

From similar studies, Lisk (1967b) concluded that the testosterone-sensitive area was limited to the anterior hypothalamic-preoptic region. Although his bilateral implants apparently resulted in greater release of testosterone into the systemic circulation than was found in the studies described above, Lisk did not find effects from bilateral posterior hypothalamic implants. It is doubtful, however, that enough animals with implants in various areas of the hypothalamus were studied to eliminate ineffective regions outside the anterior one.

The forerunner of these investigations was a brief report by Fisher in 1956 on the immediate activation of copulatory responses in a small proportion of intact rats following acute intracerebral injections of a testosterone salt. In this study, and others showing regular behavioral restoration in castrates of various avian species with testosterone implants (Barfield, 1969; Hutchison, 1967; Gardner and Fisher, 1968) attention was focused mainly on the preoptic region.

The results of experimental production of lesions in the anterior hypothalamic-preoptic continuum support the conclusion that this region is testosterone-sensitive, although, as mentioned above, lesion experiments do not in themselves provide conclusive evidence. Brookhart and Dey (1941) working with guinea pigs, and Soulairac and Soulairac (1956) with rats, found that anterior hypothalamic lesions depress sexual behavior in the absence of testicular atrophy. In a more recent study, Heimer and Larsson (1966/1967) described complete elimination of mating behavior following large lesions in the preoptic-anterior hypothalamus of male rats. The behavior could not be restored by 20 days' administration of large doses of testosterone. The depressive effect of preoptic lesions on male sexual behavior was confirmed by Lisk (1968). Lott (1966) has claimed that the general debilitating effect of large preoptic lesions is responsible for their sexual behavior-inhibiting effect. Indeed, more discrete lesions in the medial or lateral preoptic appeared to have no effect (Lott, 1966) or the effect was reversible with testosterone (Heimer and Larsson, 1966/1967).

While little is yet known of the postulated hypothalamic testosterone receptor for sexual behavior, there is evidence that it differs from the testosterone receptor in the hypothalamic median eminence which is believed to be involved in mediating the feedback regulation of gonadotropin secretion (Davidson and Sawyer, 1961b). Thus, systemic administration of cyproterone (an antiandrogenic compound) (Neumann, 1966; von Berswordt-Wallrabe and Neumann, 1967) or its implantation in crystalline form in the median eminence (Bloch and Davidson, 1967) apparently prevents access of testosterone to the feedback receptor, with the result that gonadotropin secretion is increased. However, while investigating contradictory claims on the effects of cyproterone on the sexual behavior of normal male rats (Steinbeck *et al.*, 1967; Zucker, 1966b; Beach and Westbrook, 1968), we found that this steroid actually has a stimulatory effect on the behavior of castrates. This facilitory effect has been demonstrated by chronic systemic administration of the free and the acetylated forms from the day of castration (Bloch and Davidson, 1971) and by hypothalamic implantation of crystalline cyproterone (free alcohol) in testosterone-treated long-term castrates (Fig. 4). When both cyproterone and testosterone are administered simultaneously to castrates, no antiandrogenic effect on sexual behavior is observed (Fig. 5; Whalen and Edwards, 1969). We have also found cyproterone to have rather potent "androgenic" effects on the growth of the penile spines, though when given in conjunction with testosterone propionate to castrates, which is highly sensitive to androgen, it is markedly antiandrogenic for this response (Table IV). This reduced spine growth would be expected if, as is presumed, cyproterone is a competitive inhibitor of testosterone at the receptor level. The behavioral response is less androgen-sensitive than is spine growth (Smith et al., 1971). Thus, the effects of cyproterone on behavior cannot be explained, as can the effects on the penis, in terms of a mild androgenic effect resulting in antiandrogenicity in the presence of exogenous androgen. Since the behavioral response differs in this respect from all other androgen-dependent responses which have been studied, we have postulated that these distinct phenomena reflect a difference in the nature of the respective androgen receptors (Davidson and Bloch, 1969). The possibility therefore emerges of differences between the two androgen receptors in the hypothalamus, which subserve the gonadotropin feedback mechanism and male sexual behavior, respectively.

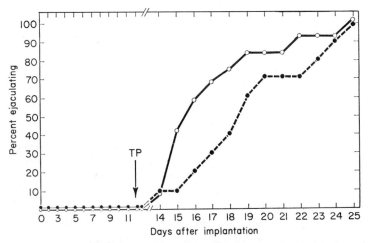

Fig. 4. Cumulative percentages of long-term castrate rats with double intrahypothalamic (anterior and posterior midline) cyproterone acetate (−) (N = 12) or cholesterol implants (−−) (N = 10) showing the ejaculatory pattern of behavior before and after onset of daily injections of 100 μg testosterone propionate (TP). Implantation was performed 2 months following castration. [From data of Bloch and Davidson (1971).]

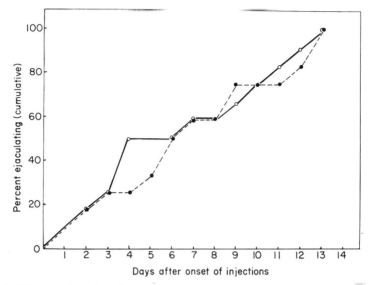

Fig. 5. Effects on behavior of 100 μg testosterone propionate (TP) (0) and TP with 10 mg cyproterone acetate (●), administered sc daily to long-term castrates having ceased to manifest mating behavior. [From Bloch and Davidson (1971).]

3. Peripheral Action of Testosterone

The apparent primacy of the testosterone-sensitive hypothalamic mechanism does not negate the possible importance of other targets of the hormone. The suboptimal quality and frequency of mating responses in testosterone-implanted adults (Davidson, 1966c) may be the result of failure of the experimentally administered testosterone to deliver the hormone to the relevant cells via the appropriate pathways. An equally likely interpretation, however, is that extracerebral tissues may require testosterone for implementation of optimal behavior, a possibility to which we must now direct attention.

Following castration in the adult rat, the overall size of the penis and the cornified papillae on the glans declines (Beach and Levinson, 1950). Both of these changes can be reversed by testosterone treatment. The similar though larger "spines" of the male cat are likewise androgen-dependent (Aronson and Cooper, 1967).

For the adult the functional consequences of these morphological effects of androgen are by no means clear, although absence of androgen in the prepuberal and especially neonatal period has profound behavioral implications, which are due in part to irreversible changes in the penis (Beach and Holz, 1946; Mullins and Levine, 1969). A relatively large percentage of cats and rats continue to show apparently complete patterns of mating behavior long after the regressive

TABLE IV. Androgenic and Antiandrogenic Effects of Cyproterone Acetate on Cornified Papillae of the Rat's Glans Penis[a]

Treatment	N	Ventral prostate weight (mg)	Seminal vesicle weight (mg)	Penile papillae (spines/section)[b]
Experiment 1: Injected from day of castration[c]				
Vehicle	12	59.5 ± 4.4	116.7 ± 3.5	17.4 ± 3.9
Cyproterone acetate (10 mg/day)	12	83.9 ± 3.2	125.0 ± 4.5	69.7 ± 3.0
Experiment 2: Long-term castrates[d]				
Testosterone propionate (100 µg/day)	12	308.5 ± 35.8	351.5 ± 21.5	89.0 ± 1.5
Testosterone (100 µg/day) cyproterone acetate (10 mg/day)	12	32.8 ± 2.9	78.6 ± 5.3	44.2 ± 3.0

[a]From Bloch and Davidson (1971).

[b]Mean spines/section in normal adults = ~ 90–100.

[c]Cyproterone was administered daily for 2 weeks before, and 5 weeks after castration. Animals were tested twice weekly for mating behavior, and cyproterone-treated castrates showed significantly higher levels of responding than the oil-injected castrates on all tests. Note the marked stimulation of penile papillae. The effect of cyproterone on ventral prostate weight was minimal, since mean weights in untreated animals of this age are in excess of 450 mg.

[d]Long-term castrates were treated for 2 weeks with testosterone or testosterone and cyproterone. Results of daily behavioral tests are shown in Fig. 5.

changes in the penis have occurred, including complete atrophy of spines (Aronson and Cooper, 1967). The importance of sensory afferents in male copulation is indicated by the "genital disorientation" and failure of intromission found in cats after section of the dorsalis penis nerve (Aronson and Cooper, 1969). Similar results were obtained in male rats (Adler and Bermant, 1966). Whatever the receptors for sensory feedback are, however, we have no way of knowing whether they, or the nerves themselves, are androgen-sensitive.

According to an early concept, the swelling of the seminal vesicles with secretions was believed to create the tension or sensory input which was directly related to sexual desire. There is no real evidence for the truth of this assertion, and Wilson and Beach (1963) in fact showed that male rats which had their seminal vesicles removed showed no demonstrable impairment of mating behavior.

There is surprisingly little experimental evidence on the effects of testosterone on the capacity for erection. Failure of erection in the mating test situation has been reported in castrated cats (Rosenblatt and Aronson, 1958). Since erection has neural representation at many levels, including widespread regions of the CNS (MacLean and Ploog, 1962), this failure yields little information about the site of androgen action. Although we know little of the changes in genital reflexes which may be caused by castration, preliminary work on rats in this laboratory (Rodgers and Davidson, 1968) indicates that there is a slow decline in erectile response to penile stimulation following postpuberal castration. Hart has conducted important studies on evocation of sexual reflexes, including erection, by stimulation of the penis in spinally sectioned rats (1967) and dogs (1968b). These reflexes were markedly facilitated following administration of large doses of testosterone. Of particular interest is the finding of Hart and Haugen (1968) that implantation of crystalline testosterone in the caudal spinal cord of rats was clearly stimulatory to certain of the spinal sexual reflexes ("long flips"), although they found no significant effect on erections.

Still undetermined is the extent of correlation between the spinal reflexes studied by Hart in paraplegic rats and dogs and the apparently similar events which occur in natural mating behavior. His work is, however, clearly suggestive of a secondary site of action of testosterone at the spinal level, a factor which might explain, at least in part, the behavioral deficiencies of rats with hypothalamic testosterone implants. Further work on reflexes in conjunction with observations of mating behavior in intact animals is needed if we are to succeed in finally differentiating the multiple effects of androgen on the numerous processes which comprise the complex patterns of male sexual behavior.

C. Cellular Mechanisms

Though there is yet no definitive evidence pinpointing the gonadal hormones' sites of action, the question remains as to what physicochemical changes these receptor cells undergo following hormone action. Does the hormone modify membrane potentials, directly activate or inhibit firing in the neurons, or change thresholds to afferent input? These and other related questions have not yet been answered.

As long as we do not know precisely which cells are receptors and as long as we cannot measure changing hormone concentration via physiological input and output relationships, the mechanisms of hormonal action at the cellular level will remain unknown. However, despite the fact that research in this area must depend on often tenuous correlations between cerebral and behavioral events, a few promising approaches to this study have been developed. These include: (1) study of the pattern of uptake of hormones by CNS regions (e.g. Michael, 1962; Stumpf, 1968), (2) electrophysiological recording of neuronal responses to hormone administration (e.g., Kawakami and Sawyer, 1959; Lincoln and Cross, 1966; Ramirez et al., 1967), and (3) the neuropharmacological approach, in which effects of drugs on behavior which can be correlated with neurochemical changes are sought (Soulairac and Soulairac, 1963; Meyerson, 1964). Space is inadequate here for an appropriate evaluation of the efforts of the investigators who are pioneering in this area. Whether or not they will be able to elucidate these areas of cellular psychobiology is, in any case, a question that cannot yet be answered.

V. DIFFERENTIATION OF SEXUAL BEHAVIOR

An area which has received much investigative attention in recent years is the determination or "organization" of sexual behavior mechanisms by hormonal influences during early development. Although it has been amply reviewed (e.g., Young et al., 1964; Phoenix et al., 1967; Levine and Mullins, 1966), the importance of this field to psychoendocrinology is so great that at least an outline of the main results and problems must be included in this chapter. The original, and still basic experimental findings relevant to differentiation of sexual behavior are twofold. (1) Administration of testosterone in a single dose to the newborn rat (Barraclough and Gorski, 1962; Harris and Levine, 1965) or in multiple doses to the pregnant guinea pig (Phoenix et al., 1959) prevents development in the young of the capacity to respond to ovarian hormones with the manifestation of female sexual behavior. (2) Neonatal castration of male rats, on the other hand, produces animals which, when adult, respond to ovarian hormone administration with lordosis behavior closely resembling that of normal female rats (Grady et al., 1965).

From these and other investigations the concept has emerged that the developing animal of both sexes has, by manifesting female sexual behavior, the inherent potential to respond to ovarian hormones. In males this potentiality is suppressed by the action of endogenous testicular androgen secreted shortly after birth in the rat and prenatally in animals like the guinea pig which undergo more complete development *in utero*. The resemblance of this process to that operative in differentiation of male and female reproductive tracts (Burns, 1961) is fairly obvious. It is worth noting that the mechanisms which differentiate male from female sexual behavior do not result in *absolute* behavioral dimorphism between the sexes. Mounting, which is usually regarded as a typically male event, is a common element in the mating pattern of the females of many species (Beach, 1968). Lordosis, on the other hand, is extremely rare as a spontaneous occurrence in the male. However, the potential to display lordosis behavior is present in males, and high lordosis quotients may be obtained from male rats following serial administration of high doses of estrogen (Davidson, 1969a). In male and female rats, the differential responses to ovarian hormones within "female" sexual behavior may be characterized as (1) a low sensitivity to estrogen stimulation, (2) a more variable response, and (3) apparently complete unresponsiveness to the facilitatory effects of progesterone following estrogen priming (see Table V). Since the sensitivity to progesterone is apparently suppressed by neonatal testosterone, neonatally castrated male rats do show progesterone-facilitation of lordosis in adulthood (Davidson and Levine, 1969), and neonatal testosterone treatment suppresses that response in females (Clemens *et al.*, 1969b).

The concept of an early testosterone influence operating in a suppressive fashion on a basic propensity for development of female behavioral mechanisms has successfully survived a considerable amount of intensive and often repetitive research. Other notions arising from the original research have not, however,

TABLE V. Effects of Progesterone on Estrogen-induced Lordosis in Adult Male Rats, Commencing either 1 week after Postpuberal Castration or 5.5 Months after Castration on the First Day of Life[a]

EB (μg/day)	Progesterone (mg)[b]	N	Days after onset of EB injections		
			2	4	8
Adult castrates					
2	0	6	2 ± 2	14 ± 7	34 ± 15
2	0.5	5	7 ± 5	30 ± 8	20 ± 12
2	0	8		39 ± 7	39 ± 12
2	5.0	8		24 ± 8	32 ± 7
Neonatal castrates					
2	0	7	10 ± 1	40 ± 17	63 ± 15
2	0.5	7	17 ± 8	77 ± 11	94 ± 3

[a]Data from Davidson (1969a) and Davidson and Levine (1969).

[b]Progesterone was administered in all cases 4–6 hours before testing. Results are expressed as mean lordosis quotient (lordosis/mounts × 100) ± standard error.

fared as well, particularly those related to the "organization" of male behavior. Since the neonatally castrated male rat is incapable of responding to testosterone in adulthood with ejaculatory or, to a large extent, intromission behavior, and perinatally androgenized female guinea pigs and rats show mounting behavior under those circumstances (Phoenix et al., 1959; Harris and Levine, 1965), it was assumed that early androgen, in addition to suppressing female potentiality, also organized male behavior patterns. However, it was shown long before by Beach and Holz (1946) that neonatal orchidectomy irreversibly impairs penile development in the rat, which, even after massive testosterone treatment in adulthood, presumably makes normal intromission and ejaculatory behavior impossible (Mullins and Levine, 1969). Furthermore, mounting is a normal component of the female as well as the male mating pattern, and Whalen believes that mount frequency is basically unaffected in rats of either sex by postnatal hormonal manipulations (Whalen et al., 1968). It is now known that perinatal testosterone treatment not only promotes phallic development in the female offspring, but also facilitates the appearance of intromission patterns following treatment of the adult with testosterone (Nadler, 1969). Combined prenatal and postnatal "androgenization" results in the development of females whose androgen-induced behavior approaches that of normal male guinea pigs (Gerall, 1963) or rats (Ward, 1969; Whalen and Robertson, 1968).

Unexpectedly, neonatal estrogen also suppresses lordosis (Levine and Mullins, 1964; Whalen and Nadler, 1963) and stimulates the development of male behavior patterns (Levine and Mullins, 1964) in female rats. These findings are not relevant to the normal developmental situation; the prenatal or neonatal ovary probably does not secrete estrogen and is not involved in the differentiation process (Beach, 1945; Adams-Smith, 1967).

In conclusion, it appears well established that prenatal androgen in the guinea pig and neonatal androgen in the rat exercise a primary influence in suppressing the potentiality for development of female behavior patterns in genetic males, although subsidiary prenatal effects in the rat are not yet entirely ruled out (Gerall and Ward, 1966). The mechanism operates presumably via an organizing effect of early androgen on the developing hypothalamus (Nadler, 1968). Although androgen certainly exerts an early organizational action on male behavior, we can as yet neither pinpoint that action in time nor distinguish between effects peripherally on the developing genitalia and those on the CNS.

There is evidence, however, that androgen does have some "organizing" influence on sex dimorphic behavioral characteristics which do not require a fully developed penis. Aggressive behavior, which is exhibited more by male than female rats, is suppressed by neonatal castration and cannot be reinstated by replacement with androgen, whereas a similar suppression of fighting in weanling castrates is completely reinstated by androgen (see Chapters 1 and 7).

VI. HORMONES AND HUMAN SEXUALITY

Among the lay public, factual knowledge of the relationships between reproduction, hormones, and sex behavior is rare. Unfortunately, the confusion is hardly less great in the medical-scientific community, a result in part of two factors: the tremendous complexity of psychosociocultural factors that influence human sexual behavior, and the severe lack of relevant, scientifically valid experimental data. Of course, such experimental techniques as gonadal ablation followed by replacement therapy are excluded in normal healthy subjects, and even where nonhazardous procedures are involved, experimental data are lacking because of social taboos. In order to study human sexuality, therefore, we must gather information from clinical reports on patients suffering from a variety of physical or psychological disorders. Because of the lack of effective control procedures or serious attempts to quantify the results, and because data collected during patient-doctor interviews often have questionable validity, these reports are seldom very illuminating.

Under these circumstances, the conclusion of Kinsey *et al.* (1953) that there are no specific effects of the gonadal hormones on human sex behavior and that the nonspecific effects of all hormones are mediated by general metabolic conditions seems premature at the very least. Furthermore, as pointed out by Whalen (1966), the failure to find true analogies between the hormonal control of animal and human sexual behavior stems, in part, from the fact that facets of human and animal sexuality that are not analogous are often compared. In these reports undefined and perhaps undefinable terms such as libido are frequently used, and seldom are the various components of sexuality appropriately identified (Whalen, 1966). In the remainder of this chapter we shall evaluate the extent to which valid conclusions about the role of hormones in human sexuality can be drawn.

When we ask the simple question "Is copulation possible in humans in the absence of the gonads?" we find an interesting difference from the situation described in our earlier discussions on mating in lower animals. In subprimate species, orchidectomy is followed by variable but often prolonged retention of mating capacity, and ovariectomy by complete and immediate abolition of the behavior. In humans, while orchidectomy seems to have similar sequelae, the ovaries are, on the other hand, not at all essential for any major aspect of female sexual behavior.

Castration of males is one of the earliest surgical techniques man has performed on members of his own as well as other species. Human males are known to have been castrated ever since the dawn of history for such diverse purposes as to supply safe companions or guards for ladies in ancient Egypt and Rome; to subdue captives; to punish enemies or criminals; to prolong the usefulness of choir boys in the medieval church, and for other religious reasons (see Tauber, 1940). In modern times orchidectomy has been performed to treat such conditions as genital tuberculosis, malignancy or traumatic injury and as a legal measure, either for eugenic reasons or to deter sex offenders. Despite all this experience, little precise, detailed, and scientifically valid information exists on the behavioral effects of orchidectomy.

The results of the fairly extensive study by Bremer (1959), on several hundred men legally castrated in Norway, confirm the main conclusions of a number of other such studies. First, the response was notably variable. Some men showed a fairly rapid and complete decline in sexual behavior following the operation, while others continued to have intercourse for years thereafter. Since the psychological factor of the fear of impotence would tend to operate inversely on sexual ability, the evidence on retention of potency is particularly convincing, and there are many reports of such retention for periods of years. Because of possible unwillingness to admit impotence, however, it is necessary that these claims be carefully validated. As to the ensuing steady decline in potency, Kinsey et al. (1953) relate this to the general overall decline in sexual ability resulting from the aging process in men. This argument would not be applicable, of course, to the relatively rapid postcastration changes which can occur, though these might well be psychological in origin. Unfortunately, there is little if any systematic information on the rate of decline or the physiological factors affecting the loss of behavioral responses.

In the practice of clinical endocrinology it is generally accepted that androgen treatment increases potency in hypogonadal or castrated men (Lloyd, 1968). The incidence of spontaneous erection which is reported to decrease after castration or in hypogonadism (Miller et al., 1938; Yamamoto and Seeman, 1960; Bremer, 1959) increases again following institution of testosterone therapy (Miller et al., 1938; Lloyd, 1968). Carefully controlled large-scale studies on the effects of testosterone on erection and other aspects of sexuality have not been performed. Variations of as much as 100% in plasma testosterone levels among different individuals were reportedly not correlated with differences in sexual behavior (Kobayashi et al., 1966), a finding which is consistent with the previously mentioned studies on rodents. We can conclude from the above information that there is considerable similarity between the hormonal control of sexual behavior in men and in subhuman male mammals.

The fact that removal of ovarian secretions by menopause or premenopausal oophorectomy need have no deleterious effect on sexual activity of women contrasts dramatically with the situation in subprimate females. Even in simian species, although the few published reports suggest rather variable effects of ovariectomy (Michael, 1969), mating behavior is often completely lost in the female subhuman primate. Failure to demonstrate gross changes following disappearance of ovarian secretions does not, however, imply that the sexual life of the human female is totally uninfluenced by hormones. A fairly widely held claim is that adrenal androgen is the "libido hormone" in women (Money, 1965). This concept is based first on the results of testosterone administration to women, which is reputed to stimulate sexual responsiveness (Foss, 1951; Salmon and Geist, 1943). However, the fact that testosterone in the doses administered in these studies causes clitoral hypertrophy vitiates the worth of this evidence (Carter *et al.*, 1947; Kupperman and Studdiford, 1953). Doses of androgen which produce clitoral hypertrophy would be clearly supraphysiological and indeed this change may be responsible for the reported increase in "libido".

Other evidence used to support the role of adrenal androgen in sexual behavior comes from the findings on hypophysectomized (Schon and Sutherland, 1960) and adrenalectomized (Waxenberg *et al.*, 1959) women. Unlike oophorectomy, these treatments are reported to decrease sexual desire. It seems extremely difficult, however, to control for the psychological effects of radical surgery, and in any case the validity of conclusions drawn on patients with advanced metastatic cancer is open to serious question. One must conclude that there is no adequate evidence that the effects of androgen on feminine sexual behavior represent any important physiological function under normal circumstances. Even in the case of increased adrenal androgen output, as is found in congenital adrenal hyperplasia, the evidence is tenuous (Money, 1965). It would not be an insuperable task to collect valid evidence: Everitt and Herbert's recent report (1969) on the lowered sexual receptivity of corticosteroid (dexamethasone)-treated monkeys indicates one approach to the problem.

While there is no solid evidence to indicate that hormones are essential for any major aspect of sexual behavior in women, the above considerations do not eliminate a modulatory role for hormones. If ovarian steroids do have more subtle effects, these should become evident from careful study of psychosexual variables in relation to different phases of the menstrual cycle. The well-known study of Benedek and Rubenstein (see Benedek, 1952) suggested that a number of changes in the quality of the sexual impulse occur throughout the cycle. On the basis of psychoanalytic investigations, they concluded that women show an active extroverted heterosexual drive in the first (estrogen-dominated) half of the cycle, peaking around midcycle, while after ovulation there was a changeover to more introverted states of mind, with dream material becoming weighted with themes of pregnancy and mother-child relations. Of course, the significance of these studies depends in large part on the validity of the particular psychiatric methods used, and the state of the women undergoing therapy.

A number of studies have been performed attempting to correlate frequency of coitus and orgasm with stage of the menstrual cycle. Peaks in sexual activity have most often been found just before and just after menstruation [see refs. in Kinsey *et al.* (1953), p. 610]. Apart from the difficulty of obtaining reliable data from retrospective reports or even calendar-type records (McCance *et al.*, 1937). these peaks could be the result of (1) conscious or subconscious fears of conception and (2) avoidance of the period of menstrual flow. It is therefore of some interest that a recent well-conducted study (Udry and Morris, 1968), in which daily reports were collected from women not taking oral contraceptives, indicated peak incidences both of coitus and orgasm around midcycle with a trough in the premenstrual period. If substantiated, these results show some residuum in the human female of the phenomenon of estrus around the time of ovulation which is so ubiquitous in animals and is also found, albeit to a lesser extent, in subhuman primates (Michael, 1969).

The other important consequence of the study of Udry and Morris (1968) is the possibility that a decrease in libido during the late luteal phase is the result of peak progesterone secretion. While there is no clear evidence for an inhibitory effect of physiological amounts of progesterone on sexual behavior in women, evidence for such an effect has now been reported in rhesus monkeys (see II, B2). Since monkeys do appear to occupy a position intermediate between subprimate species and humans in respect to hormonal control of female sexual behavior, this inhibitory effect of progesterone suggests that it is important to investigate possible behavioral effects of the progestational oral contraceptive agents. Recent preliminary findings of Michael (1969) suggest changes in several measures of male sexual behavior indicative of decreased receptivity in the female following combined or sequential administration of mestranol with chlormadinone acetate or ethynodiol to female rhesus monkeys.

In women, the earlier reports on psychological effects of oral contraceptives claimed that there was either no change, or an actual improvement in "libido" (see Pincus, 1965, p. 285). Of course, distinguishing such psychological factors as freedom from fear of pregnancy, etc., from any real psychophysiological effects of these steroids is tremendously difficult, and there is great variability among women in the various "side effects" of these antifertility agents. However, it is noteworthy that a recent study reported loss of libido in a rather high proportion of a group of women taking highly progestational "pills" (Grant and Mears, 1967).

In conclusion, it is not possible to confirm or deny Kinsey's negative evaluation of the role of hormones in human sexuality (Kinsey *et al.*, 1953). Nevertheless, although conclusive evidence is no more available at the time of writing than it was 18 years ago, an open-minded attitude to this problem seems as appropriate today as it should have been then. Finally, it must be emphasized that what we have considered relates only to changes in hormonal status of the adult human. The profound effects of neonatal hormonal manipulation in animals suggest that whatever effects can be demonstrated in adult humans may represent only the tip of the iceberg. Apart from the work of Money (1961, 1965), possible influences of iatrogenic or pathogenic deviations in the prenatal or neonatal milieu on human sexual behavior have been almost totally neglected. Like most pioneers, Money has had to work with a rather inadequate armamentarium, and there is little we can yet conclude as to the influences of endocrine anomalies in early life on the development of "deviant" sexual patterns in the adult. Since experimental work cannot easily be done in this area, the only hope for answers to our questions is from large scale followup studies, combined with the development of careful scientific methods of studying human sexuality.

Acknowledgements

The studies reported from this laboratory were supported by NIH Grant HD 00778.

References

Adams-Smith, W. N. (1967). *J. Embryol. Exp. Morphol.* **17**, 1.
Adler, N. T. (1969). *J. Comp. Physiol. Psychol.* **69**, 613.
Adler, N. T., and Bermant, G. (1966). *J. Comp. Physiol. Psychol.* **61**, 240.
Anderson, L. L. (1969). *In* "Reproduction in Domestic Animals" (H. H. Cole and P. T. Cupps, eds.), 2nd ed., pp. 541-568. Academic Press, New York.
Armstrong, D. T. (1968). *Recent Progr. Horm. Res.* **24**, 255.
Aron, C., Asch, G., Asch, L., Roos, J., and Luxembourger, M. M. (1965). *Pathol. Biol.* **13**, 603.
Aron, C., Asch, G., and Roos, J. (1966). *Int. Rev. Cytol.* **21**, 139.
Aron, C., Roos, J., and Asch, G. (1968). *Neuroendocrinology* **3**, 47.
Aronson, L. R., and Cooper, M. L. (1967). *Anat. Rec.* **157**, 71.
Aronson, L. R., and Cooper, M. L. (1969). *In* "Reproduction and Sexual Behavior" (M. Diamond, ed.), pp. 51-82. Indiana Univ. Press, Bloomington.
Backhaus, D. (1958). *Zuchthyg. Fortpfistor. Besam. Haustiere.* **2**, 281.
Ball, J. (1934). *Amer. J. Physiol.* **107**, 698.
Ball, J. (1941). *Psychol. Bull.* **38**, 533.
Bard, P. (1939). *Res. Publ. Ass. Res. Nerv. Ment. Dis.* **19**, 190.
Bard, P. (1940). *Res. Publ. Ass. Res. Nerv. Ment. Dis.* **20**, 551.
Barfield, R. J. (1969). *Horm. Behav.* **1**, 37.
Barraclough, C. A., and Gorski, R. A. (1962). *J. Endocrinol.* **25**, 175.
Beach, F. A. (1942). *Endocrinology* **31**, 679.
Beach, F. A. (1945). *Anat. Rec.* **92**, 289.
Beach, F. A. (1947). *Physiol. Rev.* **27**, 240.
Beach, F. A. (1958). *In* "Biological and Biochemical Bases of Behavior" (H. F. Harlow and C. N. Woolsey, eds.), pp. 263-283. Univ. of Wisconsin Press, Madison.
Beach, F. A. (1966). *Science* **153**, 769.
Beach, F. A. (1967). *Physiol. Rev.* **47**, 289.
Beach, F. A. (1968). *In* "Reproduction and Sexual Behavior" (M. Diamond, ed.), pp. 83-131. Indiana Univ. Press, Bloomington.
Beach, F. A., and Fowler, H. (1959). *J. Comp. Physiol. Psychol.* **52**, 50.
Beach, F. A., and Holz, A. M. (1946). *J. Exp. Zool.* **101**, 91.
Beach, F. A., and Holz-Tucker, A. M. (1949). *J. Comp. Physiol. Psychol.* **42**, 433.
Beach, F. A., and Levinson, G. (1950). *J. Exp. Zool.* **114**, 159.
Beach, F. A., and Merari, A. (1968). *Proc. Nat. Acad. Sci. U.S.* **61**, 442.
Beach, F. A., and Westbrook, W. H. (1968). *J. Endocrinol.* **42**, 379.
Beach, F. A., Westbrook, W. H., and Clemens, L. G. (1966). *Psychosom. Med.* **28**, 749.

Benedek, T. (1952). "Studies in Psychosomatic Medicine. Psychosexual Functions in Women." Ronald Press, New York.
Bermant, G. (1967). *Psychology Today* 3, 28.
Beyer, C., Vidal, N., and McDonald, P. G. (1969). *J. Endocrinol.* 45, 407.
Blandau, R. J. (1945). *Amer. J. Anat.* 77, 253.
Bloch, G., J., and Davidson, J. M. (1967). *Science* 155, 593.
Bloch, G. J., and Davidson, J. M. (1968). *Physiol. Behav.* 3, 461.
Bloch, G. J., and Davidson, J. M. (1971). *Horm. Behav.* 2, 11.
Boling, J. L., and Blandau, R. J. (1939). *Endocrinology* 25, 359.
Boling, J. L., Young, W. C., and Dempsey, E. W. (1938). *Endocrinology* 23, 182.
Bremer, J. (1959). "Asexualization." Macmillan, New York.
Bronson, F. H. (1968). *In* "Reproduction and Sexual Behavior" (M. Diamond, ed.), pp. 341-361. Indiana Univ. Press, Bloomington.
Brookhart, J. M., and Dey, F. L. (1941). *Amer. J. Physiol.* 133, 551.
Brooks, C. McC. (1935). *Amer. J. Physiol.* 113, 18.
Bruce, H. M. (1959). *Nature (London)* 184, 105.
Burns, R. K. (1961). *In* "Sex and Internal Secretions" (W. C. Young, ed.), Vol. I, pp. 76-161. Williams & Wilkins, Baltimore, Maryland.
Carpenter, C. R. (1942). *J. Comp. Psychol.* 33, 113.
Carr, W. J., and Caul, W. F. (1962). *Anim. Behav.* 10, 20.
Carr, W. J., Loeb, L. S., and Dissinger, M. L. (1965). *J. Comp. Physiol. Psychol.* 59, 370.
Carter, A. C., Cohen, E. J., and Shorr, E. (1947). *In* "Vitamins and Hormones" (R. S. Harris and K. V. Thimann, eds.), pp. 317-391. Academic Press, New York.
Cheng, P., and Casida, L. E. (1949). *Endocrinology* 44, 38.
Cheng, P., Ulbert, L. C., Christian, R. E., and Casida, L. E. (1950), *Endocrinology* 46, 447.
Clemens, J. A., Minaguchi, H., Storey, R., Voogt, J. L., and Meites, J. (1969a). *Neuroendocrinology* 4, 150.
Clemens, L. G., Hiroi, M., and Gorski, R. A. (1969b). *Endocrinology* 84, 1430.
Corson, S. A., and Corson, E. O. (1968). *Proc. Int. Symp. Psychotropic Drugs in Intern. Med.,* Excerpta Med. Int. Congr. Ser. No. 182, p. 147.
Cross, B. A. (1966). *In* "Neuroendocrinology" (L. Martini and W. F. Ganong, eds.), Vol. 1, p. 217. Academic Press, New York.
Davidson, J. M. (1965). *23rd Int. Congr. Physiol. Sci.,* Abstracts, p. 647.
Davidson, J. M., (1966a). *In* "Neuroendocrinology" (L. Martini and W. F. Ganong, eds.), Vol. I, pp. 565-611. Academic Press, New York.
Davidson, J. M. (1966b). *Anim. Behav.* 14, 266.
Davidson, J. M. (1966c). *Endocrinology* 79, 783.
Davidson, J. M. (1966d). Unpublished data.
Davidson, J. M. (1969a). *Endocrinology* 84, 1365.
Davidson, J. M. (1969b). *Advan. Biosci.* 1, 119-139.
Davidson, J. M. and Bloch, G. J. (1969). *Biol. Reprod. Suppl.* 1, 1, 67.
Davidson, J. M., and Levine, S. (1969). *J. Endocrinology* 44, 129.
Davidson, J. M., and Sawyer, C. H. (1961a). *Acta Endocrinol. (Copenhagen)* 37, 385.
Davidson, J. M., and Sawyer, C. H. (1961b). *Proc. Soc. Exp. Biol. Med.* 107, 4.
Davidson, J. M., Smith, E. R., Rodgers, C. H., and Bloch, G. J. (1968a). *Physiol. Behav.* 3, 227.
Davidson, J. M., Rodgers, C. H., Smith, E. R., and Bloch, G. J. (1968b). *Endocrinology* 82, 193.
Davidson, J. M., Smith, E. R., Brown-Grant, K., Brast, N., and McKinnon, P. (1970). Unpublished data.

Dempsey, E. W., and Rioch, D. M. (1939). *J. Neurophysiol.* **2**, 9.
Denamur, R. (1963). *Dairy Sci. Abstr.* **27**, 193.
Desjardins, C., Kirton, K. T., and Hafs, H. D. (1967). *Proc. Soc. Exp. Biol. Med.* **126**, 23.
Dominic, C. J. (1966). *Naturwiss.* **53**, 310.
Drori, D., and Folman, Y. (1964). *J. Reprod. Fert.* **8**, 351.
Endroczi, E., and Lissak, K. (1962). *Acta Physiol.* **21**, 203.
Everett, J. W. (1948). *Endocrinology* **43**, 389.
Everett, J. W. (1952). *Ciba Found. Colloq. Endocrinol. Proc.* **4**, 167.
Everett, J. W. (1961). *In* "Sex and Internal Secretions" (W. C. Young, ed.), Vol. I, pp. 497-555. Williams & Wilkins, Baltimore, Maryland.
Everitt, B. J., and Herbert, J. (1969). *Nature (London)* **222**, 1065.
Feder, H. H., and Ruf, K. B. (1969). *Endocrinology* **84**, 171.
Feder, H. H., Resko, J. A., and Goy, R. W. (1966). *Amer. Zool.* **6**, 597 (abstract).
Feder, H. H., Goy, R. W., and Resko, J. A. (1967). *J. Physiol. (London)* **191**, 136.
Fisher, A. E. (1956). *Science* **124**, 228.
Fletcher, I. C., and Lindsay, D. R. (1968). *Anim. Behav.* **16**, 410.
Ford, C. S., and Beach, F. A. (1951). "Patterns of Sexual Behavior," Harper, New York.
Foss, G. L. (1951). *Lancet* **1**, 667.
Gardner, J. E., and Fisher, A. E. (1968). *Physiol. Behav.* **3**, 709.
Gerall, A. A. (1963). *J. Comp. Physiol. Psychol.* **56**, 92.
Gerall, A. A., and Ward, I. L. (1966). *J. Comp. Physiol. Psychol.* **62**, 370.
Goy, R. W. (1968). Personal communication.
Grady, K. L., Phoenix, C. H., and Young, W. C. (1965). *J. Comp. Physiol. Psychol.* **59**, 176.
Grant, E. C. G., and Mears, E. (1967). *Lancet* **2**, 945.
Grosvenor, C. E., Maiweg, H., and Mena, F. (1969). *Horm. Behav.* **1**, 111.
Grunt, J. A., and Young, W. C. (1952). *Endocrinology* **51**, 237.
Grunt, J. A., and Young, W. C. (1953). *J. Comp. Physiol. Psychol.* **46**, 138.
Hamburg, D. A. (1966). *Res. Publ. Ass. Res. Nerv. Ment. Dis.* **43**, 251.
Harrington, F. E., Eggert, R. G., Wilbur, R. D., and Linkenheimer, W. H. (1966). *Endocrinology* **79**, 1130.
Harris, G. W., and Levine, S. (1965). *J. Physiol. (London)* **181**, 379.
Harris, G. W., and Michael, R. P. (1964). *J. Physiol. (London)* **171**, 275.
Harris, G. W., Michael, R. P., and Scott, P. P. (1958). *Neurol. Basis Behav. Ciba Found. Symp. 1957* (G. E. W. Wolstenholme and C. M. O'Connor, eds.), pp. 236-254. Little Brown, Boston, Massachusetts.
Hart, B. (1967). *Science* **155**, 1283.
Hart, B. (1968a). *J. Comp. Physiol. Psychol.* **66**, 719.
Hart, B. (1968b). *J. Comp. Physiol. Psychol.* **66**, 726.
Hart, B. L. (1969). *Horm. Behav.* **1**, 65.
Hart, B. L. (1970). *Horm. Behav.* **1**, 93.
Hart, B. L., and Haugen, C. M. (1968). *Physiol. Behav.* **3**, 735.
Hartman, C. G. (1962). "Science and the Safe Period." Williams & Wilkins, Baltimore, Maryland.
Heimer, L., and Larsson, K. (1966/1967). *Brain Res.* **3**, 248.
Hori, T., Ide, M., and Miyake, T. (1968). *Endocrinol. Jap.* **15**, 215.
Hutchison, J. B. (1967). *Nature (London)* **216**, 591.
Kagan, J., and Beach, F. A. (1953). *J. Comp. Physiol. Psychol.* **46**, 204.
Kawakami, M., and Sawyer, C. H. (1959). *Endocrinology* **65**, 652.
Kinsey, A. C., Pomeroy, W. B., Martin, C. E., and Gebhard, P. H. (1953). "Sexual Behavior in the Human Female." Saunders, Philadelphia, Pennsylvania.

Kobayashi, T., Lobotsky, J., and Lloyd, C. W. (1966). *J. Clin. Endocrinol. Metab.* 26, 615.
Kuehn, R. E., and Zucker, I. (1968). *J. Comp. Physiol. Psychol.* 66, 747.
Kupperman, H. S., and Studdiford, W. E. (1953). *Postgrad. Med.* 14, 410.
Land, R. B., and McGill, T. E. (1967). *J. Reprod. Fert.* 13, 121.
LeBoeuf, B. J. (1970). *Horm. Behav.* 1, 127.
Lehrman, D. S. (1961). *In* "Sex and Internal Secretions" (W. C. Young, ed.), pp. 1268-1382. Williams & Wilkins, Baltimore, Maryland.
LeMagnen, J. (1952). *Arch. Sci. Physiol.* 6, 295.
Levine, S., and Mullins, R. F., Jr. (1964). *Science* 144, 185.
Levine, S., and Mullins, R. F., Jr. (1966). *Science* 152, 1585.
Lincoln, D. W., and Cross, B. A. (1966). *J. Endocrinol.* 37, 191.
Lindsay, D. R. (1965). *Anim. Behav.* 13, 75.
Lisk, R. D. (1960). *Can. J. Biochem. Physiol.* 38, 1381.
Lisk, R. D. (1962). *Amer. J. Physiol.* 203, 493.
Lisk, R. D. (1967a). *In* "Neuroendocrinology" (L. Martini and W. F. Ganong, eds.), Vol. II, pp. 197-239. Academic Press, New York.
Lisk, R. D. (1967b). *Endocrinology* 80, 754.
Lisk R. D. (1968). *Exp. Brain Res. (Berlin)* 5, 306.
Lisk, R. D. (1969). *Trans. N. Y. Acad. Sci.* 31, 593.
Lloyd, C. W. (1968). *In* "Clinical Endocrinology" (E. B. Astwood, ed.), Vol. 2, pp. 665-674. Grune & Stratton, New York.
Long, J. A., and Evans, H. M. (1922). *Mem. Univ. Calif.* 6, 1.
Lott, D. F. (1966). *J. Comp. Physiol. Psychol.* 61, 284.
McCance, R. A., Luff, M. C., and Widdowson, E. E. (1937). *J. Hyg.* 37, 571.
McDonald, P. G., Vidal, N., and Beyer, C. (1970). *Horm. Behav.* 1, 161.
McGill, T. E. (1970). *Horm. Behav.* 1, 211.
McGill, T. E., Corwin, D. M., and Harrison, D. T. (1968). *J. Reprod. Fert.* 15, 749.
MacLean, P. D., and Ploog, D. W. (1962). *J. Neurophysiol.* 25, 29.
Maes, J. P. (1939). *Nature (London)* 144, 598.
Masters, W. H., and Johnson, V. E. (1966). "Human Sexual Response," p. 366. Little, Brown, Boston, Massachusetts.
Matthews, L. H. (1939). *Proc. Roy. Soc. Ser. B.* 126, 557.
Meites, J., and Turner, C. W. (1942). *Endocrinology* 31, 340.
Meyerson, B. J. (1964). *Acta Physiol. Scand. Suppl.* 63, 24, 1.
Michael, R. P. (1962). *Excerpta Med. Found. Int. Congr. Series* No. 47, 650.
Michael, R. P. (1965). *Brit. Med. Bull.* 21, 87.
Michael, R. P. (1969). *In* "Metabolic Effects of Gonadal Hormones and Contraceptive Steroids" (H. A. Salhanick, D. M. Kipnis, and R. L. Van de Wiele, eds.), pp. 706-721. Plenum, New York.
Michael, R. P., and Keverne, E. B. (1968). *Nature (London)* 218, 746.
Michael, R. P., and Scott, P. P. (1964). *J. Physiol. (London)* 171, 254.
Michael, R. P., Saayman, G., and Zumpe, D. (1967). *J. Endocrinol.* 39, 309.
Miller, N. E. (1969). *Science* 163, 434.
Miller, N. E., Hubert, G., and Hamilton, J. B. (1938). *Proc. Soc. Exp. Biol. Med.* 38, 538.
Money, J. (1961). *In* "Sex and Internal Secretions" (W. C. Young, ed.), Vol. II, pp. 1383-1400. Williams & Wilkins, Baltimore, Maryland.
Money, J. (1965). *Ann. Rev. Med.* 16, 67.
Moore, N. W., Barrett, S., Brown, J. B., Schindler, I., Smith, M. A., and Smyth, B. (1969). *J. Endocrinol.* 44, 55.
Morris, D. (1969). "The Naked Ape." McGraw-Hill, New York.

Mullins, R. F., Jr., and Levine, S. (1969). *Commun. Behav. Biol.* **3**, 1.

Nadler, R. D. (1968). *J. Comp. Physiol. Psychol.* **66**, 157.

Nadler, R. D. (1969). *Horm. Behav.* **1**, 53.

Nadler, R. D. (1970). *Physiol. Behav.* **5**, 95.

Nequin, L. G., and Schwartz, N. B. (1971). *Endocrinology* **88**, 325.

Neumann, F. (1966). *Acta Endocrinol. (Copenhagen)* **53**, 53.

Palka, Y. S., and Sawyer, C. H. (1966). *J. Physiol. (London)* **135**, 251.

Parkes, A. S., and Bruce, H. M. (1961). *Science* **134**, 1049.

Phoenix, C. H., Goy, R. W., Gerall, A. A., and Young, W. C. (1959). *Endocrinology* **65**, 369.

Phoenix, C. H., Goy, R. W., and Young, W. C. (1967). *In* "Neuroendocrinology" (L. Martini and W. F. Ganong, eds.), Vol. 2, pp. 163-196. Academic Press, New York.

Pincus, G. (1965). "The Control of Fertility." Academic Press, New York.

Powers, J. B. (1970). *Physiol. Behav.* **5**, 831.

Powers, J. B., and Zucker, I. (1969). *Endocrinology* **84**, 820.

Ramirez, V. D., and McCann, S. M. (1965). *Endocrinology* **76**, 412.

Ramirez, V. D., Komisaruk, B. R., Whitmoyer, D. I., and Sawyer, C. H. (1967). *Amer. J. Physiol.* **212**, 1376.

Riss, W., and Young, W. C. (1954). *Endocrinology* **54**, 232.

Rodgers, C. H., and Davidson, J. M. (1968). Unpublished data.

Rosenblatt, J. S., and Aronson, L. R. (1958). *Behaviour* **12**, 285.

Roth, L. L., and Rosenblatt, J. S. (1968). *J. Endocrinol.* **42**, 363.

Saginor, M., and Horton, R. (1968). *Endocrinology* **82**, 627.

Salmon, U. J., and Geist, S. H. (1943). *J. Clin. Endocrinol. Metab.* **3**, 235.

Sawyer, C. H. (1959). *J. Exp. Zool.* **142**, 227.

Sawyer, C. H. (1960). *In* "Handbook of Physiology," (H. W. Magoun, ed.), Vol. II, p. 1225. Amer. Physiol. Soc., Washington, D. C.

Sawyer, C. H. (1963). *Anat. Rec.* **145**, 280 (abstract).

Sawyer, C. H., and Everett, J. W. (1959). *Endocrinology* **65**, 644.

Schon, M., and Sutherland, A. M. (1960). *J. Clin. Endocrinol. Metab.* **20**, 833.

Schwartz, N. B. (1969). *Recent Progr. Horm. Res.* **25**, 1.

Schwartz, N. B., and Talley, W. L. (1965). *J. Reprod. Fert.* **10**, 463.

Shelesnyak, M. C. (1931). *Anat. Rec.* **49**, 179.

Smith, E. R., Weick, R. F., Rodgers, C. H., and Davidson, J. M. (1971). Androgen responsiveness of various anatomical, physiological and behavioral parameters. Unpublished data.

Soulairac, A., and Soulairac, M. L. (1956). *Ann. Endocrinol.* **17**, 731.

Soulairac, A., and Soulairac, M. L. (1963). *J. Physiol. (Paris)* **55**, 339.

Spies, H. G., and Niswender, G. D. (1971). *Endocrinology* **88**, 937.

Staples, R. E. (1967). *J. Reprod. Fert.* **13**, 429.

Steinbeck, H., Elger, W., and Neumann, F. (1967). *Acta Endocrinol. (Copenhagen) Suppl.* **119**, 63 (abstract).

Stumpf, W. E. (1968). *Science* **162**, 1001.

Taleisnik, S., Caligaris, L., and Astrada, J. J. (1966). *Endocrinology* **79**, 49.

Tauber, E. S. (1940). *Psychosom. Med.* **2**, 74.

Thomas, T. R., and Neiman, C. N. (1968). *Endocrinology* **83**, 633.

Udry, J. R., and Morris, N. M. (1968). *Nature (London)* **220**, 593.

Vandenbergh, J. C. (1969). *Endocrinology* **84**, 658.

Van der Lee, S., and Boot, L. M. (1956). *Acta Physiol. Pharmacol. Neer.* **5**, 213.

von Berswordt-Wallrabe, R., and Neumann, F. (1967). *Neuroendocrinology* **2**, 107.

Walton, A. (1952). *Ciba Found. Colloq Endocrinol. Proc.* **3**, 47.

Ward, I. L. (1969). *Horm. Behav.* 1, 25.

Warren, R. P., and Aronson, L. R. (1956). *Endocrinology* 58, 293.

Waxenberg, S. E., Drellich, M. G., and Sutherland, A. M. (1959). *J. Clin. Endocrinol. Metab.* 19, 193.

Whalen, R. E. (1966). *Psychol. Rev.* 73 , 151.

Whalen, R. E. (1969). Personal communication.

Whalen, R. E., and Edwards, D. A. (1969). *Endocrinology* 84, 155.

Whalen, R. E., and Nadler, R. D. (1963). *Science* 141, 273.

Whalen, R. E., and Nakayama, K. (1965). *J. Endocrinol.* 33, 525.

Whalen. R. E., and Robertson, R. T. (1968). *Psychonom. Sci.* 11 319.

Whalen, R. E., Edwards, D. A., Luttge, W. G., and Robertson, R. T. (1968). *Physiol. Behav.* 4, 33.

Whitten, W. K. (1956a). *J. Endocrinol.* 13, 399.

Whitten, W. K. (1956b). *J. Endocrinol.* 14, 160.

Whitten, W. K. (1966). *Advan. Reproductive Physiol.* 1, 155-177.

Wilson, J., and Beach, F. A. (1963). *Proc. Nat. Acad. Sci. U.S.* 49, 624.

Wilson, E. O., and Bossert, W. H. (1963). *Recent Progr. Horm. Res.* 19, 673.

Wilson, J. R., Adler, N., and Leboeuf, B. (1965). *Proc. Nat. Acad. Sci. U.S.* 53, 1392.

Yamamoto, J., and Seeman, W. (1960). *Psychiat. Res. Rep. Amer. Psychiat. Ass.* 12, 97.

Young, W. C. (1961). *In* "Sex and Internal Secretions" (W. C. Young, ed.), Vol. II, pp. 1173-1239. Williams & Wilkins, Baltimore, Maryland.

Young, W. C., Goy, R. W., and Phoenix, C. H. (1964). *Science* 143, 212.

Zarrow, M. X., and Clark, J. H. (1968). *J. Endocrinol.* 40, 343.

Zeilmaker, G. H. (1966). *Acta Endocrinol. (Copenhagen)* 51, 461.

Zucker, I. (1966a). *J. Comp. Physiol. Psychol.* 62, 376.

Zucker, I. (1966b). *Endocrinology* 35, 209.

Zucker, I. (1967a). *J. Endocrinol.* 38, 269.

Zucker, I. (1967b). *J. Comp. Physiol. Psychol.* 63, 313.

Zucker, I. (1968). *J. Comp. Physiol. Psychol.* 65, 472.

Zucker, I., and Goy, R. W. (1967). *J. Comp. Physiol. Psychol.* 64, 378.

Zumpe, D., and Michael, R. P. (1968). *J. Endocrinol.* 40, 117.

4

Hormones and Maternal Behavior in Mammals

M. X. Zarrow, Victor H. Denenberg, and Benjamin D. Sachs

I. INTRODUCTION

Maternal behavior is a complex series of events and is the last link in a chain starting with a successful mating. The many behavioral and physiological phenomena involved insure the maintenance and perpetuation of the species. Yet in spite of the obvious importance of maternal behavior, intensive investigations by a variety of researchers on this problem have occurred only within the past decade, although some excellent research was carried out by a few scattered investigators as long as 40 years ago. Even though chemical factors are obviously of importance, the role which hormones play in influencing the various aspects of maternal behavior has not as yet been fully elucidated. Indeed, the descriptive studies of psychologists and ethologists have shown clearly the complexity of the phenomenon called "maternal behavior" and, in certain instances, findings have indicated a less than dominant role for the hormonal substrate. However, too many contradictions exist and not many generalizations can be made as yet. To some extent this may be due to species differences as well as incomplete knowledge.

The present review will be limited to those species where hormonal studies have been carried out in detail and will discuss the data with the idea of determining what generalizations may be made at this time. For earlier reviews of this subject and for discussions in depth of the biological and behavioral factors involved in maternal behavior, the reader is directed to the reviews of Wiesner and Sheard (1933), Beach (1948, 1951), Lehrman (1961), Richards (1967), Rosenblatt (1967a), Zarrow *et al.* (1968), and the volume edited by Rheingold (1963).

II. NEST BUILDING

A. The Rabbit

1. *General Description*

One of the first behavioral expressions of pregnancy in the rabbit is nest building. This is generally present in a two-phase sequence. The animal first builds a straw nest followed 1 to 5 days later by what we have called the "maternal nest" (Zarrow *et al.*, 1962b). The maternal nest differs from the straw nest in that the doe actively pulls hair from her body and incorporates this hair with the straw or other nesting materials. The straw is usually hollowed out first and then lined with the body hair and after the young are born the nest is frequently covered over with the hair. Correlated with the construction of the maternal nest is an actual loosening of the rabbit's body hair so that it is easier for the doe to pull out the hair (Sawin *et al.*, 1960). Thus, a large well-insulated nest within which to deposit the young is fabricated by the mother.

The maternal nest appears to be unique to pregnancy and pseudopregnancy, while the straw nest has been observed to be built by nonpregnant females and by males. However, there has never been a report of a maternal nest built except under conditions of pregnancy, pseudopregnancy, or experimental manipulation involving the hormones of pregnancy.

In attempting to relate endocrine manipulations to subsequent behavior it is convenient and almost necessary to have unequivocal behavioral endpoints. The

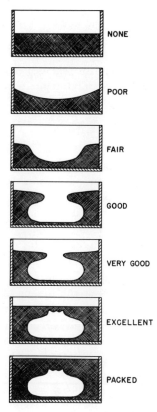

Fig. 1. Graded types of nests built by the rabbit. Only if hair from the animal's body is incorporated into the straw nest can it be considered a maternal nest. [From Sawin and Crary (1953).]

occurrence of the maternal nest (a discrete event) and the loosening of the hair (a continuous event) have been utilized as our two endpoints to study the effects of hormone manipulations.

Before discussing these more fully, however, some other characteristics of maternal behavior in the rabbit should be noted. One can roughly quantify the maternal nest by rating its quality (Sawin and Crary, 1953). The rating scale is diagramed in Fig. 1 and ranges from a flat nest with no hollowed-out area in which to place the young to a nest which is well hollowed out and completely covered over, thus offering maximum warmth and protection for the young (Sawin and Crary, 1953; Ross et al., 1956). Other behavioral patterns occurring during pregnancy and continuing after the young are born have been described by Sawin and Curran (1952) as involving "maternal protection" and "maternal interest." The former describes the doe's behavior toward an attendant who inspects the cage and nest box of the female. Rabbits range in their behavior from a high degree of timidity when approached by the attendant to vigorous, aggressive attacks upon the attendant. The degree of maternal interest may be rated on a 5-point scale ranging from 0 (no interest in the young) to 4+ (interest in the young to the point of aggressively fighting off any attempt to approach the nest or manipulate the young). This measure differs from maternal protection in that the maternal interest refers to the behavior of the doe when approached by the attendant. The interest ratings specifically refer to the response to manipulation of the nest or young. Sawin and Curran (1952) presented evidence that these two behavioral characteristics are relatively independent.

Another characteristic of maternal behavior is that of nursing the young. This can be scored simply by examining a neonate to see if the belly is distended and if the milk can be seen through the skin. It is thus possible to obtain a score based on the percentage of a litter which a mother nurses.

Two significant negative features of maternal behavior are scattering and cannibalism. Scattering is defined as the finding of one or more of the young outside of the nest or nest box rather than in the nest. Cannibalism is defined as eating of part or all of one or more young (Denenberg *et al.*, 1959).

Systematic analyses have been made of these various measures. An analysis of changes in nest quality over four litters has been reported by Ross *et al.* (1956). Relationships between nest quality, maternal interest, nursing, aggression, scattering, and cannibalism have been described by Denenberg *et al.* (1958, 1959). Any or all of these behaviors could have been used as endpoints against which to assess hormonal manipulation but we chose not to use them because of the tenuous nature of rating scales and because it would have been necessary to follow the mother and her litter through a number of postparturient days in order to obtain the necessary data. In planning our research strategy we felt it to be more advisable to terminate all observations at the time of parturition using the two unequivocal endpoints mentioned earlier. Ultimately, however, it will be necessary to relate the hormonal status of the organism to the other behaviors which we have described above.

2. Hair Loosening

A common observation has been that the hair of rabbits becomes relatively loose around the time of parturition, particularly in specific areas of the body. This observation has been quantified by means of a combing technique. Two selected areas of the body were used for combing: the flank, which is defined as the area of the thigh located over the femur, and the back, which is defined as the area from the base of the neck to the tail. The comb was held at a $45°$ angle

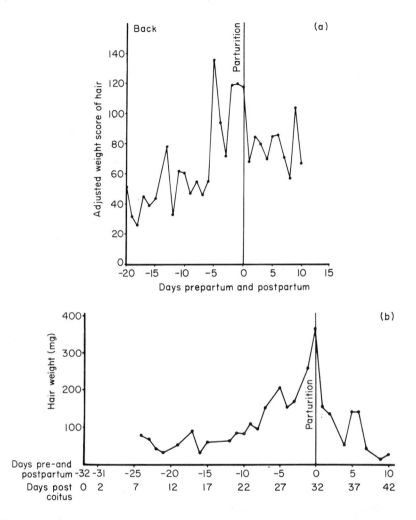

Fig. 2. Hair loosening in the pregnant rabbit. Two typical examples are presented above showing that hair loosening can occur several days prior to or at the time of parturition. [From Sawin *et al.* (1960).]

and passed over each flank area three times and over the back area six times. In each instance the hair from each pass was combined and weighed to the nearest milligram.

The first experiment established the fact that a significant degree of hair loosening occurred during gestation in the rabbit (Sawin *et al.*, 1960), with the peak occurring anywhere from 5 days prepartum to the day of parturition (Fig. 2). In addition, the pseudopregnant rabbit also exhibited a significant increase in hair loosening toward the end of pseudopregnancy. A control group of nonpregnant females failed to exhibit any increase in hair loosening over time.

Following the quantification of hair loosening and the demonstration that this is a phenomenon of pregnancy and pseudopregnancy, Farooq et al. (1963) investigated hair loosening as a function of endocrine stimulation. As found previously, normal pregnant females and pseudopregnant females both exhibited significant hair loosening. In another experiment progesterone was administered to animals from day 28 to day 35 of pregnancy in order to inhibit parturition. With a daily dose of 4 mg progesterone, parturition was duly inhibited from occurring at the expected time and none of these animals built a maternal nest. Although a significant increase in hair weight was noted, this increase was significantly less than that of controls. In another experiment, pregnant animals were given 2 mg progesterone. As with the 4 mg group an increase in hair loosening occurred, but again the increase was still significantly less than that of nonpregnant controls. Unlike the 4 mg group, however, seven of the eight animals in this experiment did build a maternal nest.

Other experiments demonstrated that hair loosening as well as nest building could be induced in castrated females given a regimen of estradiol, progesterone, and prolactin for a period of 8 weeks (Fig. 3). However, a similar regimen for 18 days failed to affect hair loosening. In order to determine whether hair loosening could be induced in the male, the same regimen which has been successful with

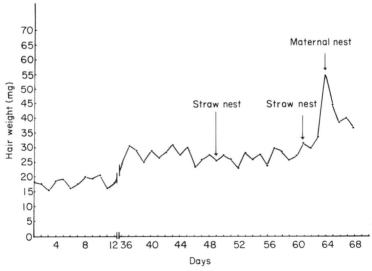

Fig. 3. Hair loosening in an ovariectomized rabbit following prolonged treatment with estradiol (5 μg, days 1-68), progesterone (1 mg, days 11-24; 2 mg, days 25-45), and prolactin (20 IU, days 46-60). Time of occurrence of construction of straw nest and maternal nest indicated in figure. [From Farooq et al. (1963).]

castrated females was used with castrated males. No evidence of an increase in hair loosening was obtained.

3. Nest Building

The building of a maternal nest normally occurs during the end of pregnancy or pseudopregnancy (Tietz, 1933; Zarrow et al., 1961). The functional value of the nest has been shown by Zarrow et al. (1963) by clipping the entire hair coat of some females on day 28 or 29 of pregnancy; 87% of young born to normal control mothers lived through weaning, while only 5.7% of the young reared with no nesting material survived.

An important question concerning maternal nest building is whether the hormones of pregnancy must act for a minimum period of time in order to initiate this behavior in the rabbit. One way to investigate this question is by castrating females at different times during pregnancy. Since removal of the corpus luteum during pregnancy (Klein, 1956) or castrating in late pregnancy (Zarrow et al., 1961) leads to maternal nest building, it is apparent that the normal length of gestation is not a prerequisite for maternal nest building. Using the Dutch belted strain, females were castrated either on day 13, 14, 15, 16, or 17 after the initiation of pregnancy. The data indicated that approximately 25% of the rabbits of a Dutch belted strain built maternal nests if castrated on the 14th day of gestation and 100% if castrated on the 17th day of gestation. Castration prior to day 14 of gestation resulted in a failure to build a maternal nest (Fig. 4). In all instances castration terminated pregnancy (Zarrow et al., 1962a).

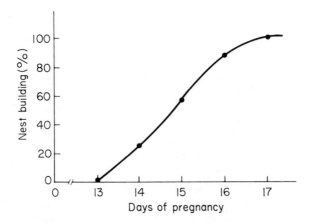

Fig. 4. Percentage of rabbits that built maternal nests following ovariectomy between days 13-17 of gestation. [From Zarrow et al. (1962a,b).]

Not only will castration after a certain critical period lead to nest building, but also complete removal of the entire conceptus mass on days 22 to 27 of gestation will do so (Zarrow *et al.*, 1962b). In addition, rabbits made pseudopregnant with human chorionic gonadotropin will build maternal nests (Zarrow *et al.*, 1961). It would therefore appear that the withdrawal of the hormones of pregnancy caused by the termination of gestation can lead to maternal nest building.

Following the above documentation that the presence of the hormones of pregnancy are essential for the manifestation of nest building behavior, Zarrow *et al.* (1963) set out to determine whether maternal nest building could be produced in a nonpregnant female by the appropriate hormonal manipulation. Castrated females were given various regimens of hormones and the occurrence of maternal nest building was noted. Three regimens were found to induce nest building 100% of the time. The first treatment involved the daily injection of 5 μg of estradiol for a period of 56 days, 1 mg of progesterone during the second and third week followed by 2 mg of protesterone for the remaining period, and 20 IU prolactin injected daily for the last 2 weeks (Zarrow *et al.*, 1962b). Within 3 or 4 days after the cessation of hormone treatment all 10 rabbits built maternal nests (Fig. 3).

Since maternal nest building occurs in the rabbit during pregnancy, a period of exposure to the proper hormones for approximately 30 days should be sufficient to induce the phenomenon. Furthermore, maternal nest building, either during pregnancy or pseudopregnancy, is associated with a decline in the circulating level of progesterone. Accordingly, a regimen was instituted in which the rabbit received 5 μg estradiol for 31 days with 2 mg progesterone on days 9-18 and 4 mg progesterone on days 19-29. Under this regimen all rabbits built maternal nests. However, if both the estrogen and progesterone treatment were stopped simultaneously, nest building failed to occur.

In an attempt to reduce even further the length of treatment, 10 rabbits were injected with 5 μg estradiol on days 1-18 and 4 mg progesterone on days 2-15. All animals built maternal nests 2 to 3 days after the cessation of progesterone treatment. Again, if treatment with estradiol and progesterone was maintained until day 18 and then simultaneously stopped, nest building failed to occur.

Castrated males were subjected to the same treatments as the castrated females. In no instance was there any evidence of nest building on the part of the males (Zarrow *et al.*, 1963).

It is apparent from the experiments described above that the onset of maternal nest building is always associated with a fall in progesterone levels, i.e., nest building occurs at parturition, near the end of pseudopregnancy, and after castration in the pregnant animal. If the fall in progesterone level triggers nest building, it then follows that the maintenance of high progesterone levels should prevent maternal nest building. Therefore, Zarrow *et al.* (1963) took 12 pregnant females and, starting on day 28, injected these females with 4 mg progesterone until day 35 of gestation. Nest building was inhibited in all but one of these rabbits. Parturition was delayed in all animals and appeared only 3-4 days after the withdrawal of progesterone. A second group of 10 pregnant rabbits was treated in a similar fashion with a dose of 2 mg progesterone. The delay as well as the subsequent onset of parturition was comparable to the former group, but 90% of these animals did build a maternal nest. The onset of nest building varied from the normal time to a slight delay of 1 or 2 days.

It is evident from these studies that the onset of maternal nest building may depend on a critical ratio between progesterone and estrogen. Therefore, either a decrease in progesterone or an increase in estrogen should result in maternal nest building. In order to test this hypothesis, 10 pregnant rabbits were given 10 μg of estradiol benzoate daily on days 20, 21, and 22 of pregnancy. Nine of these ten animals built a maternal nest between days 22 and 24 of gestation (Zarrow *et al.*, 1963).

In summary, a requirement for the manifestation of maternal nest building in the rabbit appears to be an exposure to a combination of the two female sex steroids, estradiol and progesterone. It would appear that the animal must be exposed to the two steroids for a finite length of time and that the estrogen-progesterone ratio must be such that the progesterone is in great preponderance (Zarrow *et al.*, 1963, 1965; Hafez *et al.*, 1966). Withdrawal of the progesterone, leaving a state of estrogen dominance, results in nest building. Maternal nest building fails to occur if either steroid is given alone or if a high progesterone level is maintained. Therefore, one may conclude that both estradiol and progesterone are necessary for maternal nest building but that progesterone also acts in an inhibitory manner if exposure to the hormone is prolonged. Such inhibition is not seen with estradiol.

B. The Rat

Early studies on maternal behavior in the rat have focused on nest building and retrieval of the young. In 1927, Kinder reported an increase in nest-building activity several days prior to parturition. This increase has been confirmed by numerous investigators (Sturman-Hulbe and Stone, 1929; Beach, 1937; Rosenblatt and Lehrman, 1963). In addition, a marked increase in nest building was reported at the time of parturition (Wiesner and Sheard, 1933; Obias, 1957).

This phenomenon has recently been reexamined in the authors' laboratory (Denenberg *et al.*, 1969). These investigators attempted to quantify the phenomenon of nest building in the rat by using a measure of chewing activity. The animals were given cylindrical wooden dowels made of medium grade hardwood. Each dowel was weighed when placed in the animal's cage and weighed again 24 hours later. The rat will typically chew and shred the dowel, and the decrease in weight due to the shredding activity was utilized as the index of nesting material used daily. The shredded material from the dowel is usually collected by the rat and incorporated into a nest.

The results show a marked increase in dowel shredding at the time of parturition followed by a sharp decrease (Fig. 5). Nonpregnant females and males showed no significant increase in dowel shredding scores over an equivalent period of time. These findings indicate that increased shredding during pregnancy is representative of maternal nest building. Treatment with doses of progesterone (2-8 mg/day) from day 16 to 21 after mating delayed parturition and reduced the number of females that showed a peak at parturition. In addition, when the peak shredding response did occur, it was delayed several days relative to normal parturition. Other experimental preparations involving the endocrine system included (1) pseudopregnancy, (2) ovulation, (3) estrogen treatment, (4) progesterone treatment in the ovariectomized rat, (5) combinations of the two steroids, and (6) castration during pregnancy. All of these failed to influence the dowel shredding scores. As might be expected, cold increased dowel shredding (Fig. 6), whereas heat depressed it. This study confirmed previous reports (Kinder, 1927; Richter, 1937).

The findings, as reviewed thus far, are very similar to the data on the rabbit. The rabbit's nest building behavior remains at basal level until 1 or 2 days before parturition at which time the frequency rises sharply followed by an equally sharp decline (Denenberg et al., 1963a). This is essentially the same pattern which is obtained for the rat's shredding behavior. When pregnant rabbits were given 4 mg progesterone later in pregnancy, nest building was inhibited in 11 out of 12 does. With 2 mg of progesterone 9 out of 10 pregnant animals did build a maternal nest, though the onset of nest building was delayed 1 or 2 days for some of these animals (Zarrow et al., 1963). Similarly, in these experiments progesterone acted to reduce the percentage of animals which exhibited a parturitional peak and also delayed the onset of this peak.

Even though there are several similarities between the rat and the rabbit data, there are a greater number of discrepancies. In the rabbit maternal nest building can be induced by pseudopregnancy or ovariectomy after midpregnancy (Zarrow et al., 1962a, 1965). In addition, the pregnant female can be induced to build her maternal nest earlier if she is given estradiol benzoate on days 20, 21, and 22 of pregnancy. Furthermore, maternal nest building will occur in nonpregnant female rabbits if they are castrated and given an appropriate treatment of estradiol and progesterone (Zarrow et al., 1963). All of these treatments were tried with the rat, and none succeeded in inducing a significant increase in dowel shredding. Thus, with the exception of the progesterone treatment, maternal nest building in the rat may occur relatively independently of direct hormonal control, although the phenomenon is certainly correlated

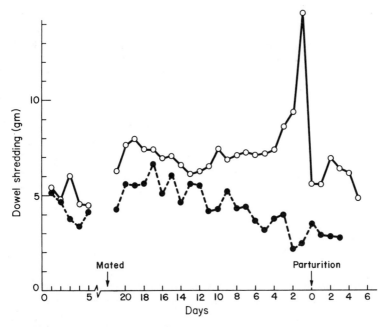

Fig. 5. Comparison of nest building in the nonpregnant and the pregnant rat. The mean amount of dowel material shredded daily is plotted for the premating, pregnancy, and the postpartum period. (○) Pregnant, $N = 104$; (●) nonpregnant, $N = 36$. [From Taylor (1965).]

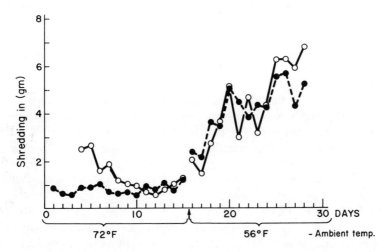

Fig. 6. The effect of temperature changes on dowel shredding in the adult rat. (●) Males, $N = 17$; (○) females, $N = 12$.

with pregnancy and expedited by gestation. Support for this conclusion is found in a study by Rosenblatt (1967b) who reported that ovariectomized or hypophysectomized female rats would eventually build a nest when presented continuously with the stimulus of 5-10-day-old pups.

C. The Mouse

The early work on nest building in the mouse failed to identify specific hormones involved in eliciting such behavior. As in the rat, nest building was attributed to a need for temperature regulation and was considered to be independent of hormonal regulations since it occurs in the hypophysectomized animal (Leblond and Nelson, 1936, 1937). Indeed, work from this laboratory indicated that the initiation of maternal activity may be due to sensitization by the young (Leblond, 1940).

Koller (1952, 1956) made an extensive investigation of nest building in the mouse. He presented mice daily with a measured amount of hay and weighed the nest 24 hours later. He described the presence of two types of nests: the sleeping nest and the brood nest. The sleeping nest is a loosely constructed nest that weighs 8-12 gm and is constructed by both males and nonpregnant females. This nest appears to be temperature-dependent and is probably utilized for protection from the cold.

The brood nest is much larger (30-50 gm) and appears only during pregnancy or following treatment with progesterone. This nest can therefore be distinguished from the sleeping nest only on the basis of size and time of appearance. Thus the maternal or brood nest in the mouse is not as unique a phenomenon as it is in the rabbit. Koller also noted that the appearance of the brood nest in the pregnant mouse coincided with the appearance of the corpora lutea of pregnancy. Treatment of intact or castrated female mice with either prolactin or estrone failed to elicit brood nest building, but progesterone at levels of 1.5-3 IU caused such behavior to appear. Progesterone treatment resulted in no nest building behavior in the intact or castrated male. Koller concluded that the regular or sleeping nest of the male and the nonpregnant female is built as a protection against the cold and that the brood nest is a part of the maternal complex stimulated during gestation by the increasing levels of progesterone available at that time. Thus it might be inferred that the regular nest is a response to ambient temperature, whereas the brood nest is the result of progesterone in a genetic female.

Lisk et al. (1969) confirmed some of Koller's findings (1952, 1956) on nest building in the mouse. They noted an increase in nest building activity at 3-4 days after mating which continued until the day before parturition. At this time a sudden drop in nest-building activity occurred followed by a return to the

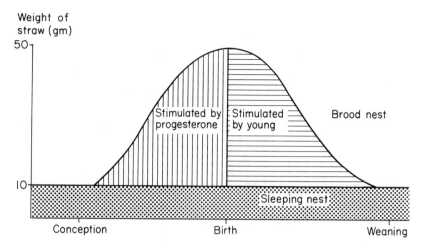

Fig. 7. A schematic diagram of nest building in the mouse during pregnancy and lactation. The weight of the nest is plotted against days of pregnancy and lactation [From Richards (1967).]

normal level of activity within a week postpartum. They also confirmed the ability of progesterone to elicit nest building by itself and observed an inhibitory action following estradiol. Some indication of a possible synergistic action of estradiol with progesterone in facilitating nest building was noted since the intact mouse exhibited a faster and greater nest building response to progesterone than did the castrated animal. This synergism is definitely dose-dependent since treatment with subcutaneous implants of 0.1-0.2 mg estradiol depressed the effect of progesterone on nest building. Lisk *et al.* (1969) also confirmed Koller's observations that neither progesterone nor estradiol has any effect on nest building in the male. This is in agreement with the findings in the male rabbit (Zarrow *et al.,* 1963) and has been interpreted by us as a basic sex difference. However, Lisk *et al.* (1969) interpret their finding as due to a decreased sensitivity to ovarian hormones in the male. Contrary to the findings of Koller (1952), Lisk *et al.* (1969) reported no correlation between nest building and ambient temperature or nest building and the estrous cycle.

A diagrammatic representation of the mechanism involved in maternal nest building has been presented in a review by Richards (1967). He points out that three separate mechanisms are involved. These include (1) the building of the sleeping nest which is independent of the gonadal hormones and is seen in both sexes; (2) the building of the brood nest which is seen in pregnancy and is produced following progesterone treatment; (3) the building of the brood nest which may occur following stimulation from the nursing young (Fig. 7).

D. The Hamster

Maternal nest building in the golden hamster appears to be comparable to that seen in the mouse. The increased use of straw shows a rise early in pregnancy with increasing amounts used as pregnancy progresses. While progesterone alone increased the level of nest building in the normal hamster, both estrogen and progesterone were required in the castrate animal indicating the need for both steroids (Richards, 1969) and thereby differing from the mouse where progesterone alone is effective (Koller, 1956). Hypothalamic implants of progesterone in an estrogenized, castrated hamster were also effective in producing maternal nest building.

The hamster (Richards, 1969) like the mouse (Koller, 1952) and the rabbit (Zarrow *et al.*, 1963) shows a sex difference in maternal nest building. When male hamsters are given the hormonal treatment described above, which was effective in producing maternal nest building in the female, no evidence of nest building was obtained in the male (Richards, 1969). It may be argued that this difference is due to the action of neonatal sex hormones upon the organization of the male and female brain. In order to test this hypothesis the following experiment was done in which (1) males were castrated in infancy and (2) females were given 500 μg of testosterone proprionate at 2-4 days of age (Richards, 1968). These animals were given the standard treatment with estrogen and progesterone in adulthood and observed for nest building. The males still did not build nests, while the females did build. Since the sex difference was not eliminated by "feminizing" the male by castration nor by "masculinizing" the female by testosterone treatment, it would appear that this difference may be independent of hormonal factors during the organization of the brain. However, this can only be regarded as a possibility. The present data are inadequate for a final evaluation.

III. RETRIEVAL OF YOUNG

The phenomenon of retrieval of the young has been known for a long time and has been well described for the rat (Wiesner and Sheard, 1933; Rosenblatt and Lehrman, 1963) as well as for the mouse and other species, excluding the rabbit.

The full pattern of maternal behavior including retrieval appears within 24 hours after delivery in rats (Rosenblatt, 1963). Rats tested for retrieval failed to retrieve any young from the 11th day before parturition until delivery, although a limited amount of retrieval has been described during the latter part of pregnancy (Wiesner and Sheard, 1933). Within 24 hours postpartum 100% of the rats retrieved the young (Fig. 8). Retrieving began to decline at about the 15th day postpartum in the lactating animal (Rosenblatt, 1969).

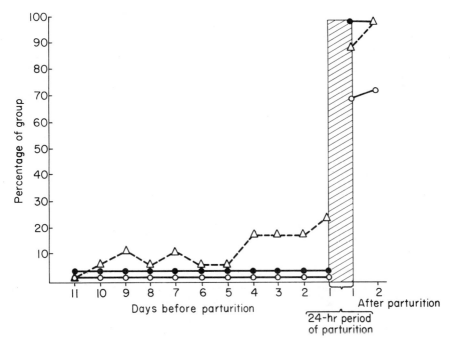

Fig. 8. Maternal behavior in the rat before and after parturition. The percentage of a group of 17 rats that retrieved (●), nursed (○), and built nests (△) during a period of 11 days before and 2 days after delivery is presented [From Rosenblatt (1965).]

Spontaneous retrieval, i.e., retrieval by a virgin rat upon first contact with a pup occurs in approximately 30% of the rat population. Induced retrieval along with the other concomitants of maternal behavior, such as nest building and crouching over the pups, has also been described following continuous exposure to pups (Cosnier and Couturier, 1966; Rosenblatt, 1967b). Cosnier and Couturier exposed their rats to pups for 4 hours daily while Rosenblatt exposed his rats continuously by removing the pups every 24 hours and replacing them with fresh pups. Essentially all the virgin rats retrieved the young. Castration or hypophysectomy had no significant effect. Retrieval was also induced in the male rat (approximately 80%) and again castration had no effect. Spontaneous retrieval has also been reported in the virgin mouse (Noirot, 1964; Gandelman *et al.*, 1970). Our own findings in the mouse (Zarrow *et al.*, 1970) agree with the findings in the rat emphasized by Rosenblatt (1969) that the virgin is responsive to the pup and that the physiological changes during pregnancy (probably hormonal) markedly increase this responsiveness. Thus there is both a nonhormonal as well as a hormonal basis to retrieval.

Recently, Plume *et al.* (1968) tested the retrieving behavior in rats using a pup, a food pellet, and a plastic toy as stimuli. The subjects included males, virgin females, pregnant females, and lactating females. The data show that lactating females retrieve the pups more often than any other group and were the only group which discriminated between retrieval of the pup and retrieval of the inanimate object. The lactating subjects also retrieved the pups significantly faster than the other subjects. The authors conclude that retrieving in lactating rats can be taken as a reflection of maternal behavior, while the lower frequency of retrieval in the nonlactating rat and her inability to distinguish between the pups and the inanimate objects indicate that this is not maternal behavior. The implication herein, that retrieving in the male or virgin female rat is not an aspect of maternal behavior, raises the question of the ancillary components of the retrieving described by Rosenblatt (1967b) and others, i.e., nest building, crouching over the young, etc. It would appear, however, that the simplest explanation would be the concept of a low level of maternal behavior existing in various species at different levels of activity and that the hormonal complex of pregnancy acts to stimulate this to the level seen in the lactating animal.

In the hamster, both the virgin females and the intact pregnant animals were reported unresponsive to the pup (Rowell, 1961). This finding has been contradicted by Richards (1966). He found that all virgin females killed and ate the young. A majority of the pregnant females ate at least one pup and then cared for the remaining pups. All the lactating mothers, except one, accepted the test young.

In general, a hormonal regulation of retrieval has not been shown except for the current studies on the presence of a blood factor shortly after parturition in the rat (see Section V) and the increased retrieval after pregnancy.

IV. PLACENTAPHAGIA

In most mammals the parturient female eats the membranes, placenta, and umbilical cord of her young. This behavior is referred to as placentaphagia. Numerous hypotheses have been put forward to account for the adaptive value of this behavior (Slijper, 1960), but its function is still unknown. One hypothesis of primary concern here is derived from the fact that the placenta is rich in hormones. Ingestion of these hormones is believed to contribute to the onset of maternal behavior and lactation.

In one investigation of this problem, newborn rats were fostered to females that had been lactating for 10 days (Denenberg et al., 1963b). When the females were permitted to eat the placentas, the foster young had longer survival times and higher body weights at weaning. Cross-fostering without permitting placentaphagia resulted in decreased survival rate and depressed body weight. No effect of placentaphagia was evident in foster mothers that had been lactating for 1 or 5 days. The salutary effects of placentaphagia on 10-day lactating mothers could be duplicated by treating foster mothers with estrogen. This finding led to the concept that placental estrogen was probably the factor involved in the stimulation of maternal behavior by placentaphagia.

In a further experiment (Zarrow *et al.*, 1967) pups were removed from mothers that had been lactating for 10 days, and the mothers were injected with various hormones. Thirty minutes later newborn pups were presented to the foster mothers without placentas. Control litters were fostered to females that did not receive hormones. The litters with prolactin-treated foster mothers had higher survival rates and body weights at weaning (Fig. 9). Progesterone increased survival rates, but did not affect body weight. Administration of estrogen with prolactin acted to increase survival rates, but not significantly beyond the effect obtained by prolactin alone. Both estrogen and prolactin have been identified in placentas but the mechanism by which these hormones exerted their effects in this experiment is still an open question.

Grota and Eik-Nes (1967) gave evidence suggestive of a hormonal conse-quence of eating placentas. They examined postpartum female rats and found that plasma progesterone reached peak concentrations 4 days after parturition. This peak was reduced significantly if litters were removed from the females after parturition. Reduction in plasma progesterone, approaching statistical significance, also resulted if the mothers were prevented from eating placentas at parturition. In a separate experiment, injection of hypophysectomized females with prolactin yielded significantly higher concentrations of plasma progesterone

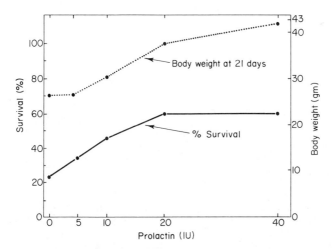

Fig. 9. Increased survival and body weight in the fostered rat pup subsequent to a single treatment of the foster mother with prolactin but without placentaphagia [From Zarrow *et al.* (1967).]

at 1-8 hours after treatment. The overall results were interpreted as suggesting that placentaphagia and exposure to the litters is essential to maternal progesterone secretion, and that progesterone contributes importantly to the onset of maternal behavior. No conclusion was drawn concerning the hormonal mechanisms intervening between placentaphagia and progesterone accumulation, but Grota and Eik-Nes implicated prolactin.

Placental prolactin is possibly the effective agent in stimulating progesterone secretion. However, it appears likely that prolactin taken orally would be ineffective. This protein hormone would probably be digested into hormonally ineffective moieties. Conceivably, placental estrogens could act, as do orally active estrogens, to stimulate pituitary prolactin, which in turn would stimulate ovarian progesterone secretion. Thus the placental estrogens could act indirectly as a stimulus to the initiation of lactation (Meites and Turner, 1944a, b; Meites et al., 1963) by acting directly on the pituitary as well as the hypothalamus in causing increased prolactin secretion.

Despite the evidence for a hormonal effect of placentaphagia in rats, no role for placental ingestion has been discovered for the normal reproductive cycle of any species. Wiesner and Sheard (1933) delivered female rats of their pups by caesarean section, the pups being separated from their placentas and cleaned by the experimenters. Later tests indicated apparently normal maternal behavior, although the caesarean-delivered pups rarely survived. Subsequent studies (Labriola, 1953; Moltz et al., 1966; Grota et al., 1967) have used additional controls and made additional observations, but they have not found significant decrements in maternal behavior or pup welfare resulting from delivery by caesarean section, whether or not placentas were fed to the mothers. It is possible that the caesarean surgery stimulates hormone secretions that mimic the effect of normal parturition and placentaphagia, but this is speculative at present. The complexity of the problem can be exemplified by another experiment (Grota et al., 1967). Caesarean-delivered rats were found to have a higher chance of survival to weaning if they were fostered without, rather than with, their placentas attached. Furthermore, the effect of placental presence or absence varied as a function of the rate of presentation of the pups to their foster mother.

The difficulty in finding support for a role of placentaphagia in normal maternal-young interaction does not rule out the possibility that placental hormones have other effects on the mother. Some alternate hypotheses were tested by Sachs (1969a,b). He prevented female rats from eating placentas during an otherwise normal delivery. These mothers were compared with control females for latency to postpartum estrus, duration of estrus, quality of estrus, and number of uterine implantation sites resulting from copulation during estrus. None of these variables was affected by the prevention of placentaphagia.

Richards (1967) has pointed out that eating of the placenta could not be essential to the normal initiation of maternal behavior because the neonate emerges before the placenta, and the young is often nursing before the placenta is delivered. If the eating of placentas does have an effect on maternal behavior, it may be to act as an insurance factor when the situation is less than optimal, as in the cross-fostering experiment of Denenberg et al. (1963b). However, it must be considered that placentaphagia may have adaptive values not directly related to maternal behavior. For example, it has long been suggested (Slijper, 1960) that protection from predators and nest hygiene are among the functions served by the placentaphagia. In this connection, Fraser (1968) has noted an interesting correlation. Among ungulates, those species that do not eat placenta are the ones that leave the birth site soon after delivery; the placentaphagic species tend to stay at the same place for several hours or days after parturition. The latter species are the ones that would presumably need greater protection from predator-attracting stimuli and from potential sources of infection. Significantly, the placenta may remain undigested after being eaten by ungulates, suggesting that at least in these animals the adaptive value of eating the placenta can be served even if it is not digested.

V. HORMONES AND MATERNAL BEHAVIOR

A. Female Sex Steroids

This subject has already been discussed above and will be briefly reviewed here. The original work on retrieval tended to point to a nonspecific hormonal effect while nest building appeared to be temperature-regulated. The situation in the rabbit wherein the maternal nest is qualitatively different from the straw nest built by the male or female at times other than during the prepartum or partum period presented us with a species well suited for study. In this species it has been clearly shown that the castrate female can be induced to build maternal nests by treatment with estradiol and progesterone in a manner comparable to that seen in pregnancy (Zarrow et al., 1961). In the mouse the brood nest has been observed to occur during gestation and differs quantitatively from the sleeping nest. Treatment with progesterone has induced the formation of the brood nest by the mouse (Koller, 1952, 1956; Lisk et al., 1969). In the hamster, both estradiol and progesterone appear to be necessary for the maternal nest (Richards, 1969). In the case of the rat, efforts to induce nest building by estrogen and/or progesterone have failed (Denenberg et al., 1969).

Moltz and Wiener (1966) had demonstrated an important role for ovarian hormones in the initiation of maternal behavior in primiparous rats. Prepartum ovariectomy significantly impaired the maternal care given by these animals, but multiparous females were not significantly affected by ovariectomy. This interesting interaction between endocrine effect and maternal experience was confirmed by Moltz et al. (1969). They administered progesterone to female rats prepartum and then, of necessity, delivered the females of their young by caesarean section. Again, multiparous females were relatively unaffected by the experimental treatments, but fewer than 50% of the primiparous females initiated normal maternal behavior. The results were interpreted in terms of progesterone acting to protect the central nervous system (CNS) structures underlying maternal behavior from the hormones that normally activate these structures in the perinatal period. The activating hormones were assumed to be estrogen and prolactin.

Rosenblatt (1969) points out that this interpretation has the virtue of being similar to the theory proposed for the induction of lactation by progesterone after parturition, thereby permitting a single theory for the two functions.

According to evidence obtained by Lott and Rosenblatt (1969), the effects of ovarian hormones on the CNS structures mediating maternal behavior begin as early as day 10 of the 22-day gestation period. In a series of experiments they studied the effects of pregnancy, and of termination of pregnancy with or without ovariectomy, on the sensitivity of female rats to induction of maternal behavior by concaveation. In the concaveation procedure, test animals were continuously exposed to 5-10-day-old rat pups until maternal responses appeared. The studies of Lott and Rosenblatt indicated that (1) beginning on day 10, pregnant females are progressively more sensitive to concaveation ("pregnancy effect"), (2) cessation of pregnancy by hysterectomy accelerates this sensitivity ("termination of pregnancy effect"), and (3) the termination of pregnancy effect depends on the ovaries, for if hysterectomy is combined with ovariectomy, the increased sensitivity to concaveation is not found. The studies suggested that during pregnancy the ovarian hormones have begun to sensitize the nervous system to the stimuli provided by rat pups. Presumably the sensitization reaches a maximum at the time of parturition, accounting for the immediate maternal behavior normally demonstrated by the parturient female.

B. Prolactin

The idea of hormonal control of maternal behavior in the mammal stems from the early work of Wiesner and Sheard (1933) and Riddle et al. (1942). In both instances some doubt has arisen as to the validity of the findings. Wiesner and Sheard (1933) reported the induction of maternal behavior in the rat following the injection of a crude pituitary extract. Aside from the fact that the authors failed to use proper controls, it is impossible to know what was being injected. In 1942, Riddle and his colleagues confirmed the above findings and reported the induction of maternal behavior in the rat following treatment with either prolactin, progesterone, or deoxycorticosterone. However, both Wilson

(1961) and Lott and Fuchs (1962) failed to confirm the above results with prolactin.

Though it is apparent that a contradiction exists in the findings of the more recent investigations, it has become generally accepted that prolactin is the hormone involved in the induction of maternal behavior (Barnett, 1963). In the earlier work of Riddle *et al.* (1942), 1-7-day-old pups were exposed to virgin rats for a pretest period of 10 days and the subjects were checked for retrieving, licking, and cuddling. The animals that responded with maternal behavior were discarded, and the remainder received the prolactin injections for another 10-day period along with daily testing. In some instances, subjects that failed to respond were given a 10-day test period without treatment and then placed on the treatment schedule. Lott and Fuchs (1962) repeated the above experiment using 1-2-day-old pups with and without a sensitization period. These investigators failed to confirm any of the findings of Riddle and his colleagues. It is regrettable that the latter failed to include the dosage of prolactin used.

Self-licking of the nipple line by the preparturient female rat is apparently necessary for normal development of the forthcoming litter. It has been noted (Rosenblatt and Lehrman, 1963; Roth and Rosenblatt, 1967) that as the time of parturition approached, the female localized self-licking around the nipple lines as well as the pelvic and genital regions. Birch (1956) showed that pregnant females prevented by wide rubber collars from licking themselves were unable to raise offspring through the nursing period. Although Christopherson and Wagman (1965) found no survival differences between litters born to females fitted with collars and control animals, they did find a consistent body weight deficit in litters reared by females deprived of self-licking. Roth and Rosenblatt (1965, 1966, 1967) have recently indicated that animals deprived of preparturient self-licking had significantly less functional mammary tissue than did control animals. This provides a potential explanation for both the lack of litter survival and body weight deficits in the above experiments. It appears that the self-licking seen in preparturient female rats stimulates prolactin release and hence promotes mammary development and function, much as the presence of a litter (Moltz *et al.*, 1969; Grosvenor and Mena, 1969; Grosvenor and Turner, 1957, 1958; Rothschild, 1960) maintains luteal and mammary function through prolactin release. However, self-licking of just the nipple line by the postparturient rat in the absence of stimuli from the litter does not reduce the mother's pituitary prolactin content (Grosvenor and Mena, 1969).

C. A Blood Factor in Maternal Behavior

In 1925, Stone placed a maternal and nonmaternal rat in parabiosis in an attempt to induce maternal behavior in the nonmaternal rats. Although he got negative results, this could be ascribed to the failure of the substance or substances in the blood of the maternal rat to cross the parabiotic union. Forty-three years later, Terkel and Rosenblatt (1968) reported the presence of a bloodborne factor in the rat shortly after parturition that induced maternal behavior in the virgin rat. Plasma taken from donor rats within 48 hours after parturition when the rats showed good maternal behavior significantly reduced the latent time to retrieving of young by virgin rats. Saline and plasma taken from proestrous rats were without effect while plasma from diestrous rats was inhibitory. The authors point out that the onset of retrieving in the treated rats was also accompanied by crouching over the young, licking, and nest building. Some indications of maternal behavior appeared as early as 4-8 hours after injection of the maternal plasma.

This experiment raises the question, is this bloodborne factor a hormone or a mixture of hormones? The present data do not present us with an answer to this question. It would be most convenient if the bloodborne factor is one of the known hormones, but in view of the order of magnitude necessary to get an effect following systemic injection, the amount present in plasma is too minute to be a known hormone. Nevertheless, it is most likely that the bloodborne factor is probably related in some manner to a hormone and could produce its effect by acting upon certain endocrine glands or by acting directly on the CNS. In the latter instance its synthesis may be the result of hormone action.

D. Androgens

Fisher (1956) reported the induction of maternal behavior in both female and male rats by placing sodium testosterone sulfate into restricted areas of the hypothalamus. Nest building, retrieving of young, and grooming of the young were stimulated. Increased intensity was suggested by increased speed of reaction, compulsiveness, and increased frequency of response. The behavior was elicited within 20 seconds to 5 minutes and continued without lessening for more than 90 minutes following exposure to the stimulus.

However, only about 10% of the treated rats responded even though, once an effect occurred, it could be reproduced many times. Of 130 male rats treated with the androgen, 5 showed a complete maternal response and 14 showed nesting behavior only. No reason is given for the low frequency of response nor has any confirmation of these findings appeared.

In a limited number of studies, androgens have been administered to pregnant guinea pigs (Phoenix et al., 1959, Diamond, 1966; Goy et al, 1967) and rats (Revesz et al., 1963) without apparently affecting maternal behavior, although the abortion or resorption rate was higher. However, most of these studies were not looking specifically at maternal behavior. In the rabbit, on the other hand, a disruption of maternal nest building and care of the young has been reported following injection of testosterone propionate from days 17-29 of gestation (Campbell, 1964). The above results were obtained in the New Zealand strain and have been repeated with the Dutch belted strain in our laboratory (Fuller *et al.,* 1970). Treatment with testosterone propionate comparable to that used by Campbell (1964) significantly inhibited maternal nest building and care of the litter through weaning, and increased the likelihood that the female would abort or resorb the young. Inhibition of maternal nest building appeared to require the full 12 days of the treatment since no other portion of the treatment time, including the first 9 days, was sufficient to inhibit this behavior. That a long treatment period is required is not too surprising since it has been shown that nest building in the rabbit following castration during pregnancy requires 15-17 days of gestation (Zarrow *et al.,* 1962a).

The attempt to determine the portion of the full treatment period which was directly related to maternal care revealed the importance of days 17-25 and days 27-29. The majority of females that failed to care for their young delivered on the cage floor and either cannibalized or mutilated the pups within 24 hours of birth. In some instances offspring were abandoned or not allowed to suckle even though a normal delivery utilizing the maternal nest had occurred. It was evident that death of the young was not due to a lactation problem as large quantities of milk were present in the mammary glands at postmortem examination. Since the presence of the maternal nest did not change the statistical significance of these results it is unlikely that the young died from being chilled. Three factors seem to be evidenced: the active cannibalism of young, the failure to deliver young in the nest box (scattering), and the failure to nurse the young born into the nest box. Cannibalism would seem to be an "activated" behavior, while scattering and failure to nurse young indicate the absence of activation. It may very well be that the presence of testosterone propionate during either days 17-25 or days 27-29 of gestation activates neural components important to "cannibalism" behavior or prevents ovarian steroids form inhibiting them. At the same time it is possible that scattering and failure to nurse are the result of testosterone preventing the activation of important neural target structures.

These data indicate that the maternal component of nest building may be separated from that of care and rearing of the young. Treatment for the entire period (days 17-29) resulted in a failure of 50% of the rabbits to rear their young as compared to 3.7% for the controls. Comparable results were obtained with the 17-25 days of treatment and with 1 mg testosterone propionate for days 27-29. Treatment with a higher dose (2.5 mg) failed to give comparable results and no explanation can be offered at this time. Finally, significant inhibition of nest building required the full treatment period with testosterone propionate, whereas shorter treatment periods inhibited care and rearing of the young.

VI. HYPOPHYSECTOMY

The experiments on the effect of hypophysectomy on maternal nest building in the rabbit are still equivocal. In one study, approximately 85% of the females aborted and built maternal nests following ovariectomy between 17 and 30 days of gestation, while none of 15 hypophysectomized rabbits, whether they were castrated or not, built maternal nests. The experiment is difficult to interpret since (1) difficulty was noted at labor and the whole process was extended for several days, and (2) simultaneous removal of ovaries and pituitary failed to induce nest building. Finally, the author also failed to get nest building in the hypophysectomized rabbit following treatment with estrogen and progesterone (Fuller, 1967). Anderson (1969) confirmed the above findings in that estradiol and progesterone failed to induce maternal nest building in the hypophysectomized rabbit. Replacement therapy with whole pituitary extracts and various pituitary hormones such as prolactin, STH, etc. failed to induce nest building in the hypophysectomized rabbit following treatment with estradiol and progesterone (Fuller, 1967). These results tend to indicate that a pituitary factor may be necessary for maternal nest building, but this cannot be said conclusively since too many questions remain unanswered. Nevertheless, the data confirm the earlier findings of Robson (1937, 1939) that hypophysectomy interfered with nest building in the normal rabbit and in those wherein pregnancy was maintained with gonadotropin, estrogen, and progesterone.

Early studies indicated that the pituitary gland is not essential for maternal behavior in the rat and mouse although its removal does inhibit lactation (Collip *et al.,* 1933; Leblond and Nelson, 1936, 1937; Leblond, 1940; Obias, 1957; Bintarningsih *et al.,* 1958). Hypophysectomy in the rat caused a 200-500% increase in nest building as measured by the amount of paper incorporated into nests (Richter and Eckert, 1936; Richter, 1937). Similar results were reported by Stone and King (1954) and Stone and Mason (1955). It was suggested that temperature regulation was the underlying mechanism involved in increased nest building following hypophysectomy.

In 1957, Obias presented data on maternal behavior in rats hypophysectomized on the 13th day of gestation. Six rats were found to be completely hypophysectomized and showed an imbalance in normal reproductive performance. This included prolonged gestation, prolonged parturition, decreased litter size, and many stillbirths. Nevertheless, the hypophysectomized rats showed the patterns of postpartum maternal behavior of nest building, retrieval, suckling, and protection of the young. These data indicate that the pituitary is not essential for maternal behavior and are in contradiction to the findings in the rabbit. If true, we may have a species difference with regard to placental vs pituitary role. Lehrman (1961) has suggested that the failure of the pituitary to influence maternal behavior in the rat is due to the ability of the placenta in these species to secrete the relevant hormone or hormones. This may be true but we still need more information and additional studies on the role of the pituitary and/or the placenta.

VII. THYROIDECTOMY, ADRENALECTOMY, AND GONADECTOMY

Richter and Eckert (1936) studied nest building following thyroidectomy, adrenalectomy, and gonadectomy in the rat. Nest building was increased from slight to two-fold in all instances. The reverse experiment in which thyroid extract was administered to intact rats inhibited nest building (Richter, 1943).

In the rabbit, removal of the thyroid gland resulted in abnormal gestation length, increased stillbirths, and absence of nest building (Chu, 1944). These abnormal sequelae of thyroidectomy could be prevented by feeding desiccated thyroid. On the other hand, Krichesky (1939) and Krohn (1951) reported that thyroidectomized pregnant females delivered normally and exhibited normal maternal behavior. Upon remating, the thyroidectomized rabbits built nests and reared normal young, although a higher percentage of the females died at the time of delivery. Recent studies by Fuller (1967) confirmed the findings of Krohn (1951) that the thyroid gland was not essential for maternal behavior in the rabbit but that trauma could play an inhibitory role. The latter could explain some of the contradictory findings. For example, 38% of the rabbits thyroidectomized on days 24-26 built nests, whereas 20% of the sham thyroidectomized rabbits failed to build as compared to essentially 100% for the normal pregnant rabbit. Simultaneous removal of both the thyroid and ovaries at day 17 of gestation failed to result in nest building in any of the eight rabbits. In a third experiment castrated thyroidectomized rabbits were treated with estradiol and progesterone to induce nest building: 100% of the castrated built nests, while 78-100% of the castrate thyroidectomized rabbits built nests if the double operation was done before treatment started or completed a week before progesterone withdrawal. However, if the castrate rabbits were hypophysectomized 2 days before progesterone withdrawal only 20% of the rabbits built nests. It would appear that nest building can occur in the absence of the thyroid but that the surgical trauma along with reduced thyroxine levels acts in an inhibitory manner.

As indicated above, gonadectomy does not interfere with nest building in the rat or mouse although the maternal type of nest never appears in the ovariectomized rabbit except if the operation is carried out in the pregnant animal. Thus, ovarian involvement is certainly present in the rabbit and probably in the mouse as well since the type of nest building described above could be of the nonbrood or temperature regulated type. In a group of pregnant rats which

were ovariectomized and the young removed by caesarian section, only 50%
accepted the young (Moltz and Wiener, 1966).

VIII. SUMMARY AND CONCLUSIONS

We now know enough about the hormonal control of many aspects of
maternal behavior in the rabbit. the mouse, and the hamster to be able to induce
a number of these responses with exogenous hormones. In the rat, however,
maternal behavior has not been reliably stimulated by exogenous hormones.
Recently, Terkel and Rosenblatt (1968) discovered a factor in the early
postpartum blood of the rat that can facilitate the expression of maternal
behavior in the virgin female. Identification of this factor will greatly enhance
our potential for an understanding of the chemical basis of maternal behavior in
this species.

It is likely that many of the species differences in maternal behavior may be
only of a quantitative and not a qualitative nature. Retrieval can be elicited in
the virgin mouse within a matter of minutes and without hormonal treatment. In
the rat, however, retrieval can be elicited without hormonal treatment but only
after sensitization to the rat pups for a period of approximately 7 days. These
results suggest that the potential for this aspect of maternal behavior is present
in all mammals and that the hormones act primarily to activate a neural
substrate, thereby increasing the maternal responsiveness of the parent. This
raises the questions of site of action of the hormones and the mechanism
whereby the substrate is activated.

Variations among different species also exist in the degree of sexual
dimorphism that is present for maternal behavior. Mice of both sexes will show
the full complement of maternal behavior responses, whereas in other species
(e.g., the hamster) maternal behavior is not displayed by the male either under
normal conditions or in response to exogenous hormones. In the rabbit,
maternal nest building appears only in the female and not in the male. The
problem then of species variation is illustrated by the sexual dimorphism that is
apparent in some species. This phenomenon may reflect sex differences in neural
organization but we know far too little about the neural and endocrine bases of
male nurturing behavior to permit any conclusions at this time.

The existence of these species differences points to the need for a
comparative approach; clearly no single species can serve as a model for the
study of the hormonal basis of maternal behavior in "the mammal." it is also
evident that researchers in this area need sophistication in behavioral as well as in
endocrine techniques. For example, because the phenomenon of sensitization
through repeated testing was unknown during some of the early work on the
endocrine causes of maternal behavior, certain premature and incorrect
inferences were drawn.

The timing of initiation or enhancement of maternal responses such as maternal nest building, retrieving, cuddling, crouching, licking, and nursing has long suggested the involvement of the hormones of pregnancy and lactation. Although many questions remain to be answered, a great deal of progress has been made in the past decade toward uncovering the endocrine involvement in maternal behavior. We now need to complete this attack and move on to the interaction between the endocrine and the neural components.

IX. ADDENDUM

Moltz *et al.* (1970) recently reported the hormonal induction of retrieval in the castrated virgin rat with several hormones. Retrieval time was reduced from 6-7 days for untreated rats to between 35 and 40 hours for animals treated with estradiol, progesterone, and prolactin. Treatment with just estradiol and progesterone required approximately 72 hours before retrieval was observed. It is apparent that both regimens significantly shortened retrieval time and that prolactin is probably essential as well as the sex steroids. The significant shortening of retrieval time with the steroids alone can be explained by the increased endogenous release of prolactin due to the estrogen treatment (Nicoll and Meites, 1962; Meites and Nicoll, 1965).

Our own studies (Zarrow *et al.*, 1971) also used the castrated virgin rat and a hormonal regimen that consisted of estradiol, progesterone, cortisol acetate, and prolactin. We found that the full treatment reduced the latency to retrieve from an average of 4.9 days to 1.4 days and that elimination of prolactin gave a latency of 1.8 days. Both latencies were significantly decreased in the treatment groups as compared to the controls.

The results from the two laboratories are essentially in agreement and suggest that the threshold for retrieval is significantly lowered by hormonal treatment and that the hormones involved in this aspect of maternal behavior are estradiol, progesterone, and prolactin.

Acknowledgments

This review was written during the tenure of NIH Grants HD-02068, HD-4639, HD-04048.

We should like to express our appreciation to Ronald Gandelman and Clark O. Anderson for their thoughtful comments and criticisms of the manuscript.

REFERENCES

Anderson, C. O. (1969). Ph.D. Thesis, Purdue Univ., Lafayette, Indiana.
Barnett, S. A. (1963). "The Rat." Aldine, Chicago.
Beach, F. A. (1937). *J. Comp. Physiol.* 24, 339.
Beach, F. A. (1948). "Hormones and Behavior." Harper (Hoeber), New York.
Beach, F. A. (1951). *In* "Handbook of Experimental Psychology" (S. S. Stevens, ed.). Chapman & Hall, London.

Bintarningsih, Wm., Lyons, W. R., Johnson, R. E,, and Li, C. H. (1958). *Endocrinology* 63, 540.

Birch, H. G. (1956). *J. Orthopsychiat.* 27, 279.

Campbell, H. J. (1964). *Nature (London)* 204, 809.

Christopherson, E. R., and Wagman, W. (1965). *J. Comp. Physiol. Psychol.* 60, 142.

Chu, J. P. (1944). *Endocrinology* 4, 109.

Collip, J. P., Selye, H., and Thompson, D. L. (1933). *Nature (London)* 131, 56.

Cosnier, J., and Couturier, C. (1966). *C. R. Soc. Biol.* 160, 789.

Denenberg, V. H., Sawin, P. B., Fromme, G. P., and Ross, S. (1958). *Behaviour* 13, 131.

Denenberg, V. H., Petropolus, S. F., Sawin, P. B., and Ross, S. (1959). *Behaviour* 15, 71.

Denenberg, V. H., Huff, R. L., Sawin, P. B., and Zarrow, M. X. (1963a). *Anim. Behav.* 11, 494.

Denenberg, V. H., Grota, L. J., and Zarrow, M. X. (1963b). *J. Reprod. Fert.* 5, 133.

Denenberg, V. H., Taylor, R. E., and Zarrow, M. X. (1969). *Behaviour* 34, 1.

Diamond, M. (1966). *Nature (London)* 209, 1322.

Farooq, A., Denenberg, V. H., Ross, S., Sawin, P. B., and Zarrow, M. X. (1963). *Amer. J. Physiol.* 204, 271.

Fisher, A. E. (1956). *Science* 124, 228.

Fraser, A. F. (1968). "Reproductive Behavior in Ungulates." Academic Press, New York.

Fuller, G. B. (1967). Ph.D. Thesis, Purdue Univ., Lafayette, Indiana

Fuller, G. B., Zarrow, M. X., Anderson, C. O., and Denenberg, V. H. (1970). Testosterone propionate during gestation in the rabbit: effect on subsequent maternal behavior. To be published.

Gandelman, R., Zarrow, M. X., and Denenberg, V. H. (1970). *Develop. Psychobiol.* 3, 207.

Goy, R. W., Phoenix, C. H., and Meidinger, R. (1967). *Anat. Rec.* 157, 87.

Grosvenor, C. E., and Mena, F. (1969). *Horm. Behav.* 1, 85.

Grosvenor, C. E., and Turner, C. W. (1957). *Proc. Soc. Exp. Biol. Med.* 96, 723.

Grosvenor, C. E., and Turner, C. W. (1958). *Endocrinology* 63, 535.

Grota, L. J., and Eik-Nes, K. (1967). *J. Reprod. Fert.* 13, 83.

Grota, L. J., Denenberg, V. H., and Zarrow, M. X. (1967). *J. Reprod. Fert.* 13, 405.

Hafez, E. S. E., Lindsay, D. R., and Moustafa, L. A. (1966). *Z. Tierpsychol.* 6, 691.

Kinder, E. F. (1927). *J. Exp. Zool.* 47, 117.

Klein, M. (1956). *In* "L'instinct dans le Comportement des Animaux et de l'Homme" (P. P. Grassé, ed.). pp. 287-344. Masson, Paris.

Koller, G. (1952). *Verb. Deut. Zool. Ges. Freiberg*, p. 160.

Koller, G. (1956). *Zool. Anz.* Suppl. 19, 123.

Krichesky, B. (1939). *Amer. J. Physiol.* 126, 234.

Krohn, P. L. (1951). *J. Endocrinology* 7, 307.

Labriola, J. (1953). *Proc. Soc. Exp. Biol. Med.* 83, 556.

Leblond, C. P. (1940). *J. Genet. Psychol.* 57, 327.

Leblond, C. P., and Nelson, W. O. (1936). *C. R. Soc. Biol.* 122, 548.

Leblond, C. P., and Nelson, W. O. (1937). *Amer. J. Physiol.* 120, 167.

Lehrman, D. S. (1961). *In* "Sex and Internal Secretions" (W. C. Young, ed.), 3rd ed., Vol. II. pp. 1268-1382. Williams & Wilkins, Baltimore, Maryland.

Lisk, R. D., Pretlow, R. A., 3rd, and Friedman, S. A. (1969). *Anim. Behav.* 17, 730.

Lott, D. F., and Fuchs, S. S. (1962). *J. Comp. Physiol. Psychol.* 55, 111.

Lott, D. F., and Rosenblatt, J. S. (1969). *In* "Determinants of Infant Behaviour IV" (B. M. Foss, ed.), pp. 61-68. Methuen, London.

Meites, J., and Turner, C. W. (1944a). *Endocrinology* 30, 719.

Meites, J., and Turner, C. W. (1944b). *Endocrinology* 30, 726.

Meites, J., Nicoll, C. S., and Talwalker, P. K. (1963). *Advan. Neuroendocrinol. Proc. Symp.*, *1961*. pp. 238-288.

Meites, J., and Nicoll, C. S. (1965). *In* "Hormonal Steroids" (I. Martini and A. Pecile, eds.), pp. 307-316. Academic Press, New York.

Moltz, H., Robbins, D., and Parks, M. (1966). *J. Comp. Physiol. Psychol.* **61**, 455.

Moltz, H., and Wiener, E. (1966). *J. Comp. Physiol. Psychol.* **62**, 382.

Moltz, H. M., Lubin, M., Leon, M., and Numan, M. (1969). *J. Comp. Physiol. Psychol.* **67**, 36.

Moltz, H., Lubin, M., Leon, M., and Numan, M. (1970). *Physiol. Behav.* **5**, 1373.

Nicoll, C. S., and Meites, J. (1962). *Endocrinology* **70**, 272.

Noirot, E. (1964). *Anim. Behav.* **12**, 52.

Obias, M. D. (1957). *J. Comp. Physiol. Psychol.* **50**, 120.

Phoenix, C. H., Goy, R. W., Gerall, A. A., and Young, W. C. (1959). *Endocrinology* **65**, 369.

Plume, S., Fogarty, C., Grota, L. J., and Ader, R. (1968). *Psychol. Rep.* **23**, 627.

Revesz, C., Kernaghan, D., and Bindra, D. (1963). *J. Endocrinol.* **25**, 549.

Rheingold, H. L., ed. (1963). "Maternal Behavior in Mammals." Wiley, New York.

Richards, M. P. M. (1966). *Anim. Behav.* **14**, 310.

Richards, M. P. M. (1967). *Advan. Reproductive Physiol.* **2**, 53-100.

Richards, M. P. M. (1969). *Anim. Behav.* **17**, 356.

Richter, C. P. (1937). *Quant. Biol.* **5**, 258.

Richter, C. P. (1943). *Harvey Lect.* **38**, 63.

Richter, C. P., and Eckert, J. F. (1936). *Res. Pub. Ass. Res. Nerv. Ment. Dis.* **17**, 561.

Riddle, O., Lahr, E. L., and Bates, R. W. (1942). *Amer. J. Physiol.* **137**, 299.

Robson, J. M. (1937). *J. Physiol. (London)* **90**, 145.

Robson, J. M. (1939). *J. Physiol. (London)* **95**, 83.

Rosenblatt, J. S. (1965). *In* "Determinants of Infant Behaviour III" (B. M. Foss, ed.), pp. 3-45. Methuen, London.

Rosenblatt, J. S. (1967a). *In* "Childbearing—Its Social and Psychological Aspects" (S. A. Richardson and A. F. Guttmacher, eds.). Williams & Wilkins, Baltimore, Maryland.

Rosenblatt, J. S. (1967b). *Science* **156**, 1512.

Rosenblatt, J. S. (1969). *Amer. J. Orthopsychiat.* **39**, 36.

Rosenblatt, J. S., and Lehrman, D. S. (1963). *In* "Maternal Behavior in Mammals" (H. L. Rheingold, ed.), pp. 8-57. Wiley, New York.

Ross, S., Denenberg, V. H., Sawin, P. B., and Meyer, P. (1956). *Brit. J. Anim. Behav.* **4**, 69.

Roth, L. L., and Rosenblatt, J. S. (1965). *Amer. Zool.* **5**, 234.

Roth, L. L., and Rosenblatt, J. S. (1966). *Science* **151**, 1403.

Roth, L. L., and Rosenblatt, J. S. (1967). *J. Comp. Physiol. Psychol.* **63**, 397.

Rothschild, I. (1960). *Endocrinology* **67**, 9.

Rowell, T E. (1961). *Anim. Behav.* **9**, 11.

Sachs, B. (1969a). Placentaphagia and cannibalism in female rats. Presented at *Int. Etholog. Conf. 11th, Rennes, France.*

Sachs, B. (1969b). *Amer. Zool.* **9**, 1068.

Sawin, P. B., and Crary, O. D. (1953). *Behaviour* **6**, 128.

Sawin, P. B., and Curran, R. H. (1952). *J. Exp. Zool.* **120**, 165.

Sawin, P. B., Denenberg, V. H., Ross, S., Hafter, E., and Zarrow, M. X. (1960). *Amer. J. Physiol.* **198**, 1099.

Slijper, E. J. (1960). *In* "Handbuch der Zoologie" (J.-G. Helmcke, H. v. Lengerken, and D. Starck, eds.). Vol. 8 (25). Walter de Gruyter, Berlin.

Stone, C. P. (1925). *Endocrinology* **9**, 505.

Stone, C. P., and King, F. A. (1954). *J. Comp. Physiol. Psychol.* **47**, 213.

Stone, C. P., and Mason, W. A. (1955). *J. Comp. Physiol. Psychol.* **48**, 456.

Sturman-Hulbe, M., and Stone, C. P. (1929). *J. Comp. Psychol.* **9**, 203.

Taylor, R. L. E. (1965). Ph.D. Thesis, Purdue Univ., Lafayette, Indiana.

Terkel, J., and Rosenblatt, J. S. (1968). *J. Comp. Physiol. Psychol.* **65**, 479.

Tietz, E. G. (1933). *Science* **78**, 316.

Wiesner, B. P., and Sheard, N. M. (1933). "Maternal Behaviour in the Rat." Oliver & Boyd, Edinburgh.

Wilson, J. R. (1961). Maternal behavior in the rat: The effect of selected hormones. Reported at the *Western Psychol. Ass., Seattle, Washington, June 1961.*

Zarrow, M. X., Sawin, P. B., Ross, S., Denenberg, V. H., Crary, D., and Wilson, E. D. (1961). *J. Reprod. Fert.* **2**, 152.

Zarrow, M. X., Farooq, A., and Denenberg, V. H. (1962a). *Proc. Soc. Exp. Biol. Med.* **111**, 537.

Zarrow, M. X., Sawin, P. B., Ross, S., and Denenberg, V. H. (1962b). *In* "Roots of Behavior" (E. L. Bliss, ed.), pp. 187-197. Harper (Hoeber), New York.

Zarrow, M. X., Farooq, A., Denenberg, V. H., Sawin, P. B., and Ross, S. (1963). *J. Reprod. Fert.* **6**, 375.

Zarrow, M. X., Denenberg, V. H., and Kalberer, W. D. (1965). *J. Reprod. Fert.* **10**, 397.

Zarrow, M. X., Grota, J. J., and Denenberg, V. H. (1967). *Anat. Rec.* **157**, 13.

Zarrow, M. X., Brody, P. N., and Denenberg, V. H. (1968). *In* "Reproduction and Sexual Behavior" (M. Diamond, ed.). Indiana Univ. Press, Bloomington.

Zarrow, M. X., Gandelman, R., and Denenberg, V. H. (1971). *Hormones and Behavior* **2**, 343.

5

The Role of Pituitary-Adrenal System Hormones in Active Avoidance Conditioning

D. De Wied, A. M. L. van Delft, W. H. Gispen, J. A. W. M. Weijnen, and Tj. B. van Wimersma Greidanus

I. GENERAL INTRODUCTION

The present expansion of the number of publications on the relationship between changes in levels of pituitary and adrenal hormones and conditioned avoidance behavior might make it somewhat redundant to refer again to the classical studies of Selye in the introduction of a new paper on the subject. His description of the nonspecific and stereotyped character of the reaction of the pituitary-adrenal system to stress has received much attention. This response is the core of the integrated syndrome of closely interrelated adaptive reactions to nonspecific stress, termed the "general adaptation syndrome" (Selye, 1950). Not only traumatic stress, but also emotional stress can evoke the reaction of the pituitary-adrenal system.

Selye's concept contributed to the development of a "second generation" of experiments in which experimentally changed pituitary and adrenal hormone levels were used as independent variables in research on the effects of these substances on behavior. This latter line of research was also stimulated by the alterations observed in human behavior following adrenocorticotropic hormone (ACTH) and adrenocorticosteroid therapy or pituitary and adrenocortical dysfunction.

Among the first investigators of effects of pituitary-adrenal system hormones on animal behavior were Mirsky and his associates (Mirsky *et al.,* 1953). Monkeys served as subjects. They were first trained to press a bar; each bar-press produced the reinforcement (food) and a tone. Then the animals were subjected to "fear" conditioning in another apparatus. The same tone was repeatedly presented and was ended with an electric shock. During these fear-conditioning sessions the experimental animals received ACTH in gelatin. Reinstatement of the first situation led to rapid and efficient bar-pressing in the ACTH-treated monkeys but not in the control animals that displayed strong startle reactions in response to the tone. In a second experiment, ACTH administration to monkeys during extinction of an operant avoidance response led to a rapid decrease in avoidance performance. These experiments, and additional ones in different avoidance situations with monkeys and rats, led the authors to the tentative generalization that "adrenocortical hypersecretion may influence the organism in such a manner as to either decrease the effectiveness of an anxiety-producing situation or eliminate a poorly integrated defense against the anxiety provoked by the persistence of a traumatic memory." It should be noted that a "fear" theory is still prominent among the theories put forward to account for the behavioral effects of pituitary-adrenal system hormones.

No exhaustive survey of all experiments reported in the literature is intended in this chapter. As an introduction to our own studies we shall briefly discuss a few relevant experiments which were performed with the shuttlebox avoidance situation.

Murphy and Miller (1955) found that daily administration of ACTH in gelatin to rats during the acquisition phase did not modify acquisition of a conditioned avoidance response (CAR) but delayed extinction of the response. No significant differences in rate of extinction were found which might be attributed to ACTH administration during extinction. The latter results were at variance with some of the preliminary data reported in the above-mentioned study of Mirsky *et al.* that were obtained with monkeys in a different avoidance situation. No gross behavioral effects of the ACTH treatment were noticed. An interpretation of the behavioral effect in terms of "fear" and possible perceptual changes was tempting, but the authors stated that the available data did not justify such an interpretation.

Information about the role of pituitary-adrenal system hormones in avoidance behavior can also be obtained from studies with hypophysectomized and adrenalectomized animals, although many control studies are necessary as the removal of the pituitary or the adrenals affects more than ACTH and adrenocorticostcroid levels. Applezweig and Baudry (1955) and Applezweig and Moeller (1959) reported that hypophysectomy severely interfered with the acquisition of an avoidance response. The effect of ACTH administration on two (!) hypophysectomized rats during the acquisition of the shuttlebox response suggested a restoration of the ability of the animals to acquire the avoidance response (Applezweig and Baudry, 1955).

Applezweig and Moeller (1959) raised the possibility that ACTH might affect avoidance learning through some extraadrenal action. This suggestion was tested by Miller and Ogawa (1962). They used adrenalectomized rats and found that ACTH treatment during the acquisition period retarded extinction of the CAR; no effect of the treatment on acquisition itself could be seen. Unfortunately, no control group of intact animals was run in this experiment to evaluate the possible effect of the presumably high levels of endogenous ACTH in the placebo-treated adrenalectomized animals. The authors concluded that: "Since avoidance behaviour may be motivated by fear and reinforced by fear reduction, it is possible that ACTH has some direct effects on the subcortical structures involved in emotional behaviour."

These data implicated ACTH as a modifying agent in active avoidance behavior.

II. PITUITARY-ADRENAL SYSTEM HORMONES AND ACTIVE AVOIDANCE ACQUISITION

A. Pituitary-Adrenal Activity and Avoidance Acquisition

Subjecting animals to avoidance training can be expected to stimulate the pituitary-adrenal system. A rise in the activity of this system during avoidance training was indeed observed by Mason *et al.* (1957), De Wied (1965), Takeda *et al.* (1967), and other investigators. The relationship between individual differences in activity of the pituitary-adrenal system and differences in avoidance performance has been the subject of several studies. Wertheim *et al.* (1969) found a positive correlation between the reactivity of this hormonal system to ether stress and subsequent avoidance performance proficiency after extensive training of rats in a Sidman avoidance schedule. Mason *et al.* (1968) reported lowest 17-OH-corticosteroid excretion during conditioning sessions in monkeys to correlate with highest lever-pressing rate in a Sidman avoidance schedule. Corticoserone secretion rate in rats under Nembutal anesthesia was measured after a conditioning period of 15 days by Bohus *et al.* (1963). It was shown that avoidance performance was superior in animals showing the highest corticosterone secretion rate.

Van Delft (1970b) determined the activity of the pituitary-adrenal system in unanesthetized rats, bearing a cannula in the carotid artery, by measuring the plasma corticosterone level according to Glick *et al.* (1964). Blood samples were taken via the cannula before starting avoidance training. The animals were subjected to three 10-trial sessions, one session per day, in a pole-jumping situation. In contrast to what one might have predicted from the results of Wertheim *et al.* (1969), a negative correlation was found between the pretraining level of plasma corticosterone and the total number of CAR's made. The pretraining plasma corticosterone level was also negatively correlated with the total number of intertrial responses (ITR's) made during the three sessions of avoidance acquisition. Furthermore, the initial level of plasma corticosterone in cannulated animals was found to be positively correlated with the level of plasma corticosterone 10 minutes after an ether stress of 1 minute duration. From these experiments it was postulated that the learning ability of rats in the pole-jumping test as well as the corticosterone level following ether stress is associated with the pretraining level of pituitary-adrenocortical activity.

B. ACTH or Corticosteroid Administration and Avoidance Acquisition

The results of studies on the effects of ACTH or corticosteroid administration on avoidance acquisition are confusing. The daily injection of 5 mg ACTH (Murphy and Miller, 1955) or 0.5 and 1.5 IU of purified ACTH in a long-acting preparation (De Wied, 1969a) had no effect on avoidance learning in the shuttlebox. Beatty *et al.* (1970) showed in the same test situation a facilitatory effect of the administration of 12 IU of this hormone when a high shock level and 50-trial sessions were used.

Bohus and Lissák (1968) demonstrated that the injection of cortisone, 1 or 2 mg/100 gm body weight, 2 hours prior to each session did not affect the acquisition of a CAR in rats, although the intertrial activity was lowered after the steroid treatment. This reduction of ITR's was also found by Bohus and

Endröczi (1965) following injection of 2 IU ACTH/100 gm in rats 2 hours before the session, and by Bohus et al. (1968) after daily injection of 2 IU ACTH. A single injection of 2 IU ACTH/100 gm in rats increased the number of responses on the second day of avoidance acquisition, but not on the fifth day (Bohus and Endröczi, 1965).

In a Sidman avoidance procedure, administration of either ACTH (8, 10, or 12 IU) or dexamethasone (200 µg) improved avoidance performance of rats (Wertheim et al., 1967).

C. Adrenalectomy and Avoidance Acquisition

In many studies no effect of adrenalectomy on avoidance acquisition was reported (Applezweig and Moeller, 1959; Bohus and Endröczi, 1965, De Wied et al. 1968; van Delft, 1970a). However, Beatty et al. (1970) observed an ameliorating effect of adrenalectomy on shuttlebox avoidance behavior when high shock level was employed. The absence of corticosteroids in adrenalectomized animals results in an increased ACTH production and release from the pituitary under stress conditions (Hodges and Vernikos-Danellis, 1962). The increase in the ACTH level in blood under stress conditions could be blocked by the administration of 1 mg corticosterone to the animals 4 hours before stress (Hodges and Jones, 1964).

Therefore it was deemed of interest to study the effect of corticosteroids in adrenalectomized animals on the acquisition of a pole-jumping avoidance response. Dexamethasone (21-sodium phosphate) (20 µg) was injected subcutaneously into male rats of about 120 gm during different periods after adrenalectomy (Table I). The steroid was administered at the end of the day after the session. Daily injection of 2.5 µg aldosterone, and saline as drinking fluid, were used as substitution therapy. As can be seen from Table I, no effect of dexamethasone administration during any period, on the number of CAR's or ITR's could be observed.

TABLE I. The Effect of Dexamethasone Phosphate Treatment on the Rate of Acquisition of a Pole-Jumping Avoidance Response and on the Intertrial Responses during Acquisition[a]

Treatment from day 8 to 12 after adrenalectomy before conditioning	Treatment from day 14 to 16 after adrenalectomy during conditioning	Total no. CAR's	Total no. ITR's	N
Placebo	Placebo	13.8 ± 1.7^{b}	10.6 ± 2.5	12
	Dexamethasone	13.6 ± 1.6	9.2 ± 1.9	12
Dexamethasone (20 µg)	Placebo	12.7 ± 1.9	9.7 ± 3.5	12
	Dexamethasone	13.2 ± 1.8	11.6 ± 2.3	13

[a]Three acquisition sessions were given on days 14 to 16 after adrenalectomy.

[b]Mean ± standard error of the mean.

When corticosterone or dexamethasone were applied to adrenalectomized animals 4 hours before each session, an increase in the number of avoidance responses and changes in the number of ITR's could be observed as indicated in Table II and Fig. 1. This increase in the number of avoidance responses could not be found after injection of 20 μg dexamethasone in sham-operated animals, although some tendency to a difference seemed to exist. It is relevant to note that avoidance conditioning in the two experiments was started, respectively, 14 and 2 days after adrenalectomy.

D. Discussion

In our experiments the rate of acquisition of rats in the pole-jumping test was negatively correlated with the pretraining level of corticosterone in the cannulated animal. The variability in the pretraining corticosterone levels in cannulated rats may reflect different reactions to the cannulation. This might also hold for other types of stress.

Our results on the relationship between plasma corticosterone levels and avoidance acquisition seem to be at variance with the results of Bohus *et al.* (1963) and Wertheim *et al.* (1969). The discrepancy may be explained by assuming that the pretraining activity of the pituitary-adrenal system bears no relation to the activity of this system following prolonged avoidance training.

It is still difficult to represent an integrated picture of the role of the pituitary-adrenal system hormones in the acquisition of avoidance behavior. The

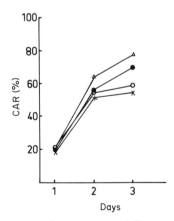

Fig.1. Percentage of conditioned avoidance responses (% CAR) in 3 days of pole-jumping avoidance acquisition of adrenalectomized animals. The acquisition started 2 days after adrenalectomy and the treatments were applied 4 hours before each session. (x) Placebo, $N = 20$; (o) 100 μg corticosterone, $N = 17$; (●) 1000 μg corticosterone, $N = 17$; (△) 20 μg dexamethasone phosphate, $N = 10$.

TABLE II. The Effect of Treatment with Corticosterone or Dexamethasone Phospate, Four Hours before Each Session, on the Acqusition of a Pole-Jumping Avoidance Response and on Intertrial Responses during Acquisition[a]

Treatment		Total number of CAR's	Total number of ITR's	N
Sham	Placebo	13.1 ± 2.0[b]	10.1 ± 2.0	9
	Dexamethason (20 µg)	15.7 ± 1.7	13.7 ± 4.5	9
Adrenalectomy	Placebo	12.4 ± 1.1[c]	8.8 ± 1.6	20
	Corticosterone (100 µg)	13.4 ± 1.4	5.8 ± 0.9	17
	Corticosterone (1000 µg)	14.5 ± 1.0	7.5 ± 1.5	17
	Dexamethasone (20 µg)	16.3 ± 1.5	13.0 ± 1.9	10

CAR's: $p < 0.10$, $p < 0.025$
ITR's: $p < 0.05$, $p < 0.05$

[a] Acquisition started 2 days after adrenalectomy or sham operation.
[b] Mean ± standard error of the mean.
[c] Wilcoxon two-sample test.

evidence for an effect of ACTH or corticosteroids on active avoidance performance is contradictory. In many studies neither adrenalectomy (Applezweig and Moeller, 1959; Bohus and Endröczi, 1965; De Wied *et al.*, 1968; van Delft, 1970a) nor the administration to adrenalectomized animals of ACTH (Miller and Ogawa, 1962; Beatty *et al.*, 1970) or of dexamethasone (this study), or the administration of cortisone to intact animals (Bohus and Lissák, 1968) resulted in a change in the number of CAR's during acquisition. However, other studies showed an effect of adrenalectomy or administration of ACTH or corticosteroids to intact or adrenalectomized animals on performance in different kinds of avoidance behavior (Bohus and Endröczi, 1965; Wertheim *et al.*, 1967; Beatty *et al.*, 1970; van Delft, 1970a). Differences in the schedule of administration of ACTH or corticosteroids in normal or adrenalectomized animals may have contributed to the discrepancies reported. In addition, the behavioral tasks used to evaluate the effects of these hormones are sufficiently different so that different behavioral mechanisms may be involved.

In summary it seems justified to say that normal functioning of the pituitary-adrenal system is not essential for proficient avoidance learning. However, it is evident that the activity of the pituitary-adrenal system is in some way associated with the behavior of animals in avoidance situations.

III. HYPOPHYSECTOMY
AND ACTIVE AVOIDANCE ACQUISITION

From the foregoing discussion (Section II,D) it is clear that normal functioning of the pituitary-adrenal system is not essential for the acquisition of a conditioned avoidance response. However, removal of the pituitary gland has been shown to retard the acquisition of a shuttlebox avoidance response as mentioned in Section I (Applezweig and Baudry, 1955; Applezweig and Moeller, 1959). In contrast, Bélanger (1958), using a somewhat different procedure, found avoidance acquisition of hypophysectomized rats nearly as good as that of control rats. An important difference between the schedule used by Bélanger and that employed by Applezweig and associates was the conditioned stimulus-unconditioned stimulus (CS-US) interval. Whereas Applezweig *et al.* used 2 seconds, Bélanger allowed 10 seconds between CS and US onset. Accordingly, the behavioral deficiency of the hypophysectomized rats might be explained by the fact that the response of the hypophysectomized rat to the CS is slower. The results obtained by Applezweig and associates were further investigated by us with rats in which only the anterior pituitary had been removed (De Wied, 1964). These rats were also inferior to sham-operated controls in acquiring a shuttlebox avoidance response.

A. ACTH and Avoidance Acquisition of Hypophysectomized Rats

An adrenal maintenance dose of ACTH (1.5 U/2 days) restored the rate of avoidance acquisition of adenohypophysectomized rats toward normal levels (De Wied, 1964). So the preliminary data of Applezweig and Baudry (1955) could be confirmed with anterior lobectomized animals. ACTH was administered subcutaneously as a long-acting zinc phosphate complex preparation as in most of our studies with ACTH or related peptides. When the hypophysectomized male rats were treated with a hormone replacement therapy consisting of cortisone, testosterone, and thyroxin, avoidance learning was significantly improved. Since this treatment resulted in an improvement of the general physical state of the adenohypophysectomized rat, it could be inferred that a general debilitation of the hypophysectomized organism might be responsible for the inability of adenohypophysectomized rats to acquire the avoidance response in the shuttlebox situation. However, subsequent experiments indicated that this hypothesis was not tenable. These experiments were performed with rats in which the whole pituitary was removed and which, like the adenohypophysectomized rat, show severe deficit in avoidance learning. It was found that synthetic ACTH β 1-24 in a dose of 20 μg, which maintains the size of the adrenal cortex of the hypophysectomized rat, restored the rate of avoidance acquisition in a way similar to that of the natural ACTH A_1 peptide used in previous experiments in adenohypophysectomized rats.

B. ACTH-Related Peptides
and Avoidance Acquisition of Hypophysectomized Rats

An amount of α-melanocyte stimulating hormone (MSH) equivalent to that of ACTH exerted a similar action on avoidance acquisition without affecting adrenal weight. Experiments with ACTH analogs subsequently showed that the decapeptide ACTH 1-10 and the heptapeptide ACTH 4-10 facilitated avoidance learning in hypophysectomized rats in a similar fashion as ACTH β 1-24 (De Wied, 1969a). These findings, obtained with peptides which do not stimulate the adrenal cortex (Lebovitz and Engel, 1964; Schwyzer, 1969), proved that this action of ACTH is based upon an extraadrenal effect.

Further studies were performed to determine whether these peptides acted on locomotor or sensory capacities, on endocrine or metabolic functions, or whether they improved the general health or condition of the hypophysectomized rat. Studies on motor capacities of hypophysectomized rats in a runway revealed that the speed of escaping the electrified grid floor was markedly decreased in these animals. Treatment with ACTH 4-10 somewhat improved the speed with which the animals escaped this unavoidable shock but could not account for the marked improvement in avoidance responding of hypophysectomized rats treated with the heptapeptide (De Wied, 1969b). The response of hypophysectomized rats to electric shock was studied and the electric shock threshold (EST) level was found to be significantly lower in the operated animals as compared to that of intact controls of the same weight. This responsiveness to lower shock intensities might indicate that sensory functioning is modified. The decapeptide ACTH 1-10 did not affect the threshold of hypophysectomized rats indicating that the stimulatory effect of this peptide and other analogs on avoidance acquisition cannot be due to an effect on sensory capacities of the hypophysectomized organism (Gispen et al., 1970a).

Is the effect of the ACTH analogs the result of an influence on endocrine or metabolic functions or on the general health and condition of the hypophysectomized rat? Chronic treatment of hypophysectomized rats with ACTH 4-10 did not affect loss of body weight of these animals nor did it influence adrenal or testes atrophy which occurs as a result of hypophysectomy. Thymus weight was not affected and plasma corticosterone was not detectable. Also, peptide treatment did not influence the decreased insulin levels present in hypophysectomized rats, and plasma glucose levels in hypophysectomized rats treated with the heptapeptide or placebo were similar to that of sham-operated controls. A slight decrease in plasma free fatty acids was the only metabolic effect found with ACTH 4-10 in hypophysectomized rats (De Wied, 1969b). Experiments with intact animals indicated that ACTH analogs do not act via stimulation of thyroid gland activity (De Wied and Pirie, 1968). From these studies it is clear that the behavioral effect of the ACTH analogs is not mediated by endocrine or metabolic activities.

C. A New, Recently Isolated Pituitary Peptide and Avoidance Acquisition of Hypophysectomized Rats

It was postulated that peptides closely resembling ACTH 4-10 normally operate in the formation of new behavior patterns. Such peptides with neurogenic activities may be synthetized by the pituitary gland and released upon adequate stimulation to affect central nervous structures involved in learning processes. In order to test this hypothesis, a study was undertaken with the aim of isolating relatively small peptides related to the aforementioned compounds from the pituitary (De Wied et al., 1970). The starting material was a fraction with high MSH activity from hog pituitaries obtained from Schally et al. (1962). The material was separated by ion exchange chromatography (Lande et al., 1965) and Sephadex G-25 (Upton et al., 1966). Fractions were tested for their ability to reinstate acquisition of shuttlebox avoidance in hypophysectomized rats. Several fractions appeared to be active. Purification of a fraction of a rather low molecular weight by paper chromatography in two systems (De Wied et al., 1970) yielded a pure peptide with marked behavioral activity.

Amino acid analysis of this fraction indicated that the peptide contained six to eight amino acids. Since neither histidine nor tryptophane or arginine could be detected, it followed that it was not related to ACTH 4-10. Further analysis of the peptide suggested that it is more related to vasopressin. The potency of the isolated peptide appeared to be at least 10 times higher than that of the heptapeptide ACTH 4-10 and it is of interest to mention that lysine vasopressin is markedly less active than the isolated peptide or ACTH 4-10 in stimulating the rate of acquisition of the avoidance response of hypophysectomized rats. Structure analysis of this polypeptide might be accomplished in the near future.

Whether this peptide is produced by the pituitary gland and is involved in conditioned avoidance behavior can be proven only by the demonstration of its presence in the pituitary and by determining a relationship between release of this factor from the anterior pituitary and the acquisition of avoidance behavior.

D. Biochemical Aspects of Hypophysectomy and Avoidance Acquisition*

In recent years a close association between ribonucleic acid (RNA) synthesis [review: Glassman (1969); Glassman and Wilson (1970)] and/or protein synthesis (Hydén and Lange, 1968; Bochoch, 1968) in the brain and learning processes of animals has been claimed. It is thought that during learning certain neuronal synapses are changed in order to consolidate the acquired information (Barondes, 1965). As a first step in this consolidation, biochemical changes in the nerve cells seem to be necessary (Glassman, 1969).

It has been demonstrated in rats that the metabolism of macromolecules is disturbed in peripheral organs, such as muscles and liver, following hypophysectomy (Korner, 1965, 1968; Tata and Williams-Ashman, 1967). The lack of growth hormone in hypophysectomized rats causes a marked decrease in RNA and protein synthesis in the liver. Presumably less RNA components (messenger RNA (mRNA) and ribosomes) are present in the cytoplasm of liver cells of these rats than required for a normal rate of protein synthesis (Forster and Sells, 1969). In fact, several authors have reported a lowered content of polysomes in the cytoplasm of the liver cell as a result of hypophysectomy (Korner, 1965; Staehelin, 1965; Brewer et al., 1969). Such a decreased content could account for the low rate of incorporation of radioactively labeled amino acids into protein as was reported by Korner (1964). Although the effect of hypophysectomy on macromolecular metabolism in the brain has not been intensively studied, some evidence for an altered metabolism in the brain has been reported. The incorporation of amino acids into proteins in cell-free systems from brain

*The experiments reported in this section have been performed in collaboration with P. Schotman and H. S. Jansz of the Laboratory of Physiological Chemistry, Medical Faculty, University of Utrecht. The authors highly esteem this cooperation.

tissue was decreased following hypophysectomy (Dunn and Korner, 1966), and both RNA and protein content seem to be reduced in the brain by removal of the pituitary (De Vellis and Inglish, 1968; Cheek and Graystone, 1969). It was of interest, then, to study whether the metabolism of macromolecules in brain is indeed under the influence of the pituitary and, if so, if the poor conditioning of hypophysectomized rats is in some way related to changes in macromolecule metabolism.

The brain stem was chosen as an object of study because evidence in the literature suggested a marked effect of hypophysectomy on morphology and metabolism of this region, especially in young rats (Diamond, 1968; Gregory and Diamond, 1968; Libertun et al., 1969). Moreover, Glassman and Wilson (1970) suggested a relationship between RNA synthesis in this area and the acquisition of conditioned avoidance behavior. In most of the studies on the effect of hypophysectomy on macromolecule metabolism, the effect on polysomes was investigated. At first our interest was focused upon polysomes in the brain stem.

1. Hypophysectomy and Polysomes in the Brain Stem of Rats

Male rats weighing approximately 120 gm were used. Three weeks following hypophysectomy, rats were decapitated and the brain stems of three rats were pooled together and homogenized. Polysomes were isolated and separated on linear sucrose gradients [see for experimental details Gispen et al. (1970b)]. In comparison to preparations of brain stem of intact rats (120 gm), hypophysectomized rats contained less polysomes in their brain stem (Fig. 2).

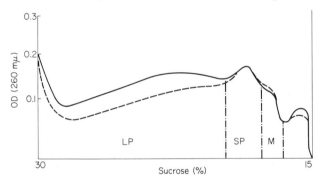

Fig. 2. Optical density pattern of polysomes isolated from brain stems of either intact (—) rats or hypophysectomized (– –) animals 3 weeks after operation. LP, large polysomes; SP, small polysomes; M, monomers.

In order to quantify the observed effect the mean optical density of the region of the large polysomes was divided by the mean optical density of the region of the monosomes. As a result of hypophysectomy this optical density ratio was significantly lowered (Gispen et al., 1970b). This decrease in polysomes is accompanied by a decreased incorporation of radioactive uridine into nuclear, cytoplasmic, and polysomal RNA (Gispen and Schotman, 1970; Gispen *et al.*, 1970b). It was therefore concluded that the effect of hypophysectomy on RNA metabolism in the brain stem is highly comparable to that found in the liver. These results suggest that RNA metabolism in the brain stem is under the influence of the pituitary.

2. Avoidance Acquisition of Hypophysectomized Rats and Polysomes in the Brain Stem

A possible relationship between the poor performance of hypophysectomized rats in conditioned avoidance training and biochemical changes in their brain stem was subsequently investigated. Recently, evidence has been presented which suggested an increase in the number of large polysomes in rat brain as a result of training (Dellweg *et al.*, 1968). Glassman also reported changes on the polysomal level in mouse brain during the acquisition of a CAR. With this in mind, studies were performed to see if there were differences on the polysomal level between hypophysectomized rats which mastered the task in shuttlebox conditioning as a result of peptide treatment and hypophysectomized rats which were treated with placebo suspension and did not reach the learning criterion.

In the first experiment the effect of ACTH 1-10 treatment per se on the polysome pattern in the brain stem of hypophysectomized rats was studied. Male rats weighing 150-160 gm were hypophysectomized and 1 week after the surgery the treatment began. ACTH 1-10 zinc phosphate (20 μg/0.5 ml sc every other day for 10 days) and placebo suspension were administered without the training procedure in the shuttlebox. The day after the last injection the animals were decapitated and the brains of three similarly treated animals were pooled together and homogenized. Polysomes were isolated and separated on linear sucrose gradients. The peptide treatment itself had no detectable influence on polysomes in the brain stems of hypophysectomized rats (Gispen and Schotman, 1970). There also was no detectable effect of ACTH 1-10 treatment on labeled uridine incorporation in nuclear and cytoplasmic RNA in the brain stem after 70 minutes of incorporation (Schotman and Gispen, 1970).

3. Avoidance Acquistion of Peptide-Treated Hypophysectomized Rats and Polysomes in the Brain Stem

In the next experiment, peptide treatment (ACTH 1-10, β-MSH) was given in combination with 10 days shuttlebox training (see for details, De Wied *et al.*, 1970, Gispen and Schotman, 1970). The peptide-treated hypophysectomized rats showed a superior performance over the placebo-treated rats. The day after the last training session the animals were decapitated and polysomes were isolated from their brain stems. As can be seen from Figs. 3 and 4, and Table III

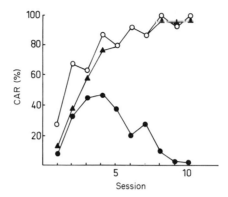

Fig. 3. Effect of treatment with ACTH 1-10 or β-MSH on the acquisition of a CAR of hypophysectomized rats in the shuttlebox. (●) Placebo; (○) ACTH 1-10; (▲) β-MSH.

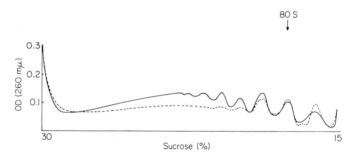

Fig. 4. Optical density pattern of polysomes isolated from brain stems of placebo-treated (−−) or ACTH 1-10-treated (−) hypophysectomized rats which have been conditioned in the shuttlebox.

TABLE III. The Effect of Conditioning in the Shuttle Box of Hypophysectomized Rats Treated with Zinc Phosphate Suspension, on the Polysome Pattern in the Brain Stem

	Small polysomes	Large polysomes	Total no. CAR's	N
	monomers	monomers	(100 trials)	(groups of 3)
Hypox	1.16 ± 0.04^a	1.08 ± 0.09		3
Hypox + placebo + shuttlebox	1.24 ± 0.07	1.13 ± 0.11	24 ± 2	3

[a]Mean ± standard error of the mean.

the brain stems of those rats which reached the learning criterion as a result of peptide treatment, contained more polysomes than the brain stem of placebo-treated rats which did not reach the criterion. The increase in isolated polysomes cannot be the result of peptide treatment. This possibility had already been investigated in the foregoing experiment, with negative results. The difference in the pattern might have been caused by the different amount of electric shock received by the peptide-treated rats and the placebo-treated groups, since the peptide-treated rats avoided the US much more than did the placebo-treated rats. Environmental stimulation (electric shock, light, sound, etc.) can affect the metabolism of macromolecules in the brain as was found by several authors [review: Glassman (1969)]. Moreover, the change in the pattern could reflect a decrease in polysome content in brain stems of placebo-treated rats instead of an increase in content in the peptide-treated rats. A control experiment, however, did not provide evidence in support of the alternative explanations. Table IV shows the optical density ratios of the polysome patterns isolated from brain stems of hypophysectomized rats treated with placebo and trained in the shuttlebox for 10 days.

The results clearly demonstrate that there is no influence of the conditioning procedure itself on the optical density pattern. Thus the change observed in the foregoing experiment could neither be caused by the peptide treatment nor by differences in stimulation during conditioning, but should be associated with the acquisition of a CAR in long-term shuttlebox conditioning is accompanied by an increase in polysomes in the brain stem of peptide-treated hypophysectomized rats. These results were so intriguing that it was decided to extend the experiment by treating hypophysectomized rats with a pituitary peptide of natural origin (see Section III,C). This peptide shows the same behavioral action as the ACTH analogs. Again there was a marked increase in large polysomes in

TABLE IV. Relation between Polysome Pattern in the Brain Stem and the Rate of Acquisition of a Shuttlebox Avoidance response in Hypophysectomized Rats Following Treatment with ACTH$^{1-10}$ or β—MSH

	Small polysomes	Large polysomes	Total no. CAR's	N
	monomers	monomers	(100 trials)	(groups of 3)
Hypox placebo	1.63	1.02	23 ± 2^a	2
	1.22	1.25		
Hypox ACTH$^{1-10}$	1.35	1.67	79 ± 3^b	1
Hypox β—MSH	1.32	1.50	73 ± 2^b	1

[a] Mean ± standard error of the mean.
[b] $P < 0.05$ (U test).

the brain stems of those rats which reached the acquisition criterion (Gispen and Schotman, 1970). At the same time livers of rats of both groups were isolated. Each liver was homogenized 1 : 2 in the homogenization buffer and 5 ml homogenate was used as a source of liver polysomes. The polysomes were isolated with the same procedure as was used for the brain stem polysomes, except that the postmitochondrial supernatant was incubated with sodium deoxycholate in a concentration of 1% (Gispen *et al.*, 1970b). The isolated polysome fraction appeared to contain many small monomers and a small number of large polyribosomal aggregates [see also Korner (1965); Staehelin (1965); Wurfbain-Moolenburgh (1968)]. The shuttlebox training in combination with peptide treatment had no effect on the polysome content of the liver. Accordingly, the change in polysome pattern in the brain stem that was found in peptide-treated hypophysectomized rats, which reached the learning criterion, seems to be specific for the brain.

4. *Discussion*

Acquiring a response is a process which of course will have molecular and electrophysiological consequences for the brain. Many experiments suggest changes in RNA and/or protein metabolism during learning. However, it is difficult to speculate on the meaning of the changes that we found. The increase in large polysomes could have been the result of an increase in the stability of the mRNA-ribosome connection. Zomzely *et al.* (1968) suggested that electrical activity of the nerve cell could parallel changes in stability of brain polysomes. These stability changes would be caused by the changes in ionic environment which accompany electric activity of the nerve cell. No real evidence, however, was presented to support this hypothesis. We assume that the increase in polysome content might be caused by an increase in mRNA and/or ribosomes in the cytoplasm, since other authors have shown that acquiring new behavior is accompanied by an increase in RNA synthesis (Hydén, 1967; Glassman and Wilson, 1970). The learning process itself might stimulate certain neurons or neuronal networks.

Physiological stimulation under various conditions affects brain macromolecule metabolism [see for review Glassman (1969)]. For example, light stimulation has been reported to cause a marked increase in polysomes in the brain of light-deprived rats (Appel *et al.*, 1967). Physiological stimulation has also been reported to increase RNA content. However, rats that were trained to acquire a particular behavioral response not only showed the increase in RNA synthesis, but also a modified population of RNA molecules in the brain as was concluded from base composition analysis (Hydén, 1967; Shashoua, 1968, 1970; Machlus and Gaito, 1969). Thus, participation of neurons in a learning process might be a special stimulation for these neurons. This stimulation could cause the observed changes in RNA and protein metabolism (Hydén, 1967; Bochoch, 1968; Glassman, 1969).

Presumably, biochemical changes are steps in the consolidation of information in the brain (Barondes, 1965; Glassman, 1969). The information need not be coded in a protein or peptide, as is supposed by several investigators; it is more likely that the protein or peptide will change the properties of the neuronal and synaptic membranes (Flexner and Flexner, 1969). Such a change in membranes could account for new functional synaptic connections or for modified synapses. Therefore, it may well be that the modified RNA metabolism, taking place during the acquisition of new behavioral patterns, is not specific to the particular information content being stored, but may be required for the consolidation process in general (Shashoua, 1970).

Hypophysectomy caused a marked alteration of RNA metabolism in the brain. This alteration is not specific for the brain but could be detected in the entire organism. Since it is likely that macromolecule metabolism is a step in consolidation of newly acquired information, this alteration might even interfere with the acquisition of new behavioral patterns. The poor performance of the hypophysectomized rat in long-term shuttlebox conditioning could be the result of a disturbed RNA metabolism in the neuronal circuits involved in acquiring the task. If hypophysectomy is performed after the animal has acquired the response, hypophysectomy does not interfere with the maintenance of the learned behavior. This was concluded from experiments by De Wied (1964) who found that after rats had acquired the task in a shuttlebox, removal of the adenohypophysis had only a minor effect on the extinction of the CAR. These adenohypophysectomized rats met the acquisition criterion in a reacquisition training period in the same way as sham-operated rats. Once the consolidation of the stimulus-response relationship has taken place, the adenohypophysis is no longer essential.

ACTH 1-10 treatment improved the performance of hypophysectomized rats markedly. As mentioned elsewhere in this chapter, the mechanism of action of this peptide is thought to be at the membrane or synapse level. In hypophysectomized rats the peptide might be a substitution for normally circulating relatively small pituitary peptides which could have a direct effect on central structures (De Wied et al., 1970). In such a way the peptide might restore the membrane properties of certain neurons to normal. There does not seem to be a direct effect of the peptide treatment on polysomes and RNA synthesis. These results are difficult to interpret. It might be that the lack of pituitary factors is responsible for the dramatic effect on performance by an action at the membrane level in the brain also. A lowered polysome content in the brain reflects a lack of circulating hormones regulating protein synthesis and may therefore interfere with the consolidation process. The improvement of the performance in hypophysectomized rats following administration of synthetic

ACTH analogs or pituitary peptides might be caused by their suggested normalizing effect on the membrane level. The resulting increased polysome content of the brain stem could then just be the reflection of stimulation in the brain by the acquisition process itself, via a permissive action of the peptides on the membrane.

IV. PITUITARY-ADRENAL SYSTEM HORMONES AND ACTIVE AVOIDANCE EXTINCTION

In the previous sections we have been concerned primarily with hormonal influences on the acquisition of a CAR both in the shuttlebox and in the pole-jumping situation. Somewhat ambiguous data were reported with respect to the role of this system in acquisition of an avoidance response. It should be noted that the earliest report of any influence of the hormones elaborated by the pituitary-adrenal system on behavior involved extinction of the avoidance response (Section I). The next part of this chapter will be devoted to the effects of peptides and steroids on extinction of avoidance behavior.

A. ACTH and Avoidance Extinction

In a first experiment the effect of purified ACTH on extinction of shuttlebox avoidance behavior was studied (De Wied, 1966). Also, in these experiments with male rats, long-acting zinc phosphate complex preparations of peptides were administered subcutaneously every other day. The first injection was given following the last acquisition session. Chronic administration of purified porcine ACTH led to inhibition of extinction. The effect was dose-dependent and lasted as long as the treatment was maintained. Whereas extinction of placebo-treated rats took place in about 10 days, the highest dose of ACTH almost completely prevented extinction of the avoidance response.

This result did not agree with the preliminary effect reported by Mirsky *et al.* (1953) and did not agree with the lack of an ACTH effect obtained by Murphy and Miller (1955). New experiments were required to elucidate the behavorial effect of ACTH.

B. Steroids and Avoidance Extinction

1. Chronic Treatment

The treatment with the highest dose of ACTH resulted in a marked rise in the activity of the adrenal cortex as indicated by high circulating levels of corticosterone. For this reason the influence of corticosterone in various dose levels on the rate of extinction of the shuttlebox avoidance response was studied (De Wied, 1967; De Wied *et al.,* 1968). Corticosterone was administered subcutaneously every day during the extinction period. Treatment with 0.2 and 1.0 mg corticosterone had an effect opposite to that of ACTH, in that it facilitated the rate of extinction of the avoidance response. The effect was dose-dependent.

Since these amounts of corticosterone inhibit the release of ACTH as a consequence of the negative feedback action of glucocorticosteroids, the facilitatory effect of corticosterone on extinction of the avoidance response might be explained by blockade of pituitary ACTH release. However, when corticosterone was given to hypophysectomized rats extinction was also facilitated, indicating that this steroid can exert an effect independently of pituitary ACTH (De Wied, 1967). Other steroids like dexamethasone 21-sodium phosphate and aldosterone were also tested in order to investigate the extent to which the effect on extinction of conditioned avoidance behavior was correlated with the glucocorticoid activity. The data obtained from these experiments suggested that glucocorticoid rather than mineralocorticoid activity was responsible for the facilitatory effect on extinction of the CAR (De Wied, 1967).

2. Acute Treatment

In a structure-activity relationship study (van Wimersma Greidanus, 1970a,b) dexamethasone, corticosterone, progesterone, 19 norprogesterone, pregnenolone, 4-pregnene-3-one, hydroxydione (Viadril), estradiol, testosterone, and cholesterol were tested for their effects on extinction of a pole-jumping avoidance response in acute experiments. This conditioning procedure was employed since it is less time consuming than the shuttlebox procedure. Ten conditioning trials are given each day for 4 days. On the fifth day extinction trials are run.

The crystalline steroids were dissolved in heated 96% ethanol, diluted afterward with 0.9% sodium chloride, and administered subcutaneously in two different dose levels immediately after this first extinction session. The effect of the steroid was studied 4 hours after injection in a second extinction session of 10 trials.

Corticosterone (subcutaneously administered in doses of 0.1 and 0.5 mg), dexamethasone (0.2 and 1.0 mg), progesterone (0.2 and 1.0 mg), 19 norprogesterone (0.2 and 1.0 mg), and pregnenolone (0.2 and 1.0 mg) facilitated extinction of the pole-jumping avoidance response in a dose-dependent way. All these steroids act in an equipotent manner, while 4-pregnene-3-one appeared to have only a weak effect. The latter caused significant facilitation of extinction following injection of the high dose (1.0 mg) only (Fig. 5). Cholesterol showed no effect on extinction of the pole-jumping avoidance response at all, neither did

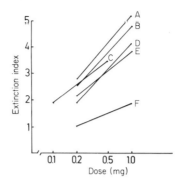

Fig. 5. Effects of several steroids on extinction of a pole-jumping avoidance response. The extinction index represents the difference between the number of CAR's following placebo treatment minus the number of CAR's following administration of either the high or the low dose of steroid. (A) Dexamethasone; (B) progesterone; (C) 19-norprogesterone; (D) pregnenolone; (E) corticosterone; (F) 4-pregnene-3-one.

hydroxydione which is used in higher doses as an anesthetic agent. Testosterone and estradiol were also inactive in facilitating extinction of the pole-jumping avoidance response. From these results it is clear that of the tested steroids only the pregnene (or pregnadiene)-type steroids facilitated extinction of conditioned avoidance behavior. The cholestene, androstene, estratriene, and pregnane types were ineffective. Common features of the active steroids are their double bond(s) in ring A or B and their keto group or hydroxy group at C-3 (see Fig. 6). The keto group at C-20 is important for the strength of the effect, but not essential. The action of the steroids on extinction of conditioned avoidance behavior is not directly correlated with their glucocorticoid activity. For example, progesterone and pregnenolone facilitate extinction of CAR in a similar way as corticosterone. It is interesting that the secretion of progesterone by the adrenal gland is controlled by ACTH, at least in ovariectomized rats (Resko, 1969) and that acute stress caused an increase in the concentration of pregnenolone and progesterone in the adrenal gland (Holzbauer and Newport, 1967).

Not all the steroids which have been shown to be effective in facilitating extinction of a CAR need to have a physiological role during avoidance behavior. In the male rats that we used, only corticosterone might be relevant in this respect.

The data obtained from the avoidance experiments with steroids brought also further evidence against the hypothesis that the corticosteroid effect on extinction of avoidance behavior solely depends on a blockade of pituitary-ACTH release. Bohus had found that implantation of cortisol in the median eminence region of the hypothalamus which inhibits ACTH release, facilitated

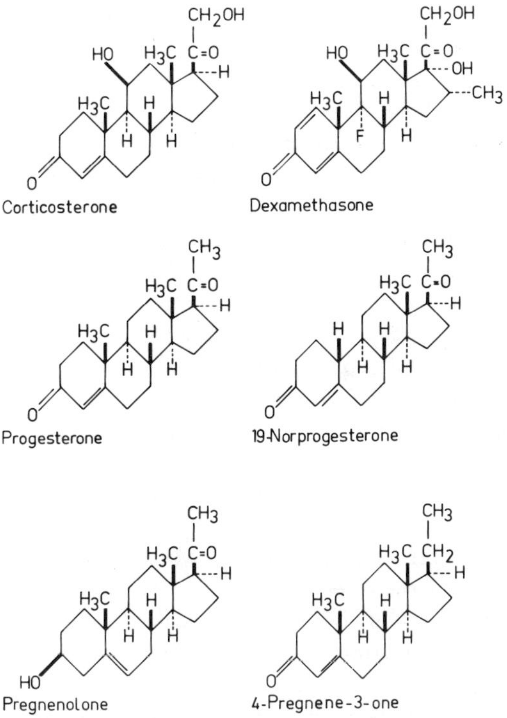

Fig. 6. Chemical structure of those steroids which facilitated extinction of the pole-jumping avoidance responses.

extinction of shuttlebox avoidance behavior. The more the release of ACTH was suppressed, the stronger the effect. However, cortisol implantation in the mesencephalic reticular formation which hardly reduced ACTH release, markedly facilitated extinction of the avoidance response. Accordingly, corticosteroids may have multiple effect on extinction of the avoidance response: through inhibition of ACTH release and through direct action on the central nervous system (CNS) (Bohus, 1968).

C. ACTH Analogs and Avoidance Extinction

Concerning ACTH, further proof of the fact that the influence of this peptide was independent of its effect on the adrenal cortex was obtained when it was shown that synthetic α-MSH as well as purified β-MSH affected extinction of the avoidance response in a fashion similar to ACTH (De Wied, 1966; De Wied and Bohus, 1966).

The two MSH preparations were administered as long-acting zinc phosphate complexes every other day in a dose of 6 μg. Both peptides significantly delayed extinction of the avoidance response. Another long-acting peptide preparation, protamine-zinc insulin, in an amount of 2 IU every other day, was inactive (De Wied, 1966).

The naturally occurring ACTH molecule consists of 39 amino acids, the first 24 of which are essential for steroidogenesis. The question arose whether the behavioral effects of ACTH were dependent on the same sequence (see Fig. 7). Since synthetic ACTH and fragments of this peptide had become available, a structure-activity study could be undertaken (De Wied, 1966).

The pole-jumping test was used again for this study. Rats which made 10 or more CAR's during the 3 days of acquisition, were used for extinction trials and run for another 3 days. All peptides were administered subcutaneously, again as long-acting preparations. The treatment was started on the third day of acquisition immediately after conditioning was completed. Substances were given only once.

Synthetic ACTH β 1-24, like the porcine preparation, delayed the rate of extinction of the pole-jumping avoidance response in a dose of 10 μg. The N terminal part of ACTH, ACTH 1-10, likewise inhibited extinction of the avoidance response, but the C-terminal part, 11-24, was inactive in this respect. Therefore, the active part of the ACTH molecule affecting avoidance behavior had to be located in the N-terminal part of the ACTH molecule.

Further studies with ACTH analogs in which the peptide chain was progressively shortened at the amino end revealed that the amino acids 1-3 were not necessary for the effect (De Wied et al.,1968). Whereas ACTH 4-10 possessed full behavioral activity, the effect of the 5-10 analog was considerably reduced (De Wied, 1966). This result compared well with those of Ferrari and associates (Ferrari et al., 1963). They reported that intracisternally injected ACTH produced a unique behavioral syndrome in several animal species. The animals first became apathetic and showed diffuse muscular tremors, they were also drowsy and yawned frequently. Then they start to stretch "in the way they usually do when they awake from physiological sleep." According to the authors, "stretching and yawning are two physiological acts that might be considered as an effort of the body to delay the onset of sleep and a mechanism to reinforce wakefulness after sleep." It is of interest that not only ACTH could elicit this "stretching syndrome," but MSH and the sequence 4-10 of the ACTH molecule as well (Ferrari et al., 1963). In a later study the induction of sexual excitement was reported also (Bertolini et al., 1969).

D. ACTH Analogs with a D-isomer Amino Acid and Avoidance Extinction

During the foregoing studies it was found that the amino acid sequence ACTH 1-10, in which the phenylalanine in the 7th position had been replaced by β-MSH (human):

```
1     2     3     4     5     6     7     8     9     10    11    12    13    14    15    16    17    18    19    20    21    22
Ala - Glu - Lys - Asp - Glu - Gly - Pro - Tyr - Arg - Met - Glu - His - Phe - Arg - Try - Gly - Ser - Pro - Pro - Lys - Asp
```

β-MSH (pig):

```
1     2     3     4     5     6     7     8     9     10    11    12    13    14    15    16    17    18
H - Asp - Glu - Gly - Pro - Tyr - Lys - Met - Glu - His - Phe - Arg - Try - Gly - Ser - Pro - Pro - Lys - Asp - OH
```

β-MSH (beef):

```
1     2     3     4     5     6     7     8     9     10    11    12    13    14    15    16    17    18
H - Asp - Ser - Gly - Pro - Tyr - Lys - Met - Glu - His - Phe - Arg - Try - Gly - Ser - Pro - Pro - Lys - Asp - OH
```

α-MSH:

```
           1     2     3     4     5     6     7     8     9     10    11    12    13
CH₃CO - Ser - Tyr - Ser - Met - Glu - His - Phe - Arg - Try - Gly - Lys - Pro - Val - NH₂
```

ACTH 1-10:

```
      1     2     3     4     5     6     7     8     9     10
H - Ser - Tyr - Ser - Met - Glu - His - Phe - Arg - Try - Gly - OH
```

ACTH 1-24:

```
      1     2     3     4     5     6     7     8     9     10    11    12    13    14    15    16    17    18    19    20    21    22    23    24
Ser - Tyr - Ser - Met - Glu - His - Phe - Arg - Try - Gly - Lys - Pro - Val - Gly - Lys - Lys - Arg - Arg - Pro - Val - Lys - Val - Tyr - Pro
```

Fig. 7. Amino acid sequence of some ACTH-like peptides.

the *d*-isomer exhibited an opposite effect on extinction of the shuttlebox avoidance response, in that it facilitated extinction (Bohus and De Wied, 1966). In another experiment the peptide was administered subcutaneously in a dose of 10 μg every other day during the extinction period. The *D*-peptide facilitated extinction of the avoidance response as long as it was injected. Extinction took place rapidly and was demonstrable as early as 1 day after injection of the peptide. After the treatment was stopped, the behavior of the peptide-treated animals gradually returned to that of placebo-treated controls within 4-5 days (De Wied, 1969a).

Since the effect of the *D*-form peptide might have been the result of an antagonistic action against naturally occurring peptides such as ACTH or MSH, this peptide should be inactive in animals deprived of these hormones. Rats were therefore trained to criterion in the shuttlebox and subsequently hypophysectomized or sham-operated (Bohus and De Wied, 1966). Hypophysectomized rats were treated with a substitution therapy consisting of cortisone, testosterone, and thyroxin. Two weeks after surgery they were retrained to criterion and subjected to extinction trials for 6 days. The *D*-form peptide appeared to have an even greater effect on facilitation of extinction in hypophysectomized than in intact animals.

Accordingly, the effect of the *D*-form peptide could not be explained by a direct antagonistic action against structurally related *L*-form peptides of natural origin.

E. ACTH Analogs and Escape Behavior

To assess whether alterations in motor and/or sensory function could explain the marked behavioral difference between the two closely related peptides, escape behavior was studied, in a runway equipped with a grid floor, under chronic treatment with the two peptides or placebo. The speed with which a rat traversed the electrified grid floor of the runway served as the index of escape behavior. Five trials a day were given for 14 days. After a few days animals had learned to escape the shock and they maintained a high escape speed during the whole experiment.

No difference in escape latency between rats treated with either peptide or placebo was found. This suggested that the behavioral effect of the two peptides was not due to influences on motor and/or sensory capacities or to changes in escape motivation (Bohus and De Wied, 1966).

F. ACTH Analogs and Open Field Behavior

To obtain information about the effect of the two peptides on untrained behavior, the influence of these compounds on the behavior of rats in an open field was studied 18 hours after a single injection of 10 μg of either of the two peptides or a placebo. Behavior in this test was observed during a 3-minute period. Ambulation, rearing, and grooming frequencies, as well as the number of fecal boluses produced, were scored.

None of these measures was significantly affected by treatment with the peptides as compared with placebo injection (Bohus and De Wied, 1966). In subsequent studies observations were made during repeated sessions but, again, no effect of peptide administration (every 48 hours) on the general activity level of the animals was observed (Weijnen, 1968; Weijnen and Slangen, 1970).

G. Structure-Activity Relationship Studies with D-Form ACTH Analogs

Since these studies were performed, a number of structural analogs of the D-form peptide have become available. It was found that ACTH 4-10 (7-D-phe) had the same effect as ACTH 1-10 (7-D-phe). The heptapeptide markedly facilitated extinction of the shuttlebox avoidance response. The effect disappeared when the amino acid sequence was shortened. ACTH 7-10 (7-D-phe) failed to facilitate extinction of the avoidance response. In fact it significantly delayed extinction of the avoidance response. No explanation of this can be given at present. It is of interest to note that the decapeptide in which the amino acid tyrosine in the second position had been replaced by the D-isomer also exhibited facilitatory effects on extinction of the avoidance response. The effect, however, was not as strong as with ACTH 1-10 (7-D-phe). The phenylalanine in the 7th position therefore seems to be more important than the tyrosine in the second position for facilitation of extinction (De Wied, 1969a).

H. Acute Administration of ACTH Analogs and Avoidance Extinction

In more acute experiments the effects of ACTH 1-10 and of ACTH 1-10 (7-D-phe) on extinction of conditioned avoidance behavior has been observed. Long-acting preparations are not used in these studies; the peptides are just dissolved in saline. In the pole-jumping test the facilitatory activity of ACTH 1-10 (7-D-phe) on extinction was investigated in the same way as described earlier for the structure-activity relationship study on the effect of steroids on extinction of the avoidance response. Rats were trained in the pole-jumping box for 4 days and on the fifth day extinction trials were run. Animals which made eight or more CAR's on the first extinction session, were subcutaneously injected with 100 μg of the peptide and the effect was studied 4 hours later in a second extinction session. As seen from Fig. 8, ACTH 1-10 (7-D-phe) markedly facilitated extinction of the avoidance response within 4 hours following administration.

In order to investigate more acute effects of ACTH 1-10 on extinction, rats

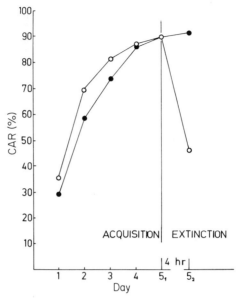

Fig. 8. Effect of 100 μg ACTH 1-10 (7-D-phe) (○) on extinction of a pole-jumping avoidance response. (●) Placebo.

were trained in the pole-jumping box for 3 days. On the fourth day extinction trials were run. All animals which reached the 80% criterion were injected subcutaneously with 100 μg of the peptide and the effect was studied in a second and a third extinction session at 2 and 4 hours after injection of the decapeptide. As seen from Fig. 9, ACTH 1-10 significantly delayed extinction of the avoidance response. This effect was more marked at 4 hours than at 2 hours after injection (van Wimersma Greidanus and De Wied, 1970, 1971).

It is of interest to note that much more of the peptides is needed in this 4-hour period of observation than of the long-acting preparations in a 48-hour period.

I. ACTH Analogs and Avoidance Extinction. Site of Action

Several attempts were made to localize the site of action of the ACTH-like peptides in the CNS. As an initial experiment it was decided to make use of rats bearing lesions in the thalamic area. This area was chosen because a number of observations (Vanderwolf, 1964; Thompson, 1963; Rich and Thompson, 1965; Cardo, 1965; Delacour et al., 1966) suggested that thalamic structures are involved in acquisition and retention of conditioned avoidance behavior. Lesions were made bilaterally with the aid of a stereotaxic apparatus with high frequency cauterization.

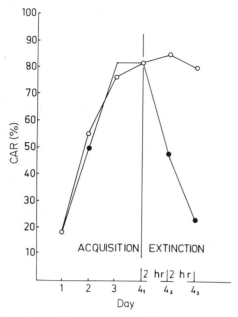

Fig. 9. Effect of 100 μg ACTH 1-10 (○) on extinction of a pole-jumping avoidance response. (●) Placebo.

Animals were trained for 14 days in the shuttlebox to induce a relatively high resistance to extinction. Large lesions in the midline thalamic reticular area produced severe deficits in avoidance learning and in escape behavior. Smaller lesions in this area interfered with avoidance acquisition but not with escape behavior (Bohus and De Wied, 1967a).

Bilateral destruction of the nuclei parafasciculares did not affect avoidance learning, but extinction of the avoidance response in the shuttlebox was markedly facilitated. These animals were used to study the effect of an ACTH analog. α-MSH was chosen and was administered in a dose of 10 μg as a long-acting preparation every other day during the extinction period. Extinction of lesioned rats was rapid as compared to that of sham-operated rats. Treatment with α-MSH failed to affect the rate of extinction of avoidance response of rats bearing lesions in the nucleus parafascicularis (Bohus and De Wied, 1967b).

Further attempts to localize the action of ACTH analogs in the CNS were done by implantation of these peptides in various subcortical structures (van Wimersma Greidanus, 1970b). For these experiments the same test situation was used as described before in the studies concerning the acute effects of the peptides on extinction of conditioned avoidance behavior (Section IV,H).

To implant the peptide into various parts of the brain of freely moving conscious rats, a stainless steel plate equipped with 12 holes was used. Tubes of

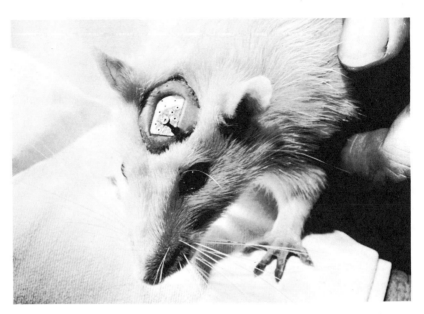

Fig. 10. Conscious rat with plate fixed on the skull and needle inserted into the brain.

the same material protruding 2.5 mm from the lower side of the plate were attached to the holes in the plate. The plate was placed on the rat skull under ether anesthesia and fixed with dental cement. Through the tubes needles of different lengths containing peptide material at the tip could be directed into the brain (Hulst and De Wied, 1967; van Wimersma Greidanus and De Wied, 1969). Figure 10 shows the plate *in situ*. Animals were allowed to recover from the operation until they had regained their preoperative weight.

Before the operation animals had been trained in the pole-jumping box for 4 days. After operation animals were reconditioned and subsequently run for extinction trials. When at least 8 out of 10 CAR's were scored, the actual experiment began. Either a needle containing peptide material or an empty control needle was implanted into the brain through one of the 12 holes. Extinction trials were run 4 hours after application of the ACTH 1-10 (7-D-phe) or one, 2, 3, and 4 hours after ACTH 1-10 implantation.

It appeared that ACTH 1-10 exerted an inhibiting effect on extinction of the avoidance response when this peptide was implanted in the nucleus parafascicularis and adjacent areas, e.g., the nucleus posteromedianus thalami and the nucleus lateralis habenulae. Implantation of ACTH 1-10 in the cerebrospinal fluid also resulted in inhibition of extinction of the pole-jumping avoidance response. Implantations of this peptide in other brain structures did not modify avoidance extinction (nucleus ventralis thalami, nucleus anterior medialis thalami, nucleus reticularis thalami, nucleus posterior thalami, nucleus reuniens, the fasciculus retroflexus, and forebrain structures such as globus pallidus and putamen) (van Wimersma Greidanus and De Wied, 1970, 1971).

Implantations of the D-form peptide revealed that application of ACTH 1-10 (7-D-phe) to the nucleus parafascicularis and adjacent ventrocaudal and caudal structures in the central gray, the corticotectal tract, the posterior thalamic nuclei, and the rostral reticular formation facilitates the rate of extinction of the avoidance response. No effects on avoidance extinction were noticed following implantation with this D-form peptide in the medial and ventral part of the thalamus, the nucleus accumbens, the nucleus interstitialis striae terminalis, the fornix, and the hippocampus (van Wimersma Greidanus and De Wied, 1971). It is worth noting that earlier experiments (van Wimersma Greidanus and De Wied, 1969; van Wimersma Greidanus, 1970b), in which the site of action of dexamethasone 21-sodium phosphate, corticosterone, and progesterone on extinction of conditioned avoidance behavior was investigated, also pointed at the same sites of the brain. So this region, where mesencephalon and diencephalon shade off into each other at the posterior thalamic level, seems to be important for the inhibitory and facilitatory effects of locally applied peptides and steroids on extinction of the CAR.

J. Discussion

The locus of action of the peptides as well as of the corticosteroids on extinction of avoidance responses appeared to be in the rostral mesencephalic/caudal diencephalic area at the thalamic level, in particular in the posterior thalamus and more specifically in the nuclei parafasciculares (Fig. 11). That this area, which belongs to the thalamic reticular system, is involved in extinction phenomena, was shown by the implantation studies (see Section IV,I).

This was supported by the results of experiments with animals bearing lesions in this part of the brain. Medial thalamic damage tended to destroy a preoperatively established CAR (Vanderwolf, 1964), while lesions destroying portions of the diffuse thalamic nuclei profoundly disturbed the CAR (Thompson, 1963; Rich and Thompson, 1965; Bohus and De Wied, 1967a). Cardo showed that the nonspecific thalamic nuclei like the nucleus parafascicularis and centrum medianum could play an important role in the maintenance of conditioned avoidance behavior. Lesions which destroyed these nuclei, did interfere with CAR, while electrical stimulation of this area led to better performance. The parafascicular/centrum medianum complex is thought to have an important integrative function (Cardo, 1965, 1967). Delacour (1970) suggested that the role of the parafascicular/centrum medianum complex could involve an interaction between defensive motivation and some mechanism of

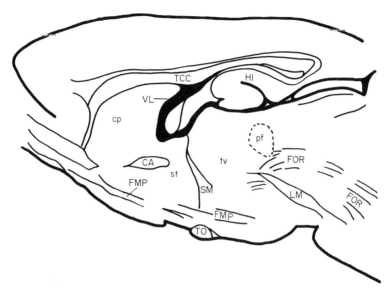

Fig. 11. A diagram of a sagittal section (L 1160 μ) of the rat brain after König and Klippel (1963). CA, commissura anterior; cp, nucleus caudatus putamen; FMP, fasciculus medialis prosencephali; FOR, formatio reticularis; HI, hippocampus; LM, lemniscus medialis; pf, nucleus parafascicularis; SM, stria medullaris thalami; st, nucleus interstitialis striae terminalis; TCC, truncus corporis callosi; TO, tractus opticus; tv, nucleus ventralis thalami; VL, Ventriculus lateralis.

avoidance responding in certain avoidance paradigms. However, some complex food-reinforced tasks could also be affected by similar lesions. The parafascicular/centrum medianum complex receives the main part of the fibers from the reticulothalamic and tegmentothalamic tract. These afferent fibers split at the thalamic level into several routes, each conducting a stream of impulses. A subcortical commutation exists in this area where signals from ascending pathways are concentrated and finally converge before being redistributed in a divergent way (Gastaut, 1958; Papez, 1937, 1956).

On the other hand, there are connections between the brain stem and basal forebrain which play a role in the organization of behavioral reactions (Korányi and Endröczi, 1970). A mesodiencephalic activating circuit is suggested by them which included the mesencephalic reticular formation, the thalamic midline nuclei, striopallidal connections, the basal septum area including Broca's diagonal band, the medial forebrain bundle, and the brain stem reticular core (Endröczi and Korányi, 1969).

This ascending activatory system might influence the forebrain which is known to be involved in complex behavioral mechanisms and in the regulation of pituitary functions. On the other hand, the descending inhibitory pathways of basal forebrain origin terminate at brain stem and thalamic level. This system plays an important role in the control of sensory input. Stimulation of this system induces, among other things, extinction of conditioned responding. It also elicits inhibition of mono- and polysynaptic reflex activity in the ascending activating system. Both ascending and descending systems are interconnected at the subcortical as well as the cortical level.

The peptides and steroids act in a rather limited area. This may be due to the fact that the posterior thalamus is a structure where all incoming impulses converge. In this area, implantations and lesions are, however small, rather effective in disturbing the output of this system by interfering with impulse-transmission processes.

The way in which peptides and steroids affect neural processes is unknown. It is reported by Sawyer and associates (Sawyer et al., 1968; Beyer and Sawyer, 1969) that ACTH injection (2 U) produced an elevation in electrical background activity in the arcuate nucleus. This excitatory effect in the nucleus arcuatus could also be evoked in adrenalectomized rats, indicating that there is a direct action of ACTH on the arcuate cells. A drop in the background activity was observed in the basolateral thalamus, the zona incerta, and the nucleus interpeduncularis. No effect was found in the medial forebrain bundle. The influence of β-MSH on evoked potentials in the spinal cords of cats (Krivoy and Guillemin, 1961) and of ACTH on inhibitory neurons in the spinal cord of rabbits (Korányi and Endröczi, 1967) and on transmission in sympathetic ganglia of the cat (Koltai and Minker, 1966) suggest that these peptides affect neural neural processes through a direct action on transmission in neural elements, or by influencing the biochemical or vascular environments on these elements.

Effects of steroids on the electrical activity of the brain have been described by many authors. Testosterone and hydrocortisone affect the cortical arousal reaction following stimulation of the mesencephalic reticular formation in rats (Soulairac et al., 1963). Progesterone, pregnenolone, and the metabolites 5β-pregnane-3,20-dione and 3α-hydroxy-5β-pregnane-20-one inhibit the cortical arousal reaction following stimulation of the mesencephalic reticular formation in rats (Gyermek et al., 1967). Spontaneous electrical activity of neuronal units in the hypothalamus and their responsiveness to photic, acoustic and sciatic stimuli were changed following hydrocortisone administration in rats and cats (Feldman et al., 1961; Slusher et al., 1966; Feldman and Dafny, 1970; Steiner, 1970). Progesterone induces a decrease in the electrical background activity of the diencephalon of female rats (Beyer et al., 1967). Cortical arousal reactions following sensory stimuli are blocked following progesterone administration (Komisaruk et al., 1967). Barraclough and Cross (1963) and Cross and Silver (1965) demonstrated that high plasma levels of progesterone, either of exogenic or endogenic origin, blocked the electrical response of neurons in the lateral hypothalamus following stimulation of the cervix uteri. High doses also blocked the response to other sensory stimuli. The alterations in threshold levels of neurons for sensory stimuli and changes in impulse transmission might therefore be involved in the acute behavioral effects observed following peptide or steroid administration.

V. PITUITARY-ADRENAL SYSTEM HORMONES
AND ANALOGS: SOME NOTES
ON THEIR BEHAVIORAL EFFECTS

The survey of a substantial part of the research performed by the authors of this chapter warrants an attempt to a general evaluation of the behavioral results. The choice of the discussed material has been selective. Attention was concentrated on available data concerning active avoidance behavior, leaving aside, for instance, the accumulating data on passive avoidance or conditioned emotional behavior.

The use of the shuttlebox and pole-jumping situation as a tool in the study of the effects of pituitary-adrenal hormones and their analogs on behavior has been very fruitful from a pharmacological and a physiological point of view. However, the implications for behavior are still obscure. This does not mean that hardly any behavioral effects were observed, on the contrary, but we are still far from an unambiguous interpretation of these effects. A diversity of hypotheses have been discussed by different authors to account for the behavioral effects. Some keywords in these hypotheses are: *adaptation* (De Wied *et al.,* 1968), *anxiety or fear* (Mirsky *et al.,* 1953), *arousal* (Weiss *et al.,* 1970), *internal inhibition* (Levine, 1968), *memory* (De Wied and Bohus, 1966), and *reinstatement of motivational cues* (Levine and Brush, 1967). The number of effects observed reflects our basic ignorance of the many factors which determine the performance level of the subjects in the test situations employed. We should mention that not all of these hypotheses refer to the pituitary-adrenal axis as a system that plays a role in the control of avoidance behavior. Some of them are more concerned with the action of the separate hormones and their analogs on a particular kind of behavior. Nevertheless, it is evident that there is a great need for detailed parametric studies of animal behavior in the different behavioral paradigms.

The lack of a better understanding of the many factors influencing active avoidance performance has another facet. We are sometimes tempted to forget that a similar observed change in performance following different treatments does not necessarily mean the same psychophysiological system(s) is (are) affected. We should also keep in mind that the same treatment might influence the organism in more than one way. Differentiation in theorizing is apparent for instance in the discussion of the effects of corticosteroids on extinction of shuttlebox avoidance behavior: an effect mediated by inhibition of ACTH release and a direct action on the CNS. The similar performance modification could, determined behaviorally, be quite different.

The results of attempts to manipulate behavior by changing ACTH and corticosteroid levels during active avoidance acquisition are still puzzling. Different studies on the prediction of future avoidance performance based on pretraining plasma corticosterone values also yielded inconsistent results. The interpretation of treatment effects on avoidance acquisition is complicated by possible interaction with the motivation used (foot shock). The intensity of the shock is one of the factors involved in determining avoidance performance during acquisition. In two-way avoidance situations, such as the shuttlebox, the range of optimum levels of shock with respect to speed of acquisition is quite narrow. A possible effect of the hormone treatment on the sensory input resulting from suprathreshold values of electric shock is very difficult to evaluate. This very point makes extinction studies attractive as shock is no longer applied. Treatment with ACTH during conditioning of an active avoidance response, as in the experiment of Murphy and Miller (1955), did not result in a detectable change in performance during acquisition, but led to a marked inhibition of extinction even though the treatment was discontinued. This result should warn us of the danger involved in dichotomizing the evaluations of behavioral data obtained in acquisition and extinction. Effects on extinction have to be attributed to some ACTH-induced change during acquisition, although this is not observed directly. Administration of hormones of pituitary and adrenals during extinction of active avoidance behavior has produced internally consistent results. In addition it was found that similar effects can be produced by some other peptides and steroids.

In trying to interpret the behavioral effects of pituitary and adrenal hormones and related substances, we cannot limit ourselves to results obtained with two active avoidance situations. Integrating these with the results of studies on passive avoidance and conditioned emotional behavior is necessary. In addition, results from experiments that do not involve the application of electric shock would be extremely important. However, at this time an attempt to integrate all the reported data on this subject would be premature.

Considering the results, the shuttlebox and the less time-consuming pole-jumping situation have been worthly tools in the investigation of hormonal effects on behavior. A disadvantage of the latter test in particular is the crucial role of the experimenter in the conditioning process (e.g., rats do not always leave the pole spontaneously). His acquired skill is difficult to convey in the method section of a publication. Attempts have been made to replicate data obtained in the pole-jumping situation in an apparatus equipped with a retractable jump-on ledge instead of a pole. This experiment was run automatically. No effect of peptide treatment on extinction of the active avoidance response has yet been observed (Weijnen and Slangen, 1970).

The pituitary-adrenal system has been shown to play an essential adaptive role in maintaining organismic integrity in situations where the organism is exposed to traumatic stimuli such as tissue injury, disease, infection, etc. However, it is important to note that myriad stimuli can evoke a response from the pituitary-adrenal system. This response to stimuli such as novelty, noise, fear, restraint, etc. cannot initially be differentiated from the response to tissue injury. In the past it has been difficult to assign a functional role to the pituitary-adrenal system under conditions as nonspecific as those listed above. The results discussed in this paper suggest strongly that in addition to the metabolic effects of ACTH and corticosteroids there are clearly behavioral effects of these compounds—and of related peptides and steroids—which are separable from the metabolic activity and which indicate independent activity of these hormones on the CNS. But we should conclude that there is still not sufficient unequivocal evidence either to assign to the pituitary-adrenal *system* a clear role in active avoidance conditioning under physiological conditions, or to enable us to interpret the behavioral effects in a unified way. However, research on hormonal effects on behavior is "booming" and a better insight might be gained in the near future.

It is evident that this kind of behavioral research provides valuable feedback to physiological and pharmacological thinking. Therefore we would like to come back to Selye. The motto of his book *Stress* reads:

> Our facts must be correct.
> Our theories need not be if they
> help us to discover important
> new facts.

References

Appel, S. H., Davis, W. and Scott, S. (1967). *Science* **157**, 836.

Applezweig, M. H., and Baudry, F. D. (1955). *Psychol. Rep.* **1**, 417.

Applezweig, M. H., and Moeller, G. (1959). *Acta Psychol.* **15**, 602.

Barondes, S. H. (1965). *Nature (London)* **205**, 18.

Barraclough, C. A., and Cross, B. A. (1963). *J. Endocrinol.* **26**, 339.

Beatty, P. A., Beatty, W. W., Bowman, R. E., and Gilchrist, J. C. (1970). *Physiol. Behav.* **5**, 939.

Bélanger, D. (1958). *Can. J. Psychol.* **12**, 171.

Bertolini, A., Vergoni, W., Gessa, G. L., and Ferrari, W. (1969). *Nature (London)* **221**, 667.

Beyer, C., and Sawyer, C. H. (1969). *In* "Frontiers in Neuroendocrinology" (W. F. Ganong and L. Martini, eds.), pp. 225-287. Oxford Univ. Press, London and New York.

Beyer, C., Ramirez, V. D., Whitmoyer, D. I., and Sawyer, C. H. (1967). *Exp. Neurol.* **18**, 313.

Bochoch, S. (1968). "The Biochemistry of Memory." Oxford Univ. Press, London and New York.

Bohus, B. (1968). *Neuroendocrinology* **3**, 355.

Bohus, B., and Endröczi, E. (1965). *Acta Physiol.* **26**, 183.

Bohus, B., and Lissák, K. (1968). *Int. J. Neuropharmacol.* **7**, 301.

Bohus, B., and De Wied, D. (1966). *Science* **153**, 318.

Bohus, B., and De Wied, D. (1967a). *J. Comp. Physiol. Psychol.* **64**, 26.

Bohus, B., and De Wied, D. (1967b). *Physiol. Behav.* **2**, 221.

Bohus, B., Endröczi, E., and Lissák, K. (1963). *Acta Physiol. Acad. Sci. Hung.* **24**, 79.

Bohus, B., Endröczi, E., and Lissák, K. (1963). *Acta Physiol.* **24**, 79.

Bohus, B., Nyakas, Cs., and Endröczi, E. (1968). *Int. J. Neuropharmacol.* **7**, 307.

Brewer, E. N., Foster, L. B., and Sells, B. H. (1969). *J. Biol. Chem.* **224**, 1389.

Cardo, D. (1965). *Psychol. Fr.* **10**, 334.

Cardo, B. (1967). *Physiol. Behav.* **2**, 245.

Cheek, D. B., and Graystone, J. E. (1969). *Pediat. Res.* **3**, 77.

Cross, B. A., and Silver, I. A. (1965). *J. Endocrinol.* **31**, 251.

Delacour, J. (1970). *Prog. Brain Res.* **32**, 158-170.

Delacour, J., Albe-Fessard, D., and Libouban, S. (1966). *Neuropsychol.* **4**, 101.

Dellweg, H., Gerner, R., and Wacker, A. (1968). *J. Neurochem.* **15**, 1109.

De Vellis, J., and Inglish, D. (1968). *J. Neurochem.* **15**, 1061.

De Wied, D. (1964). Unpublished data.

De Wied, D. (1964). *Amer. J. Physiol.* **207**, 255.

De Wied, D. (1965). *Int. J. Neuropharmacol.* **4**, 157.

De Wied, D. (1966). *Proc. Soc. Exp. Biol. Med.* **122**, 28.

De Wied, D. (1967). *Proc. Int. Congr. Horm. Steroids, 2nd, 1966*, pp. 945-951. Excerpta Medica, Amsterdam.

De Wied, D. (1969a). *In* "Frontiers in Neuroendocrinology" (W. F. Ganong and L. Martini, eds.), pp. 97-140. Oxford Univ. Press, London and New York.

De Wied, D. (1969b). *Excerpta Medica Found. Int. Congr. Series* No. 184, 310.

De Wied, D. and Bohus, B. (1966). *Nature (London)* **212**, 1484.

De Wied, D. and Pirie, G. (1968). *Physiol. Behav.* **3**, 355.

De Wied, D., Bohus, B., and Greven, H. M. (1968). *In* "Endocrinology and Human Behavior" (R. P. Michael, ed.), pp. 188-199. Oxford Univ. Press, London and New York.

De Wied, D., Witter, A., and Lande, S. (1970). *Prog. Brain Res.* **32**, 213.

Diamond, M. C. (1968). *Brain Res.* **7**, 407.

Dunn, A. J., and Korner, A. (1966). *Biochem. J.* **100**, 76P.

Endröczi, E., and Korányi, L. (1969). *In* "Aggressive Behaviour" (S. Garattini and E. B. Sigg, eds.), pp. 132-140. Excerpta Medica, Amsterdam.

Feldman, S., and Dafny, N. (1970). *Prog. Brain Res.* **32**, 90-100.

Feldman, S., Todt, J. C., and Porter, R. W. (1961). *Neurology* **11**, 109.

Ferrari, W., Gessa, G. L., and Vargiu, L. (1963). *Ann. N. Y. Acad. Sci.* **104**, 330.

Flexner, L. B., and Flexner, J. B. (1969). *Proc. Nat. Acad. Sci. U.S.* **60**, 923.

Forster, L. B., and Sells, B. H. (1969). *Arch. Biochem. Biophys.* **132**, 561.

Gastaut, H. (1958). *In* "Reticular Formation of the Brain" (H. H. Jasper, L. D. Proctor, R. S. Knighton, W. C. Noshay, and R. F. Costello, eds.), pp. 561-579. Little, Brown, Boston, Massachusetts.

Gispen, W. H., and Schotman, P. (1970). *Prog. Brain Res.* **32**, 236.

Gispen, W. H., van Wimersma Greidanus, Tj. B., and De Wied, D. (1970a). *Physiol. Behav.* **5**, 143.

Gispen, W. H., De Wied, D., Schotman, P., and Jansz, H. S. (1970b). *J. Neurochem.* **17**, 751.

Glassman, E. (1969). *Annu. Rev. Biochem.* **38**, 605.

Glassman, E., and Wilson, J. E. (1970). *Prog. Brain Res.* **32**, 245.

Glick, D., von Redlich, D., and Levine, S. (1964). *Endocrinology* **74**, 653.

Gregory, K. M., and Diamond, M. C. (1968). *Exp. Neurol.* **20**, 394.

Gyermek, L., Genther, G., and Fleming, N. (1967). *Int. J. Neuropharmacol.* **6**, 191.

Hodges, J. R., and Jones, M. T. (1964). *J. Physiol. (London)* **173**, 190.

Hodges, J. R., and Vernikos-Danellis, J. (1962). *Acta Endocrinol. (Copenhagen)* **39**, 79.

Holzbauer, M., and Newport, H. M. (1967). *J. Physiol. (London)* **193**, 131.

Hulst, S. G. T., and De Wied, D. (1967). *Physiol. Behav.* **2**, 367.

Hydén, H. (1967). *Progr. Nucl. Acid Res. Mol. Biol.* **6**, 187.

Hydén, H., and Lange, P. W. (1968). *Science* **159**, 1370.

Koltai, M., and Minker, E. (1966). *Acta Physiol. Acad. Sci. Hung.* **29**, 410.

Komisaruk, B. R., McDonald, P. G., Whitmoyer, D. I., and Sawyer, C. H. (1967). *Exp. Neurol.* **19**, 494.

König, J. F. R., and Klippel, R. A. (1963). "The Rat Brain. A Stereotaxic Atlas of the Forebrain and Lower Parts of the Brain Stem." Williams & Wilkins, Baltimore, Maryland.

Korányi, L., and Endröczi, E. (1967). *Neuroendocrinology* **2**, 65.

Korányi, L., and Endröczi, E. (1970). *Prog. Brain Res.* **32**, 120.

Korner, A. (1964). *Biochem. J.* **92**, 449.

Korner, A. (1965). *Recent Progr. Horm. Res.* **21**, 205.

Korner, A. (1968). *Ann. N.Y. Acad. Sci.* **148**, 408.

Krivoy, W., and Guillemin, R. (1961). *Experientia* **18**, 20.

Lande, S., Lerner, A. B., and Uptor, G. V. (1965). *J. Biol. Chem.* **240**, 4259.

Lebovitz, H. E., and Engel, F. L. (1964). *Metabolism* **13**, 1230.

Levine, S. (1968). *Nebraska Symp. Motivation* (W. J. Arnold, ed.), pp. 85-101. Univ. of Nebraska Press, Lincoln, Nebraska.

Levine, S., and Brush, F. R. (1967). *Physiol. Behav.* **2**, 385.

Libertun, C., Moguilevsky, J. A., Schiaffini, O., and Foglia, V. (1969). *Experientia* **25**, 196.

Machlus, B., and Gaito, J. (1969). *Nature (London)* **222**, 573.

Mason, J. W., Brady, J. V., and Sidman, M. (1957). *Endocrinology* **60**, 741.

Mason, J. W., Brady, J. V., and Tolliver, G. A. (1968). *Psychosom. Med.* **30**, 608.

Miller, R. E., and Ogawa, N. (1962). *J. Comp. Physiol. Psychol.* **55**, 211.

Mirsky, I. A., Miller, R., and Stein, M. (1953). *Psychosom. Med.* **15**, 574.

Murphy, J. V., and Miller, R. E. (1955). *J. Comp. Physiol. Psychol.* **48**, 47.

Papez, J. W. (1937). *Arch. Neurol. Psychiat.* **38**, 725.

Papez, J. W. (1956). *Electroencephalogr. Clin. Neurophysiol.* **8**, 117.

Resko, J. A. (1969). *Science* **164**, 70.

Rich, I., and Thompson, R. (1965). *J. Comp. Physiol. Psychol.* **59**, 66.

Sawyer, C. H., Kawakami, M., Meyerson, B., Whitmoyer, D. I., and Lilley, J. L. (1968). *Brain Res.* **10**, 213.

Schally, A. V., Lipscomb, H. S., and Guillemin, R. (1962). *Endocrinology* **71**, 164.

Schotman, P., and Gispen, W. H. (1970). Unpublished data.

Schwyzer, R. (1969). *In* "Protein and Polypeptide Hormones" (M. Margoulies, ed.), Vol. I. *Excerpta Med. Found. Int. Congr. Ser.* No. 161, 201.

Selye, H. (1950). "Stress." Acta, Inc., Montreal.

Shashoua, V. E. (1968). *Nature (London)* **217**, 238.

Shashoua, V. E. (1970). *Proc. Nat. Acad. Sci. U. S.* **65**, 160.

Slusher, M. A., Hyde, J. E., and Laufer, M. (1966). *J. Neurophysiol.* **29**, 157.

Soulairac, F. A., Gottesmann, Cl., and Thangapregassam, M. J. (1963). *J. Physiol. (Paris)* **55**, 340.

Staehelin, M. (1965). *Biochem. Z.* 342, 459.

Steiner, F. A. (1970). *Prog. Brain Res.* 32, 102.

Takeda, S., Kawa, A., Ogawa, T., Inamori, Y., Okamoto, O., and Kanehisa, T. (1967). *Acta Med. Univ. Kagoshima.* 9, 161.

Tata, J. R., and Williams-Ashman, H. G. (1967). *Eur. J. Biochem.* 2, 366.

Thompson, R. (1963). *J. Comp. Physiol. Psychol.* 56, 261.

Upton, G. V., Lerver, A. B., and Lande, S. (1966). *J. Biol. Chem.* 241, 5585.

Vanderwolf, C. H. (1964). *J. Comp. Physiol. Psychol.* 58, 31.

van Delft, A. M. L. (1970a). Thesis, Utrecht.

van Delft, A. M. L. (1970b). *Prog. Brain Res.* 32, 192.

van Wimersma Greidanus, Tj. B. (1970a). *Prog. Brain Res.* 32, 185.

van Wimersma Greidanus, Tj. B. (1970b). Thesis, Utrecht.

van Wimersma Greidanus, Tj. B. and De Wied, D. (1969). *Physiol. Behav.* 4, 365.

van Wimersma Greidanus, Tj. B., and De Wied, D. (1970). *Pfluegers Arch.* 318, 282.

van Wimersma Greidanus, Tj. B. and De Wied, D. (1971). *Neuroendocrinology* 7, 291.

Weijnen, J. A. W. M. (1968). *Proc. Conf. Brit. Psychol. Soc. London,* p. 11.

Weijnen, J. A. W. M., and Slangen, J. L. (1970). *Prog. Brain Res.* 32, 221.

Weiss, J. M., McEwen, B. S., Silva, M. T., and Kalkut, M. (1970) *Amer. J. Physiol.* 218, 864.

Wertheim, G. A., Conner, R. L., and Levine, S. (1967). *J. Exp. Anal. Behav.* 10, 555.

Wertheim, G. A., Conner, R. L., and Levine, S. (1967). *Physiol. Behav.* 4, 41.

Wurfbain-Moolenburgh, M. C. W. (1968). Thesis, Leiden.

Zomzely, C. E., Roberts, S., Gruber, C. P., and Brown, D. M. (1968). *J. Biol. Chem.* 243, 5396.

6

Pavlovian Conditioning and Adaptive Hormones

E. Endröczi

I. INTRODUCTION

A classification of learning theories on the basis of experimental methodology can be divided into two categories: one involves the so-called trial-and-error situation (problem box) introduced into the psychological laboratory by Thorndike (1898), and the other is classical conditioning developed by Pavlov (1902). Studies with the problem box led to the "law-of-effect" interpretation of learning, although Thorndike did not himself hold strictly to the view that all learning involves the "law of effect." In the "trial-and-error" situation a selection from among the initial repertory of responses of the subject occurs and the motivational state is an obvious and important determinant of the initial response. Hull's (1943) theory claimed that all instances of learning are subsumed under the "law-of-effect" and designated it in the "principle of reinforcement."

In classical conditioning the main concern is in the temporal relation between the conditional signal and the response. Close temporal occurrence of such events as conditional stimulus (CS), unconditional stimulus (US), and integration of conditioned response (CR) is considered the most important factor. Although Pavlov was aware of the necessity for having his subject motivated, his work principally involved studying the rules operating during establishment of temporary linkage between CS and CR.

According to the classification of Hilgard and Marquis (1940) conditioning can be divided into subclasses as follows: training procedures with (1) instrumental reward, (2) instrumental escape, (3) instrumental avoidance, and (4) secondary reward. Instrumental conditioning is very similar to the classical procedure; in both instances the US is some kind of noxious stimulus and the CR is an "instrument of avoidance." Instrumental reward, in contrast to instrumental avoidance, is quite a different procedure from classical conditioning; in the situation of instrumental reward the experimenter does not exercise control over establishment of temporary connections between CS and US, and the acquisition of CR depends solely on the motivational state of the animal.

Hilgard (1936) has already pointed out that procedures of classical and instrumental conditioning are essentially the same, but different responses are measured in the two experimental situations. During instrumental conditioning the response that delivers the reward is measured, whereas it is ignored during classical conditioning, and the response to the US (e.g., salivation) is ignored in the instrumental conditioning. The basic role of motivational states, as well as the importance of reward in the establishment of activity, had been recognized by Pavlov, and led to regarding problem-solving learning as being similar to classical conditioning (Loucks, 1935; Loucks and Gantt, 1938; Brogden, 1939; Culler, 1938). Also, it was already recognized that instrumental avoidance represents a modification of the paradigm used in classical conditioning in the direction of trial-and-error learning.

All procedures used in studying animal learning are principally based on the establishment of temporary connections between stimulus-response (S-R) events. With regard to the mechanisms underlying these processes, there are different views in the literature. Perceptual learning theorists refuted the importance of the S-R bond (Koffka, 1935; Kohler, 1929; Lewin, 1936; Tolman, 1934), in contrast to the view of other experimental psychologists who stressed the leading role of sensorimotor integration (S-R integration) in all learning processes (Thorndike, 1917; Skinner, 1935; Schneirla, 1946; Mowrer, 1947; Hilgard, 1948).

There are terms used both in classical and instrumental conditioning which are essentially common in meaning, and there are definitions which are misused or misinterpreted in the literature. To avoid confusion a brief account is given to clarify the terms used in this chapter.

1. Acquisition of CR means the formation of a temporary connection between conditional signal and unconditional response (CS-UR). Artificial blocking of either somatic or visceral manifestations of the UR does not prevent the development of a temporary connection between CS and UR (Crisler, 1930; Light and Gantt, 1936; Kellogg *et al.,* 1940).

2. Intersignal or intertrial activity corresponds to the goal-directed motor response of the subject occurring during a period of two consecutive signals, and can be measured both in classical (e.g., salivation) and instrumental (goal-directed locomotor activity, e.g., to the feeder or into the "safe" compartment) conditioning. In a two-way conditioned reflex situation the intertrial activity resembles exploratory activity of the animals (e.g., in the shuttlebox) and the motivational states behind these somatic manifestations cannot be separated. The intensity of intertrial activity may express the intensity of motivational state in alimentary conditioned reflex situation but it seems to be in inverse correlation to the degree of fear in the shuttlebox situation (freezing state vs spontaneous locomotor and exploring activity).

3. Internal inhibition can be divided into two subclasses: differential inhibition plays a basic role in decoding of environmental signals and it is essential in all kinds of learning. The second class of internal inhibition is a variety of the former one, and related to the extinction of a CR by a serial administration of CS in the absence of US. Both types of internal inhibition are considered as counterparts of stimulus-specific excitatory states of the central nervous system (CNS) and separate brain functions are presumed for execution of these processes.

4. Obstruction is a useful tool to study the effect of an US on the temporary connection which had been established under an opposite motivational state (e.g., electric shock-induced fear vs alimentary conditioned reflex). Thus, the association of electric shock with the CS of alimentary conditioned reflex leads to the inhibition of alimentary CR and the duration of inhibition reflects the intensity of antagonistic motivational states (fear vs hunger or thirst) as well as the degree of internal inhibition.

5. Habituation may be considered as one form of differential inhibition which results in elimination of either somatic or visceral responses by repetition of stimuli that are biologically not harmful. A typical example of habituation occurs when the exploratory activity of a naive animal disappears during the

course of repeated testing in the same environment. A large number of neurophysiological observations indicate that habituation is due to active inhibitory processes, both at peripheral sensory and central integratory levels (Hernandez-Péon, 1963; Jouvet, 1961).

A. Theoretical Interpretation of Classical vs Instrumental Learning

In *The Behavior of Organisms,* Skinner (1938) proposed a distinction between two types of CR's, as type *R* (instrumental) and type *S* (classical). His suggestion implied that instrumental responses are acquired on the basis of the principle of law of effect, whereas type *S* is acquired during CS-US pairings. According to Skinner's classification type *R* is largely skeletal, whereas type *S* involves visceromotor activities. This dual interpretation of S-R learning has been accepted and modified by many investigators (Razran, 1939; Maier and Schneirla, 1942; Schlosberg, 1937).

A quite different concept of the conditioned learning had been developed by Guthrie (1942), who made a sharp distinction between movement (e.g., leg flexion or salivary secretion elicited by the CS) and act (complexity of motor patterns involved in instrumental learning). He suggested that all learning types are the result of the association of S-R events and this association is established during a single trial. Moreover, he stated that "a stimulus pattern that is acting at the time of a response will, if it recurs, tend to produce that response." This means that all the stimulus cues become associated in an all-or-none manner with the response. According to Guthrie's concept, if once a stimulus pattern is associated with a response, it remains so associated unless a different response is organized because of the occurrence of a new stimulus pattern.

Concerning the efficiency of classical conditioning vs instrumental training for acquisition of a CR, Schlosberg (1934), Munn (1939), Brogden (1939) and Whatmore *et al.* (1946) have failed to demonstrate any difference between the two procedures. In contrast to these observations, Brogden *et al.* (1938) and Sheffield (1948) assumed that instrumental avoidance is superior to classical training under some conditions. It is a general principle of Pavlovian conditioning that when a CR had been established it cannot be removed from the brain. This statement indicates that the conditioned reflex cannot be simplified as an association of stimulus pattern with a response. Moreover, it means that once a CR had been established it can only be facilitated or inhibited and its basic elements are still represented in the brain after presentation of conflicting external stimuli or extinction by nonreinforced trials. A temporary connection can be facilitated by the need of the organism (hunger, thirst, etc.) and also specific conditional environmental stimuli; similarly, changes of internal environment may inhibit the temporary connections. It frequently occurs that drastic changes in the chemical environment do not affect either acquisition or extinction of a CR. These observations show that changes of internal environment affect learning processes by fairly specific chemical messages in which the hormones play a considerable role.

B. Reinforcement, Satiety, and Internal Inhibition

Defined in a general manner, need is a state of the organism that derives from changes of either internal or external environment. All motor and visceral activities which serve to maintain the homeostatic balance provide reinforcement for the organism. Hull (1943) stated in his *Principle of Behavior* that ". . . reinforcing states of affairs result in an increment of the habit strengths of the temporally coincident stimulus components to evoke response." Guthrie (1942) suggested that ". . . a stimulus pattern that is acting at the time of a response, will, if it recurs, tend to produce that response." From the point of view of a S-R learning theorist, Woodworth (1947) claimed that reinforcement strengthens the "expectancy" which involves registration of the sequence of stimulus events.

Drive refers to a complexity of both humoral changes and neural afferentations aroused by a particular need of the organism. A differentiation between drive and motivational state is meaningless; both terms refer to the need of the organism which can be satiated by goal directed motor patterns. As early as 1920, the goal-directed motor act as the source of reinforcement was already mentioned as a relief from drive (Kuo, 1921; Perrin and Klein, 1926). This concept was adopted by Hull (1943) in his drive reduction hypothesis. A similar opinion was stressed by Miller and Dollard (1941) who pointed out that all kinds of reinforcement involves drive reduction.

To define the drive as a type of generalized force or energy which provides the biological force as determinant of ongoing activity of the animal, is extremely difficult because of the independence of goal-directed motor activities triggered by drives as sex, hunger, fear, etc. From a psychophysiological or neurophysiological point of view drive can be considered as arousal of the CNS under the influence of changes in the chemical environment or in the response to environmental stimuli, and this state manifests itself in the form of goal-directed motor patterns in a proper situation. Arousal of the CNS implies an increased excitatory state of the brain stem and forebrain structures. If arousal can be identified with drive, then factors which induce arousal of brain stem and forebrain functions could be assumed to also induce drive (Berlyne, 1960). Moreover, if we accept the concept of specific drives or arousals in contrast to the view of a generalized drive (Hull, 1943 versus Moss, 1924), we must consider that reinforcement provided by a goal-directed act has a specific reinforcing value.

Pavlov emphasized the formation of temporary connections as functions of excitatory and inhibitory processes and stressed the importance of irradiation or concentration of these nervous activities during the course of the acquisition or extinction of the CR. From a neurophysiological point of view, brain stem and forebrain connections include reciprocity of both excitatory and inhibitory processes and separate excitatory and inhibitory circuits for specific drives and their inhibition by reinforcement are also assumed (Endröczi, 1969; Endröczi and Lissák, 1962; Lissák and Endröczi, 1965).

A distinction between nonspecific arousal (from sleep to wakefulness) and motivation-specific arousal is important; the former state is an elementary function of organized multineuronal network, unlike the latter, which are the functions of specific signals coming from either internal or external environment. Nonspecific or general arousal is not necessarily related to the need of the organism but all motivational states produce a change in nonspecific arousal and lead to integration of goal-directed motor patterns. Reinforcement is a consequence of goal-directed motor pattern and basically involved in reduction of drive or specific arousal. In other words, specific arousals are controlled and reduced by motivational specific internal inhibitory processes.

C. Intertrial (or Intersignal) Activity and Internal Inhibition

Both intertrial and intersignal activity appear in goal-directed forms and express a certain degree of motivation in the conditioned reflex experiment. In free operant conditioning the intertrial activity can be a measure of motivational state and a tool to create timing behavior or instrumental conditioning. In Pavlovian conditioning, the "intertrial" activity as a term is meaningless because of the sequence of CS-US, but the appearance of intersignal responses refers to a degree of motivational state. Pavlov (1927) clearly demonstrated that gradual suppression of intersignal activity (e.g., salivation or leg flexions) is the result of increasing differential inhibition during the course of conditioning. Studying the nature of intersignal activity in alimentary reflex conditioning in cats, it was found that suppression of intersignal activity to a zero level did not occur in the absence of a differential signal. After a long training period (30-50 days or 300-500 associations of CS with US) the cats still showed a considerable number of intersignal responses, but introduction of a differential signal in the stereotype led to a fast suppression of intersignal activity. This study provided evidence of the specific character of differential inhibition; it was observed that cats sated by feeding *ad libitum* just prior to the experimental session still displayed some degree of intersignal activity and showed CR on the presentation of conditional signal, although they did not eat. These observations raised the questions whether somatomotor manifestations are specifically related to different drives and arousals, or just under limited circumstances. The acute satiety of hunger in cats proved to be less effective in inhibiting perseveration of goal-directed motor pattern than differential signal-induced inhibition (Endröczi and Lissák, 1962; Lissák and Endröczi, 1965). The inhibition which is elicited by presentation of differential signal can be considered as situation- and goal-directed motor-specific process and it develops by alternate presentation of CS-US sequences with a nonreinforced differential signal. The situation and somatomotor specificity of differential inhibition also suggests an independent integration of goal-directed motor patterns, specific drives or arousals, and separate internal inhibitory processes involved in the drive reduction. Reinforcing value of a goal-directed motor act can be considered as a measure of intensity of the specific internal inhibition and proportional with the degree of drive reduction.

D. Nonspecific and Specific Drives, Goal-Directed Motor Pattern, and Conditioned Reflex Behavior

Environmental changes result in different degrees of exploratory activity and their intensity depends on the phylogeny and ontogenesis of the species and the motivational state (Woodworth, 1921). Pavlov (1927) described this activity as "investigatory reflex" and referred to a S-R property of this behavior. A sharp distinction between nonspecific arousal and exploratory activity is not possible and the elimination of explorative reaction by repeated exposures of the animal to the same environmental changes occurs during habituation which can be regarded as one form of internal inhibition. Exploratory activity is accompanied by different intensity of visceral reaction and its measurement is a useful tool in studying reactivity of the living organism during exposure to a new environment.

In contrast to nonspecific arousal which results from environmental changes and appears in the form of exploratory activity, specific arousals or drives can be divided into two subclasses: (1) aroused by more or less specific changes of chemical environment (hunger, thirst, sexual, maternal, nest building, hoarding, motivational states), which manifested themselves in genetically coded (innate) goal-directed motor patterns, although some degree of learned behavior is also assumed in these processes; (2) behavioral reactions evoked by those noxious stimuli which interfere with maintenance of homeostatic equilibrium and produce need to eliminate such conflicting influences of the environment (pain-evoked fear, cold- or warm-induced adaptive reactions, etc.). A differentiation between these subclasses is necessary for understanding those biological reactions which are more innate in their origin and controlled by specific changes of chemical environment than those which are triggered by external stimuli with the internal environment playing a modifying role in their appearance.

It is known that sensorimotor connections (S-R substrate at neuronal level) are ready during ontogenetical development before their use. Humoral factors play an important part in these maturational processes, although they do not create new behavior patterns. They can decrease or increase thresholds of behavioral excitation, and the sensitizing effect of hormones has been called "hormonal or humoral conditioning." Beach (1947) clearly pointed at the importance of hormonal conditioning; "susceptibility to sexual arousal in lower mammals depends heavily upon hormones from the reproductive glands, and that in higher species, particularly apes and human, the rigidity of such hormonal control is relaxed sufficiently to permit a considerable amount of sexual responsiveness and potency in the complete absence of sexual secretions." The sensitizing effect of hormones on motivated behavior includes both nonspecific and specific components; e.g., an early androgen sterilization of female rat is followed by changes in reproductive behavior which are accompanied by alterations in general arousal level and cyclic character of general motor activity (Harris, 1964).

Acquisition of goal-directed motor pattern is usually the function of one-trial learning and can be regarded as a situation-specific conditioned process. A primary condition of the acquisition of goal-directed motor pattern is the need of organism and the presence of goal-object in the situation. In the absence of limiting factors the animal will repeat the somatomotor pattern to reach the goal as long as the need persists.

In studying the acquisition of goal-directed motor pattern and its perseveration during both alimentary and avoidance conditioning in cats, it was found that the somatomotor act is highly situation-specific; after some perseverations of the same route (run to the feeder or escape in fear situation) the acquisition of a new route to the same goal-object requires a considerable number of trials and is established under a process of differential inhibition (Endröczi and Lissák, 1962; Lissák and Endröczi, 1965).

A goal-directed motor act and its visceral concomitants aroused by the need of the organism can be regarded as a basic and frequently innate form of motivated behavior. This is not an UR, although it shares some characteristics of it. The goal-directed motor pattern may be considered as "spatial frame" of a conditioned reflex if it is associated with CS and the temporary connection between them serves the "temporal frame" of conditioned reflex behavior. In contrast to the acquisition of "spatial frame," the establishment of temporary connection requires an incomparably higher number of trials than those of goal-directed motor acts.

A goal-directed motor pattern appears in the same form following reconditioning as it was acquired during the course of the initial conditioning (Korányi et al., 1963). Pavlov stated that if a conditioned reflex has been established it cannot be removed from the brain. It is possible to facilitate or to inhibit temporary connections but a goal-directed motor pattern, if once acquired, becomes permanent property of brain mechanisms.

From a non-Pavlovian point of view, classical conditioning is not necessarily related to the presence of a drive and separates the US from motivational stimuli. Both in alimentary and defensive conditioned reflex experiments the US appear to be effective in forming a temporary linkage if they arouse needs of the organism. Similarly, integration of goal-directed motor pattern as the result of either US or CR requires proper need (drive) and the need can be highly specific or rather generalized depending on the previous experience of the organism and many influences of the environment. It is known that the performance of a thirsty rat in a food-reward situation is poorer than that of water-satiated, and performance of a food-satiated but thirsty rat in a water-reward situation is better than that of one not thirsty. These and other observations support Miller's (1948) view of the interactions between drives and a possible drive generalization.

E. Exploratory Activity, Goal-Directed Motor Activity, and Drives

Pavlov's classical experiments were performed in a rigidly controlled situation and his dogs did not receive other environmental stimuli than those which were manipulated by the experimenters. He clearly described the effect of a novel stimulus on the behavior of dogs under conditioned reflex situation, and designated this behavior "orientative reflex." In free operant situation, the animals show exploratory activity which manifests itself in searching, sniffing, standing up reactions, etc. We need to distinguish this behavior from the "orientative reflex," however, although they have common origin and both will decline after continuous exposure of the animal to the same stimulus pattern. The reason for this distinction is because the "orientative reflex" occurs in the response to a novel signal or stimulus pattern in a habituated situation, in contrast to the exploratory activity which appears as the result of a new environment in the absence of any previous experience, and the intensity of exploratory activity depends on the general arousal state of the animal. Strong orientative response may occur in the expectancy state if the animal is in a motivated or conditioned reflex situation, although its exploratory activity is at zero level. The orientative reflex is not necessarily related to locomotor activity and somatic signs of attentive behavior are more characteristic for this behavioral response than for exploration which is always accompanied by a different degree of locomotor activity.

Although a careful study of the intensity of exploratory activity under different motivational states is lacking, it has been observed that, e.g., cats which show high exploratory activity in an alimentary conditioned reflex situation were more active during intersignal intervals in avoidance conditioning than the cats with weak exploration. Moreover, it was found that the cats but not rats display much less exploratory activity during first exposure to a novel situation than in later tests, which may be due to a certain degree of fear in the new environment and means that the exploratory activity cannot be regarded as a simple S-R behavioral reaction (Endröczi, 1968). Similarly, a characteristic feature of exploratory activity is that it can interfere with a previously established goal-directed motor activity; thus, hungry or thirsty rats frequently stop to eat or drink and show vivid exploratory activity for a period of seconds or minutes even in a previously habituated situation.

It is well known that animals maintained on a fixed schedule of food or water deprivation show an increased general motility around the time of feeding. This activity corresponds to the expectancy state and develops under the law of time conditioning. A decrease of general motility of the animals kept on a fixed schedule of active avoidance conditioning around the time of the daily sessions has also been observed.

Exploratory activity is usually less during the early stage of active avoidance conditioning and related to a smaller territory than in an advanced phase of training. Suppression of exploratory behavior may be attributed to the fear which reduces the general motility of the animals, and can be interpreted to a more generalized internal inhibition aroused by the first presentations of US.

F. Extinction of Conditioned Response

Elimination of CR by presentations of nonreinforced conditional signal is the result of increasing degree of internal inhibition and can be considered as an active process (Pavlov, 1927). Realization of nonreinforcement appears in a different way in alimentary conditioned reflex situation than in avoidance conditioning. Furthermore, the meaning of reinforcement is a quite different one in the two situations (nonreinforcement in avoidance situation is misused). The lack of food as goal-object in alimentary conditioning means in reality the absence of reinforcement, in contrast to the avoidance conditioning in which the absence of US will be realized by the animal only if he does not perform the goal-directed motor response. In the latter situation the reinforcing value of goal-directed motor pattern (escape or jump into the safe situation) still acts until the animal realizes the absence of US. From a non-Pavlovian point of view, the extinction of conditioned avoidance is called "negative learning." With regard to the mechanism underlying the extinction of either alimentary or avoidance response, the basic role of internal inhibition is obvious; in both situations suppression of conditional signal-induced goal-directed motor activity is the function of internal inhibition.

An irradiation of internal inhibition during extinction of alimentary CR may be observed by measurement of intertrial activity; in the early period of extinction a sharp decrease of intertrial activity had been observed in the experiments on cats (Endröczi and Lissák, 1962). In contrast to this finding, intertrial activity shows a transient increase during the early extinction of a conditioned avoidance response when the animal realizes the absence of the US. A transient generalization of drive aroused by realization of the absence of the US may be responsible for an increase of intertrial activity in the avoidance situation.

Completeness of extinction can be judged by testing the failure of the conditional signal to evoke a CR in at least three consecutive daily sessions. Recurrence of CR after a period following extinction of the response means the weakening of internal inhibition and the influence of irradiated nonspecific drive or facilitatory processes.

II. NEUROPHYSIOLOGICAL APPROACH OF CONDITIONED REFLEX BEHAVIOR

Capability of higher mammals to acquire temporary connections after removal of entire neocortex has been the subject of many investigations. Zeliony (1911, 1930) was unable to establish CR on decorticated dog with introduction of weak acid solution (as US) which had been associated with intensive sound stimulus as conditional signal. On the other hand, by using a sound stimulus as a conditional signal he could create signal-induced generalized leg flexion in decorticated dogs. More detailed observations were reported by Popov (1950) who succeeded in eliciting conditioned avoidance response in "thalamic dogs." A marked degeneration of basal ganglia and thalamic nuclei was found in the dogs which survived the operation for more than 3 years. The CR had been established by conditional signals of kinesthetic stimuli. However, there was no success in creating temporary connections by pairing visual, olfactory, or acoustic stimuli and the attempts to establish alimentary CR remained futile. Moreover, he found that conditioned avoidance responses appear in a generalized form and cannot be extinguished.

Previously established CR's, both to visual and acoustic signals, had been observed after removal of cortical structures which means that neocortical structures take a part in formation of temporary connections but after their development both facilitation and inhibition of the CR is the result of subcortical mechanisms (Ten Cate, 1934; Belenkov, 1950; Ordzonikidze and Nutsubidze, 1959). Pavlov (1927) claimed the principal importance of neocortical structures is the establishment of CR which had been confirmed by a large number of studies. On the other hand, he oversimplified the role of subcortical structures in these events and did not pay attention to the possibility that these structures all have functions necessary for establishment and performance of conditioned reflex response.

A quite different approach for understanding the neurophysiological basis of conditioned reflex was performed by Lashley (1950) who summarized the role of neocortex in elaboration of temporary connections as follows:

1. "It seems certain that the theory of well-defined conditioned reflex paths from sense organ via association areas to the motor cortex is false. The motor areas are not necessary for the retention of sensory-motor habits or even skilled manipulative patterns."

2. ". . . associative areas are not storehouses for specific memories."

3. "The equivalence of different regions of the cortex for retention of memories points to multiple representation."

Moreover, Lashley stressed that any pattern of excitation is reduplicated throughout the entire nervous network by spread of excitations, and refused the theory that excess cells might be observed as the seat of special memories. Also, he rejected the theory of behaviorists who concern all psychological activity with simple associations or chains of conditioned reflexes.

Lashley's statement does not oppose what Pavlov claimed about the role of cortical structures in elaboration of conditioned reflex activity; Pavlov interpreted irradiation and concentration of both facilitatory and inhibitory processes as spreading of excitatory and inhibitory state of the neocortex without any specific relation to its neurophysiological functions. It is known that dissociation of sensory and motor analyzers by horizontal cuttings in dogs, did not interfere with establishment of temporary connections. Similarly, the interruption of all horizontal connections of the visual analyzer did not prevent the formation of visual conditioning and discrimination (Astratyan, 1941, 1952). These observations suggested separate thalamocortical circuits for elaboration of temporary connections. However, destruction of nonspecific thalamic nuclei failed to produce remarkable changes either in establishment or retention of conditioned reflex behavior (Chow, 1954; Peters et al., 1956; Warren and Akert, 1960). Those alterations which have been found after lesions of nonspecific thalamic nuclei can be attributed to changes of motivational states which manifest themselves in a deficit of problem solving but not in the more simplified learning situations.

The role of neocortex in the establishment of temporary connections is obvious and supported by many observations. A quite different question is how much the cortical structures participate in storing of these events. Complete removal of the forebrain structures after establishment of a somatovisceral conditioned reflex response did not interfere with performance in the rat (Markel and Ádám, 1969). Both spreading depression and ablation experiments as well as observations in connection with convulsive amnesia indicate that participation of neocortical structures in elaboration of temporary connections appears in the early, labile phase of conditioning, and the storing of memory appears as a function of subcortical structures (Endröczi, 1969; Lissák, 1969).

Numerous studies have been accumulated in the literature which clearly showed a tremendous plasticity on one hand, and extreme specificity of the nervous substrate for establishment of temporary connections. Electrical stimulation of both neocortical and subcortical structures may serve as conditional signal as well as UR, and the temporary connections being established in that way are virtually lacking in motivational content (Loucks, 1935; Giurgea, 1953; Doty and Giurgea, 1961; Mowrer, 1960; Korányi and Endröczi, 1967). In the experiments on rabbits, no more than 1 mm distance between electrode pairs proved to be enough to establish a conditioned avoidance response by stimulation through one of the electrodes, and its differential signal by the other one within the pyramidal layer of dorsal hippocampus. After extinction of the CR by nonreinforced trials, a reversal of conditioning electrode to differential one showed the specificity of response being established. Similar observations were reported by conditioning and differential electrical stimulation of brain stem reticular formation when electrode pairs were placed in rostrocaudal direction (Lissák and Endröczi, 1965).

Recognition of the central role of brain stem reticular formation in sleep and wakeful state, organization of complex somatomotor and visceral activities and its participation of motivational states, drew the attention of many investigators to the study of this multineuronal network in relation to establishment of temporary connections (see Moscow Colloquium of Higher Nervous Activity, 1960; Henry Ford Symposium on Reticular Formation of the Brain, 1958). There are many observations which indicate that brain stem reticular formation plays a basic role in elaboration of conditioned reflex activity; however, its lack does not interfere with establishment of temporary connections. Thus, complete destruction of reticular core at mesencephalic level (which had been performed in two stages), did not alter learning and failed to prevent both avoidance conditioning and maze learning in cats and rats (Kesner et al., 1967; Chow and Randall, 1964). In contrast to numerous studies in which destruction of brain stem reticular formation was performed on one-stage operation, a gradual elimination of brain stem reticular formation by multistage operation did not interfere with wakeful state of the animals and did not prevent development of emotional reactions and was compatible with learning processes (Moruzzi and Magoun, 1949; Jasper, 1949; Lindsley et al., 1949; Doty et al., 1959; Adametz, 1959).

Brain Stem-Limbic Circuit, Motivational State, and Conditioned Reflex Behavior

Abundant evidence has been accumulated in the literature which indicates that rhinencephalic structures, hypothalamus, and brain stem reticular core form a functional unit through reciprocal connections, and their activities manifest themselves in different motivated behavioral reactions. Compartmentalized view of the hypothalamic function had been replaced by a more dynamic concept of the brain stem-hypothalamic-rhinencephalic circuit (Dell, 1958; Guillery, 1957; Nauta, 1962; Morgane, 1961; Deutsch, 1963; Endröczi and Lissák, 1962). One of the oldest tracts which connects basal forebrain structures (septal complex, orbitofrontal cortex, afferentations from temporoamygdaloid area, and caudate nucleus) to brain stem reticular formation has descending projections along the lateral hypothalamus and it is called a septomesencephalic tract in lower vertebrates or medial forebrain bundle in higher ones (Ban, 1964; Guillery, 1957). The medial forebrain bundle is a reciprocal trajectory and its ascending neurons are very rich in monoamines (Fuxe, 1965). Both electrophysiological and behavioral studies indicated that the descending part of the medial forebrain bundle plays an important role in the integration of motivated behavioral reactions (Olds, 1962; Morgane, 1961, 1969; Endröczi and Lissák, 1962; Endröczi, 1969). There are numerous observations which showed antagonistic influence of the midline and the lateral hypothalamic structures on the feeding and drinking behavior, and had been considered as functions of "hypothalamic centers." Poor neuronal connections between ventromedial and lateral hypothalamic nuclei do not support the view that feeding and drinking behavior is maintained by a balanced state of these centers at hypothalamic level. Both degeneration and electrophysiological studies excluded direct neuronal pathways connecting ventromedial and lateral hypothalamic nuclei (Sutin and Eager, 1969; Endröczi, 1969).

Electrical stimulation of medial forebrain bundle results in a wide scale of behavioral manifestations which simulate behavioral reactions being observed in different motivational states. Without mentioning many details of both electrophysiological and behavioral studies, the main conclusions derived from these investigations may be summarized as follows:

1. Electrical stimulation of the medial forebrain bundle, Broca diagonal band, subcommissural preoptic area, and posterior medial orbitofrontal area led to an enhanced *habituation* of a novel stimulus in the cats.

2. Stimulation of the same structure mentioned above resulted in a *suppression* of *intertrial activity* both in alimentary and conditioned avoidance reflex situations.

3. Similarly, stimulation of medial forebrain bundle led to a *facilitation* of the *extinction* of CR.

4. Bilateral lesions of the medial forebrain bundle impaired learning ability of both cats and rats in avoidance situation.

5. Electrical stimulation of these pathways produced *synchronized slow waves* in the neocortex, and bilateral destruction of subcommissural region impaired integration of spindle formation and recuiting responses evoked by low frequency stimulation of nonspecific thalamic nuclei.

The broad spectra of electrophysiological and behavioral correlates produced by lesioning or stimulation of the medial forebrain bundle system led us to conclude that this tract, by its descending connections, plays a basic role in elaboration of internal inhibitory processes on one hand, and as the consequence of the internal inhibition, serves as the reinforcement-specific control of the brain stem sensory input (Endröczi and Lissák, 1962; Lissák and Endröczi, 1965; Endröczi, 1969).

Discovery of self-stimulation contributed a great deal to alter our views of the integratory role of brain stem and limbic structures in motivated behavioral processes (Olds, 1962). Reward and punishment as psychophysiological concomitants of the negative and positive self-stimulations can be accepted as motivational factors for these phenomena; however, many observations opposed this type of interpretation. Short-term stimulation of the medial forebrain bundle eliciting positive self-stimulation may be interpreted as a rebound activity of the ascending activatory system. An artificial increase of internal inhibition without specific reinforcement value may result in an unbalanced state between descending inhibitory and ascending activatory systems, and this functional unbalanced state will be adjusted by the integration of the same goal-directed motor pattern which was dominant in the situation. Integration of a new goal-directed motor pattern will lead to a new train of impulses and this results

Table I. Schematic Illustration of Events Involved in Classical and Instrumental Conditioning

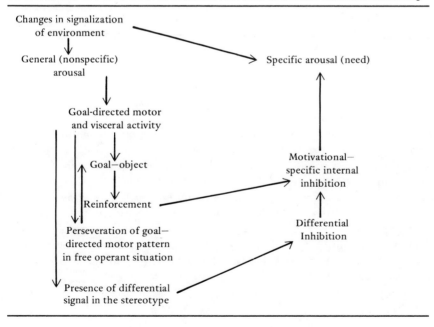

in the same unbalanced state of excitatory and inhibitory processes which initiated recurrence of goal-directed motor pattern. Perseveration of the same motor act is the result of the rebound action of the ascending activation system after cessation of stimulation in the descending inhibitory one. On the other hand, simultaneous stimulation of ascending activation projections during performance of a goal-directed motor pattern leads to long-term inhibition of this motor act (midline hypothalamic stimulation-induced inhibition of feeding and drinking) in the situation, but the animal will show the goal-directed motor response in the presence of the goal-object in another environment. The inhibition may be attributed to a rebound effect of descending inhibitory system; this action is somatomotor and situation-specific (Endröczi and Lissák, 1962; Lissák and Endröczi, 1965).

According to our concept the basal forebrain inhibitory system serves the neurophysiological basis of internal inhibition; its control on the sensory input of the brain stem and diencephalon is motivational, situational, and somato-motor-specific. Under physiological circumstances the reinforcing value resulting from goal-directed motor performance is mediated through the basal forebrain inhibition. It is obvious that reinforcement, drive reduction, and internal inhibition are different categories but they are causative in controlling motivated behavior. Moreover, there is no doubt that basal forebrain inhibition is not a tonic control for brain stem and forebrain connections but it has tremendous specificity which cannot be separated by electrical stimulation, but can be successful through excitation by humoral transmitters or chemical agents (Miller, 1966; Grossman, 1969). Separation of neuronal circuits involved either in feeding or drinking behavior by cholinergic and adrenergic stimulation suggests separate circuits for controlling basic motivational modalities.

The role of the medial forebrain bundle and the basal forebrain structures in motivated behavior has been reviewed by numerous authors (Morgane, 1961, 1969; Olds, 1962; Routtenberg, 1968; Endröczi, 1969). Conclusions derived from self-stimulation studies claim reinforcing character of stimulation in this part of the brain; our studies suggested a basic role of internal inhibition in these events. Neurophysiological observations indicated inhibitory character of basal forebrain stimulation on the mono- and polysynaptic reflex at brain stem and spinal cord level, as well as participation of this part of the brain in thalamocortical synchronization [see for review Endröczi (1969)]. Both neuroanatomical basis and functional character of the interactions between ascending activatory and descending inhibitory systems are going through changes during ontogeny and have species-dependent features. Understanding basic mechanisms underlying behavioral events within this neuroanatomical substrate needs further studies.

III. HORMONAL CONTROL
OF MOTIVATED BEHAVIORAL REACTIONS
AND CONDITIONED REFLEX PROCESSES

Changes in chemical environment may result in an unbalanced state of the central nervous excitatory and inhibitory processes which arouse specific need (drive) and lead to integration of goal-directed motor pattern. Some drives are developed in the lack or excess of specific changes of the chemical environment, and again others are aroused by mutual or simultaneous interactions of humoral and neural afferentations on the central nervous processes. A categorization between drives on the basis of their primary origin is shown in Table II.

Changes induced by external stimuli manifest themselves both in somatic and visceral reactions and the behavioral reactions elicited are dependent on the intensity of stimuli, their novelty, and on the species. Externally evoked behavioral reactions are learned processes, although they have some innate characteristics. Exploratory activity appears to be one of the basic drives; it appears in a novel situation but its recurrence can be observed following long-term habituation. This activity is associated with an optimal amount of sensory impulses which seem to be necessary to maintain an equilibrium of excitatory and inhibitory processes in the CNS. Humoral influences can modify this equilibrium and may lead to an increase or decrease of the exploratory activity.

Noxious stimuli produce a different degree of avoidance or escape reactions which are accompanied by somatic and visceral signs of fear or rage; humoral factors may increase or decrease the intensity of these behavioral reactions and

TABLE II. A Categorization between Drives on the Basis of their Primary Origin

Integration of motivated behavioral reaction		
Evoked by	Modified by	Behavioral forms and drive
External stimuli	Humoral factors	Exploratory Fear Rage Thermic adaptation
Humoral factors	External stimuli	Hunger Thirst Sex Maternal Hoarding Nest building

Table III.

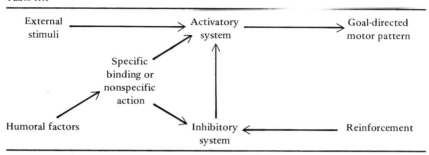

this influence of chemical messages plays a basic role in controlling emotional behavior.

Behavioral forms which are initiated by changes of chemical environment, usually innate behavioral forms, can be elicited by external stimuli if the latter become conditional signals for these behavioral reactions. Thus, in many species removal of gonadal hormones at maturity does not totally interfere with reproductive activity which is evoked by external stimuli (Beach, 1947). On the other hand, there is no doubt that the sensitizing role of gonadal hormones is important for maturation of reproductive behavioral reactions.

The influence of hormones and other humoral factors on the motivated behavioral reactions is exerted in different ways:

1. By modification of sensory input at peripheral and spinal cord level.

2. By changing of the threshold of either excitatory or inhibitory processes at the central nervous level.

3. By facilitation or inhibition of "preformed" nervous circuits which would correspond to innate behavioral patterns.

With regard to the effects of hormones on the conditioned reflex behavior, they can influence temporary connections by increasing or decreasing need of the organism to integrate a conditioned goal-directed motor pattern. A possible mechanism of these influences, which has been supported by a number of electrophysiological observations, is indicated in Table III, which includes the possibility at the same time that a single chemical agent may induce multiple or even opposite changes in the central excitatory and inhibitory processes.

Recent observations clearly indicate that certain hormones (adrenocortical and sex steroids) act on the brain at the nuclear level and change both protein synthesis as well as enzymic activity in discrete part of the CNS. Accumulation of estradiol-17β has been observed in the preoptic area, ventromedial hypothalamus and arcuate nucleus, stria terminalis and septum of both ovariectomized and androgen-sterilized rats (Eisenfeld and Axelrod, 1965; Kato and Villee, 1967; Stumpf, 1968). Similarly, selective accumulation of corticosterone was found in the hippocampus and septal area of adrenalectomized rats which showed time-dependent retention of this hormone by using highly purified cell nuclei. Nuclear retention of corticosterone was highest in the hippocampus, whereas tissue retention of other parts of the brain for corticosterone appeared to be considerable (McEwen *et al.*, 1970). Selective accumulation of corticosteroids may induce changes of enzymic activity in different brain areas, and changing excitatory and inhibitory states at neuronal level can elicit alterations in the control of gross behavioral reactions.

A. Influence of Pituitary-Adrenocortical Hormones on Conditioned Reflex Activity

Introduction of adrenocorticotropic hormone (ACTH) and corticosteroid treatment in human therapy revealed that these hormones can drastically change the excitatory state of the CNS [reviewed by Cleghorn (1952), Browne, (1952), Bleuler, (1954), Reiss, (1958), Lissák and Endröczi (1960, 1965)]. The first experimental study on the effect of adrenocortical hormones on conditioned reflex behavior was made by Liddell *et al.* (1935), who found that administration of crude adrenal extracts improved the neurotic state of goats in a conditioned situation. With regard to the possible very low quantity of corticosteroids in the extract used by the authors, these observations have more historical than scientific value.

Numerous observations have been accumulated in the literature in recent decades on the effect of adrenalectomy as well as that of administration of corticosteroids on learning; unfortunately, the data are contradictory. Almost negative findings have been reported in the response to adrenalectomy in rats (Moyer, 1958; Moyer and Moshein, 1963; Havelane and Paul, 1963).

The first observations that pituitary-adrenocortical function may be correlated to behavioral changes in conditioned reflex situation were presented by Mirsky *et al.* (1953) and Lissák *et al.* (1957) in monkeys and dogs. Mirsky *et al.* reported an increased extinction rate of fear-conditioned reflex in response to administration of ACTH in monkeys. Lissák *et al.* have found that the ratio of hydrocortisone to corticosterone as well as the total amount of corticosteroids secreted by the adrenals are correlated to passive avoidance behavior of dogs. Moreover, it was observed that hydrocortisone treatment leads to an increase of passive avoidance response. The authors claimed that corticosteroids in order of their chemical polarity exert a facilitatory influence on the internal inhibitory processes; this action manifests itself in a prolonged passive avoidance response and/or in the facilitation of extinction. In the former experimental situation internal inhibition plays a basic role as differential inhibition. During extinction which is produced by nonreinforced trials, internal inhibition is an active force to suppress goal-directed response.

Further correlations between pituitary-adrenocortical activity and conditioned reflex behavior were reported by Endröczi *et al.* (1958) in rats It was found that rats showing a greater response of pituitary-adrenocortical activity to nonspecific noxious stimuli will display a higher degree of passive avoidance learning than rats with less adrenocortical responsiveness. Similar observations have been reported by Bohus and Endröczi (1965) and Wertheim *et al.* (1967) suggest a correlation between adrenocortical activity and avoidance learning in rats. In accordance with earlier findings, de Wied (1966) found facilitation of extinction of an avoidance response following dexamethasone treatment both in adrenalectomized and hypophysectomized rats.

The effectiveness of corticosteroids to changes in conditioned reflex behavior depends on the experimental situation, the doses being administered, the species, and the chemical character of corticosteroids. Excess amount of circulating corticosteroids may influence learning ability of animals in opposite ways, depending on the experimental situation. Thus, the intravenous injection of corticosterone 10 minutes prior to the experimental sessions results in a marked suppression of the performance of active avoidance responses in a midstage of training when the animal shows no more than 30-50% level of performance. In contrast to this finding, corticosterone administration did not change learning performance if the rats were treated with 0.5 mg (i.p.) corticosterone for a week prior to the training period, or when they showed a near 100% level of avoidance. Moreover, it was found that a single large dose of corticosterone given intraperitoneally suppressed the performance level in the midstage of conditioning for 24 hours; however, an increased performance had been found on the day following corticosterone injection.

The suppressive effect of corticosterone in the active avoidance conditioned situation may be attributed to more or less degree of fear; in the former case when fear in high integration of goal-directed motor pattern is prevented by "freezing behavior"; in the latter case where fear is reduced the motivation is not sufficient to initiate escape behavioral reactions. Fear is a psychological concept and its presence or absence in conditioned reflex behavior cannot be measured, at least not on the basis of the basis of avoidance response. Our conclusion was that excess amount of corticosterone in the body results in an overwhelming inhibition which is responsible for the prevention of an integrated goal-directed motor response. Since suppression of a drive-triggered motor pattern is accompanied by a decrease of performance in active avoidance situation, this influence is highly advantageous—at least in terms of learning rate—in passive avoidance conditioning.

Intravenous injection of 50 μg/100 gm body weight resulted in a marked increase in learning of rats being deprived of food for 23 hours and kept on this fixed schedule of feeding for 3 days prior to testing passive avoidance learning. It also should be mentioned that feeding took place in the experimental situation for 3 days prior to passive avoidance. During testing (60 minutes) single electric shocks were given while attempts were made to eat (see Table IV).

TABLE IV. No. of CR and intersignal activity per daily session[a]

Days	1	2	3	4	5	6	7	8	9	10
0.3 ml physiol.	0	11	17	26	39	51	62	76	91	107
saline for 7 days prior to training (8)[b]	0	1	4	5	11	16	21	27	28	32
0.2 mg/100 gm	0	9	12	21	35	47	62	69	88	102
Compound B ip, for 7 days prior to training (8)[b]	0	1	3	3	8	15	17	24	22	26
0.3 ml physiol.	0	12	19	22	(37)[c]	48	65	81	98	(104)[c]
saline iv, on the 5th and 10th days (8)	0	2	7	7	10	13	19	27	28	28
50 μg/100 gm	0	8	17	25	(3)[d]	17	43	64	88	(101)[c]
Compound B iv, on the 5th and 10th days (8)	0	1	3	8	0	3	12	18	18	20

[a] 15 trials per day. The first line of figures in number of CR's; the second line is number of intersignal activities.

[b] No significant difference in the learning rate between the two groups.

[c] Intravenous injection, 10 minutes before testing, no significant change.

[d] Intravenous injection, 10 minutes before testing, no significant change.

The conflicting observations which have been obtained either in the active or passive avoidance situation by corticosterone treatment can be explained by the opposing effects of hormones in different experimental conditions. In the active avoidance situation (e.g., shuttlebox) signal-induced integration of the goal-directed motor pattern is the criterion of conditioned reflex; a nonspecific or tonic increase of internal inhibition, which might be interpreted as the effect of corticosterone, can elicit suppression of performance. On the other hand, in passive avoidance situation the goal-directed motor activity is opposed by the conflict of opposing drives (as the result of electric shocks), and the hunger-motivated approach behavior is under inhibitory control which seems to be supported by the corticosterone treatment. In other words, an excess increase of tonic internal inhibition as the result of corticosteroid treatment may lead to suppression of learning in active avoidance situation but just the opposite effect occurs in passive avoidance conditions. A correlation was found between high plasma corticosterone values and learning rates in passive avoidance situation, and an inverse correlation between these two parameters in active avoidance conditioning (Dupont et al., 1970). Some of these findings confirm earlier data of both ours and other authors (Endröczi et al., 1959; Lissák and Endröczi, 1960; Levine and Jones, 1965).

B. Influence of Corticosteroids on Intersignal Activity and Exploratory Behavior

Earlier observations revealed that corticosteroid treatment led to a suppression of intertrial activity both in alimentary and avoidance conditioned reflex situations in cats and rats (Endröczi and Lissák, 1962; Bohus and Korányi, 1969), and leads to better timing behavior in a Sidman-type avoidance learning (Wertheim *et al.*, 1967). The distinction between intertrial activity and exploratory motility is entirely situational. In a one-way avoidance or alimentary conditioned reflex situation the goal-directed motor activity displayed by the animal in the intertrial intervals corresponds to the intertrial response. In two-way avoidance learning (e.g., shuttlebox), the goal-object is signal-dependent. Intertrial activity cannot be considered as a drive reaction. An increase of intertrial motility could possibly represent less "fear" in the situation. In recent studies it was found that an inverse correlation exists between intertrial activity and plasma corticosterone level which had been measured in the response to 10 nonreinforced conditional signals on the 11th day of training period in a shuttle-box situation in rats (Dupont *et al.*, 1970). Moreover, it was found that rats showing high learning rate in this situation displayed relatively low corticosterone values in comparison to the high plasma values of poor performers.

Exploratory activity and responsiveness of the pituitary-adrenocortical axis upon exposure to a novel situation are inversely correlated parameters. High exploratory activity is accompanied by lower plasma corticosterone values and vice versa (Dupont *et al.*, 1970). This and other observations mentioned above provide increasing evidence that pituitary-adrenocortical function and internal inhibition form a functional unit in controlling learning; functional relationships between nervous and hormonal events are shown in Table V.

Table V.

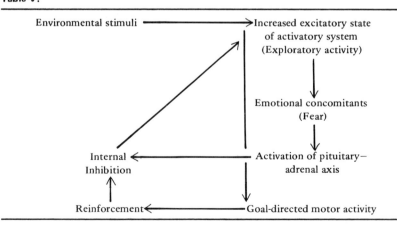

A facilitatory influence of corticosteroids on the basal forebrain inhibition has been assumed in earlier investigations (Endröczi and Lissák, 1962; Endröczi et al., 1968; Endröczi, 1969). On the other hand, it was found that both electrical and cholinergic stimulation of basal forebrain structures results in a suppression of pituitary ACTH release and inhibition of stress-induced activation of pituitary-adrenocortical axis [reviewed by Lissák and Endröczi (1965)]. It seems that adaptive endocrine processes like pituitary-adrenal axis support the reinforcing value of goal-directed motor patterns, although an increased release of pituitary ACTH is due to the unbalanced state between activational and inhibitory nervous mechanisms. In other words, corticosteroids play a role in the adjustment of the balance existing between activational and inhibitory processes at CNS level, and the balance corresponds to a "nonmotivated state" in terms of behavior, and "resting level" of the pituitary-adrenocortical function. The influence of corticosteroids is tonic in its character, and the interactions between activational and inhibitory processes are more motivational and situation-specific; the effect of corticosteroid treatment in a motivational-specific learning situation is more general than specific.

A direct effect of corticosteroids on the basal forebrain structures was studied by hydrocortisone implantation both in electrophysiological and behavioral experiments (Endröczi, 1969). Implantation of 10-15 μg hydrocortisone in the rostral preoptic area and medial forebrain bundle region led to an increased rate of the extinction of an active avoidance response in rats (Figs. 1 and 2). Other implants with cholesterol or hydrocortisone located in the midline hypothalamic nuclei did not influence the extinction of adrenalectomized animals.

In electrophysiological experiments a significant increase of basal forebrain inhibition on the brain stem sensory input was observed following intravenous injection of 50 μg/100 gm body weight corticosterone and hydrocortisone in

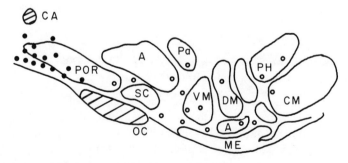

Fig. 1. CA = anterior commissure; POR = preoptic region; A = anterior hypothalamus; SC = supraoptic nucleus; OC = optic chiasm; Pa = paraventricular nucleus; VM = ventromedial nucleus; DM = dorsomedial nucleus; A = arcuate nucleus; ME = median eminence; PH = posterior hypothalamus; CM = mammillary nuclei. (●) Effective; (○) ineffective.

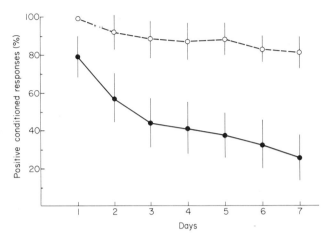

Fig. 2. Extinction of an active avoidance response in adrenalectomized rats (cholesterol) (○) and in adrenalectomized rats with cortisol implants (●) in the central nervous system.

rats. These effects appeared after a latency of 40-60 minutes. A facilitation of sensory-induced brain stem and diencephalic responses has been observed in the first 20-30 minutes after corticosteroid treatment (Endröczi *et al.*, 1968). A facilitatory effect of corticosteroids on long-latency electrical potentials of the brain stem and diencephalon has been reported by Feldman *et al.* (1961). Increased unit activity in the posterior and midline hypothalamic structures in response to corticosteroid injection was also reported by Feldman and Dafny (1968, see in Feldman, 1970). Without mentioning many details and conflicting data which have been obtained by either iontophoretic application of cortico-steroids on cell firing rate, or unit activity recordings after corticosteroid treatment, specific corticosteroid uptake and binding sites for adrenocortical hormones seem to be the highest at basal forebrain and hippocampal level and much lower in other parts of the brain.

C. Extraadrenal Action of ACTH
and Its Fragments on Conditioned Reflex Behavior

An increasing amount of data show that stimulation of the adrenal gland is not the sole action of ACTH; it also can stimulate melanocytes (Li, 1956), possess adipokinetic activity (Rosenberg, 1953), and it is highly active in increasing the liver lipid both in intact and adrenalectomized animals (Li *et al.*, 1957). Moreover, it was found that ACTH increases free fatty acids under *in vitro* circumstances (Buckle, 1962; Hollenberg *et al.*, 1961).

Li *et al.* (1964) pointed out that the smallest unit within ACTH structure that still possesses a significant adrenal-stimulating effect appears to be the heptadecapeptide acid (ACTH 1-17). Both chemistry and biology of ACTH and related peptides have been reviewed recently by Li and Oelofsen (1967).

Initial experimental evidence that ACTH administration results in an extraadrenal effect on conditioned reflex behavior was provided by Murphy and Miller (1955), as well as Miller and Ogawa (1962). ACTH injections led to a prolonged extinction rate both in intact and adrenalectomized rats. On the other hand, de Wied (1966) reported that prolonged extinction of adrenalectomized rats can be normalized by dexamethasone treatment.

Extraadrenal effects of ACTH administration cannot be compared to the action of corticosteroids in many respects; the action of ACTH is more species-dependent than that of the corticosteroids and frequently is opposite to the effect of corticosteroids. Studying the effect of both corticosteroids and ACTH on conditioned vascular responses in rabbits, it was found that large doses of hydrocortisone or corticosterone did not change the conditional signal-induced vascular reaction. The intravenous injection of 2-4 IU ACTH/kg body weight led to a marked suppression of both CR's and UR's (Korányi and Endröczi, 1965). Similar suppression of CR's was observed after ACTH administration under active avoidance conditioning in male rabbits (Korányi and Endröczi, 1965). A direct action of ACTH peptide (1-24) has been reported in relation to polysynaptic reflex activity of spinal cord in rabbits, and other spinal cord reflex responses in cats (Korányi and Endröczi, 1967; Krivoy et al., 1963). Topical application of both ACTH and ACTH 1-10 onto the surface of the cerebral cortex resulted in a diminution of amplitude of callosal-evoked potentials, which cannot be simulated by similar application of other known peptides as well as hydrocortisone (Korányi et al., 1969). Moreover, in experiments on young chickens with a relative lack of blood-brain barrier, the intravenous injection of ACTH, and its fragment ACTH 1-10, produced marked diminution of cortical potentials evoked by brain stem or optic stimulation; in addition to these electrophysiological findings, avoidance responses of chickens were markedly suppressed by intravenous ACTH or fragment 1-10 administration. Observations on the behavioral actions of ACTH and its fragments which have been obtained in rabbits and chickens oppose the results coming from rat studies (de Wied, 1966; Bohus and Korányi, 1969). It seems obvious that contradictory observations which have been obtained by ACTH administration in different species cannot be attributed to differences existing in experimental procedures and diverse effects of ACTH peptides are related to species differences.

Recent studies of the extraadrenal effects of ACTH and its fragments on human subjects showed many similarities to those which have been found in experiments on rats. The intravenous injection of 50 IU ACTH 1-24, or ACTH peptide 1-10 in a dose of 1 or 2 mg resulted in a long-lasting and marked suppression of stimulus-induced EEG responses which have manifested themselves in high amplitude slow waves and corresponded to an exaggerated habituation to the signal. Stimulus-provoked EEG synchrony had been developed by repetition of sound or flash signals several hundred times; the response showed no diminishing tendency during 3-4 months of observation period. Suppressive effect of ACTH and its fragments, which appeared to have a peak on the day following injection, may be interpreted as disinhibition and dishabituation. Saline or intravenous administration of ACTH 11-24 failed to influence the stimulus-provoked EEG synchronization. In the majority of subjects (total number of persons being investigated more than 1 month was 16) administration of both ACTH 1-24 and 1-10 evoked a different degree of euphoric state which lasted for 6-12 hours.

Without mentioning more details of the human electrophysiological studies in relation to the method being used, as well as to the effectiveness of ACTH peptides on this electrical correlate, some conclusions may be drawn from these observations.

1. ACTH 1-10, which has no potency to stimulate adrenocortical corticosteroid synthesis and secretion, showed similar action on stimulus-provoked EEG synchrony to ACTH 1-24.

2. Diminution of synchronizing activity as the result of ACTH peptide administration can be interpreted as less inhibition on the basis of the electrophysiological model used in the investigation (Endröczi et al., 1969).

3. Some psychological concomitants of peptide treatment are euphoric state, a degree of restlessness, which, in addition to changes in electrical correlates, suggest a disinhibitory or facilitatory effect of ACTH peptides. It would be difficult to interpret mechanisms underlying these processes in connection with a peptide effect on the CNS, and they need further investigations (Endröczi et al., 1969).

With regard to the observations that ACTH peptide can increase psychomotor activity in mentally healthy persons, attempts were made to influence extreme depressive states (schizophrenic patients) by treatment with daily administration of 3-6 mg ACTH 1-10 zinc phosphate (in collaboration with de Wied and Organon Research Labs, 1969). Elimination of depressive state, an increase in communication and remarkable changes in the mood could be achieved by the treatment within 5-7 days; psychiatric observations and control psychological tests were performed in collaboration with Endröczi et al., (1969). Further long-term studies are needed to completely verify and evaluate these results.

Effectiveness of hormones upon behavioral events has been observed in a large number of studies; however, their action on memory function is still obscure. Changes in memory can be attributed to an increase or decrease of attentive behavior, to altered emotionality and drive functions, as well as to changes of excitatory and inhibitory processes involved in the recall of earlier experiences. In recent experiments the administration of ACTH 1-10, but not ACTH 11-24, resulted in a marked suppression of "latent learning" or "incubation" followed by a passive avoidance test in rats. The experimental schedule of this study was as follows: 48 rats were tested for passive avoidance under 23-hour water deprivation and single electric shocks were given under drinking attempts for a period of three consecutive trials. After testing of passive avoidance learning the groups consisting of 12 rats were treated with ACTH 1-10, ACTH 11-24, corticosterone, and physiological saline. On the day following the passive avoidance test the animals were given injections (iv) with one of the materials mentioned above. Water was given to the animals in their home cage for 1 hour. The latency of the first drinking attempt in the experimental box was tested 48 hours after testing of passive avoidance learning (see Fig. 3). There was no significant difference between latencies of saline, corticosterone, or ACTH 11-24 treated groups; however, a marked lack of "latent learning" was found following treatment with ACTH 1-10 peptide. The failure of "latent learning" of this latter group may be related to an increase of exploratory activity and general motility being observed after injection of ACTH 1-10, and this assumption is in accordance with other findings which have been obtained both in human studies and animal experiments. It seems that this peptide can induce some disinhibitory effect which is accompanied by impairment of latent learning and increased excitatory state of the CNS.

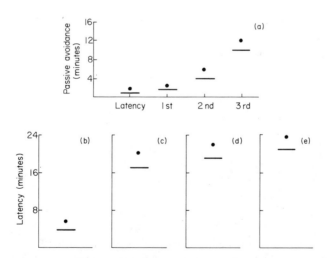

Fig. 3. Latency to drink following passive avoidance. (a) 5-day habituation; 23-hour water deprivation; 48 males rats. (b) 12 male rats treated with ACTH 1-10, 20 μg/100 grm. (c) 12 male rats treated with ACTH 11-24, 50 μg/100 gm. (d) 12 male rats treated with corticosterone (Compound B), 100μg/100 gm. (e) 12 male rats treated with physiological saline, 0.3 ml iv.

D. Some Aspects of Nonspecific and Specific Adaptive Endocrine Interactions and Their Influence on Conditioned Reflex Behavior

It is well known that thyroid hormones play a fundamental role in brain maturation and an early deficit of pituitary-thyroid function results in a "cretinoid state." There is a continually growing volume of research dealing with action of thyroid hormones on the learning behavior of adult animals (Bovet et al., 1962; Brody, 1942; Denenberg and Myers, 1958; Eayrs and Levine, 1963; Korn, 1967; Morrison and Cunningham, 1941; Sakata et al., 1966; Thompson and Kenshalo, 1954; de Wied and Pirie, 1968). A hypothyroid condition has been found to suppress both acquisition and extinction of CR's, and these studies refer to a general "weakening" of both facilitatory and inhibitory processes being involved in the establishment of temporary connections (Morrison and Cunningham, 1941; Richards and Stockburger, 1958; Sakata et al., 1966).

The contradictory findings which have been obtained with thyroxine administration may be aresult of a different amount of hormone being used in these studies, species differences, and differences in motivational states under which the learning has been tested (Bovet et al., 1962). Thus an acceleration of avoidance learning was motivational states under which the learning has been tested (Morrison and Cunningham, 1941; Thompson and Kenshalo, 1954).

Relatively few studies deal with the influence of thyroid hormones on intertrial activity during conditioning. An increase of intertrial activity of thyroidectomized rats has been observed during acquisition, and a decrease during extinction of a pole-jumping CR (de Wied and Pirie, 1968).

A direct influence of thyroid hormones on the CNS cannot be excluded in the adult; however, the passage of blood-brain barrier seems to be limited to the pituitary-stalk region. This is in contrast to the situation during the perinatal period when thyroid hormones can pass through the blood-brain barrier and affect metabolic processes at neuronal level (Eayrs, 1960). It seems that thyroid deficiency may affect central nervous processes by changes occurring in the body (microcirculation, autonomous nervous system, and metabolic processes) or by alterations of interactions between pituitary-thyroid and other pituitary-target organ functions.

In recent studies it was found that hypothyroid rats display higher exploratory rates both in $25°$ and $10°C$ environmental temperature, and in a drinking test following 23-hour water deprivation (Dupont et al., 1970). Moreover, hypothyroid rats showed a marked impairment of learning ability in the passive avoidance situation when single electric shocks were given to the rats during drinking attempts for a period of 20 minutes; the animals were kept on a fixed schedule of 23-hour water deprivation and habituated to the experimental situation for 5 days prior to testing of passive avoidance learning. Intact rats showed rapid learning in comparison to thyroidectomized animals which, despite the painful stimuli, displayed many more attempts to drink than the controls. From a behavioral point of view, a decreased learning rate of hypothyroid rats may be attributed to a reduced inhibition which corresponds to a reduction of fear, on one hand, and more exploratory activity in a novel situation, on the other. It would be difficult to interpret these behavioral findings in the light of human observations. However, basic metabolic influences of the pituitary-thyroid axis are similar in many species, although its interactions with other pituitary-target organs appear to vary during evolution.

One of the characteristic changes occurring in endocrine interactions in hypothyroid rats, is the hypofunction of the pituitary-adrenal axis. Studying the interactions between pituitary-thyroid and adrenocortical functions, a close correlation was found between thyroxine-induced increase of corticosterone-binding capacity of the rat plasma and negative feedback adjustment of pituitary ACTH secretion (Labrie *et al.,* 1968; Fortier *et al.,* 1970). The free, as opposed to total, corticosterone concentration is the variable under feedback control in the rat; in hypothyroid rats both concentration of circulating corticosterone and responsiveness of pituitary-adrenocortical axis is suppressed. An inverse correlation between plasma corticosterone concentration and intertrial activity, and a close relationship between pituitary-adrenocortical function and internal inhibition, on one hand, and a lowering of inhibition in hypothyroid state which is accompanied by a hypofunction of pituitary-adrenocortical axis, on the other, may be the basis for the assumption that both increased exploratory activity and "impaired" learning ability of thyroidectomized rats may be as a result of the concomitant hypofunction at the pituitary-adrenocortical level. In other mammals than the rat, hypothyroid state does not involve marked changes in the transcortin binding capacity of the plasma but results in a lowering of corticosteroid clearance rate and secretion of more polar corticosteroids as hydrocortisone. These events can markedly change the endocrine background which develops in hypothyroid state and lead to different behavioral manifestations.

IV. GENERAL DISCUSSION

Pavlov's contributions to our understanding of brain and behavior can be divided into two parts; first, the discovery of temporary connections and their interpretation in terms of conditioned reflex, and second, he introduced conditioning as technique into the physiological and psychological laboratories. Many students of experimental psychology believe that the theory of conditioned reflex is a rigid and outdated approach to animal behavior, which cannot be a starting point from an advanced neurobiological view. However, the development of classical Pavlovian conditioning as a technique and its combined use with other neurophysiological methods resulted in a growing body of information about neural function and learned behavior. Similarly, application of endocrine measures or controlled changes in the endocrine environment with simultaneous study of the establishment of temporary connections resulted in a vast amount of data about hormone actions on the brain and their effects on behavior.

Pavlov viewed the neuroanatomical substrate of temporary connections as a neural network which has tremendous plasticity and, at the same time, specificity to organize temporary connections between signals. He sought its location at the neocortical level. Today, as the result of an increasing amount of information as a consequence of ablating forebrain structures, there is no doubt that cortical structures are playing a role in establishment of temporary connections, as Pavlov concluded, and the excitatory and inhibitory processes which are involved in conditioned reflex events, are properties not only of cortical but subcortical structures.

Generally, speaking, temporary connections and memory functions cannot be separated; both functions show many common properties, although to study the laws which they obey requires different approaches. On the basis of our investigations, a goal-directed motor pattern which is acquired by the animal following one-trial learning can be considered as a situation conditioned reflex. This behavior pattern cannot be removed from the brain if it once has been established, but it can be facilitated or inhibited by changes of external or internal environment in the given situation. Obviously, recurrence of a goal-directed motor act implies memory of events which had been recalled by some kind of specific stimuli (conditional signal) or stimulus pattern.

Goal-directed motor pattern, memory function, and drive are factors which form a basic unit in the organization of any motivated behavior reaction. Drive as need of the organism organizes goal-directed motor patterns in the proper situation if the subject has previous experience, and this behavioral event represents the simplest form of memory. On the basis of this assumption, the three basic behavioral manifestations of living organisms—drive, goal-directed motor pattern and memory function—cannot be separated from each other. Naturally, during the course of evoluation an increasing volume of memory processes can be stored as the result of differentiation of forebrain structures, and impairment of memory function appears in hierarchical order of its stability and time.

Changes of chemical environment produce instability of the living homeostat, and under physiological circumstances readjustment of this equilibrium is mediated by the reinforcing and drive-reducing character of goal-directed behavior reactions. Reinforcing value of a goal-directed motor act cannot be measured as a physical quantity; it is an intrinsic property of a goal-directed reaction and its intensity depends on the previous experience of the individual, the goal-object and the species.

Miller (1959) formulated a "reinforcement" or "reinforcement-drive reduction" theory, and attempted to correlate reinforcement with reward as well as drive reduction. Olds (1962) suggested a rewarding effect of positive self-stimulation and supposed that this behavioral phenomenon is accompanied by subjective feelings such as pleasure. From behavioral and electrophysiological observations we have concluded that positive self-stimulation is a rebound phenomenon, and this is a consequence of a short-term artificial increase of internal inhibition in the absence of extrinsic reinforcement. A rebound integration of goal-directed motor pattern which was going on in the situation has been assumed to be the function of ascending activatory system. A corresponding reversal effect, namely, a long-term inhibition of a goal-directed motor pattern, may be evoked by stimulation of ascending activatory system (Endröczi and Lissák, 1962; Lissák and Endröczi, 1965; Endröczi, 1969). Moreover, it has been assumed that descending forebrain inhibition plays an important role in the elaboration of different forms of internal inhibitory processes, and as the result of prior activities it plays a fundamental role in decoding of environmental information.

An increasing number of observations support the view that humoral factors affect central nervous processes by changing thresholds of excitatory and inhibitory nervous circuits. More than two decades ago, Beach (1948) proposed that sexual steroids affect brain and behavior relations through changes in thresholds within the CNS. Electrophysiological investigations revealed that sexual steroids can change excitability in brain stem and diencephalic structures, and such changes are correlated with control of pituitary gonadotropin secretion and reproductive behavior.

In connection with the influence of pituitary-adrenocortical hormones we have already assumed that they affect basal forebrain inhibitory structures, and these influences play a role in negative feedback control of pituitary ACTH secretion and in the hormonal support of internal inhibition (Endröczi and Lissák, 1962; Lissák and Endröczi, 1965; Endröczi, 1969).

Behavioral manifestations occurring in the response to a lack or an excess amount of corticosteroids are situation-dependent events, In active avoidance conditioning (e.g., shuttlebox) where integration of goal-directed motor patterns requires a certain degree of differential inhibition which can be suppressed by an overwhelming tonical inhibition, an excess amount of corticosteroids may result in a suppression of CR. In the passive avoidance situation when the inhibition of a goal-directed motor pattern is the measure of temporary connections, an exaggerated activation of pituitary-adrenocortical function or exogenously increased plasma corticosteroid level may increase learning. Therefore it would

204 E. Endröczi

be difficult to conclude that pituitary-adrenocortical hormones facilitate or inhibit learning. It is certain that the pituitary-adrenocortical axis has a definite influence on avoidance behavior, although the direction of its influence depends on the motivational state of the organism and the situation under which temporary connections have been established. Therefore, a simplification of adaptation theory like the stress concept is a misleading way to understand the functional relationships between adaptive behavior and adaptive neuroendocrine processes.

References

Adametz, J. H. (1959). *J. Neurosurg.* **16**, 85.
Astratyan, E. A. (1941). *Fiziol. Zh. SSSR im. I.M. Sechenova* **30**, 13.
Astratyan, E. A. (1952). In "Problems of Higher Nervous Activity" (E. A. Astratyan, ed.), pp. 68-99. Gosisdat, Leningrad.
Ban, T. (1964). *Med. J. Osaka Univ.* **15**, 1.
Beach, F. A. (1947). *Physiol. Rev.* **27**, 240.
Beach, F. A. (1948). "Hormones and Behavior." Harper (Hoeber), New York.
Belenkov, F. A. (1950). *Bull, Exp. Biol. Med. (USSR)* **29**, 100, 182.
Berlyne, D. E. (1960). "Conflict, Arousal and Curiosity." McGraw-Hill, New York.
Bleuler, M. (1954). "Endokrinologische Psychiatrie." Thieme, Stuttgart.
Bohus, B., and Endröczi, E. (1965). *Acta Physiol.* **26**, 183.
Bohus, B., and Korányi, L. (1969). In "Recent Developments of Neurobiology in Hungary" (K. Lissak, ed.), Vol. 2, pp. 41-76. Akademia Kiado, Budapest.
Bovet, D., Bovet-Nitti, F., Bignami, G., and Orshinger, O. (1962). In "Perspective in Biology" (C. F. Cori, V. C. Foglia, L. F. Leloir, and S. Ochoa, eds.), pp. 210-221. Elsevier, Amsterdam.
Brody, E. B. (1942). *J. Comp. Psychol.* **34**, 213.
Brogden, W. J. (1939). *J. Exp. Psychol.* **25**, 232.
Brogden, W. J., Lipman, E. A., and Culler, E. (1938). *Amer. J. Psychol.* **51**, 109.
Browne, J. S. L. (1952). *Ciba Found. Colloq.* **3**, 197.
Buckle, R. M. (1962). *J. Endocrinol.* **25**, 189.
Chow, K. L. (1954). *AMA Arch. Neurol. Psychiat.* **71**, 762.
Chow, K. L., and Randall, W. (1964). *Psychonom. Sci.* **1**, 259.
Cleghorn, R. A. (1952). *Ciba Found. Colloq.* **3**, 187.
Crisler, G. (1930). *Amer. J. Physiol.* **94**, 553.
Culler, E. A. (1938). *Psychol. Bull.* **35**, 687.
Dell, P. (1958). In "Neurological Basis of Behavior" (G. E. W. Wolstenholme and C. M. O'Connor, eds.), pp. 187-203. Little, Brown, Boston, Massachusetts.
Denenberg, V. H., and Myers, R. D. (1958). *J. Comp. Physiol. Psychol.* **51**, 311.
Deutsch, J. A. (1963). *J. Theor. Biol.* **4**, 193.
De Wied, D. (1966). *Proc. Soc. Exp. Biol. Med.* **122**, 28.
De Wied, D., and Pirie, G. (1968). *Physiol. Behav.* **3**, 355.
Doty, R. W., and Giurgea, C. (1961). In "Brain Mechanisms and Learning" (J. F. Delafrasnaye, ed.), pp. 133-151. Blackwell, Oxford.
Doty, R. W., Beck, E. C., and Kooi, K. A. (1959). *Exp. Neurol.* **1**, 360.
Dupont, A., Endröczi, E., and Fortier, C. (1970). *Meeting Int. Soc. Psycho-Neuroendocrinol., 1st*, New York.

Eayrs, J. T. (1960). *Brit. Med. Bull.* **16**, 122.

Eayrs, J. T., and Levine, S. (1963). *J. Endocrinol.* **25**, 505.

Eisenfeld, A. J., and Axelrod, J. (1965). *J. Pharmacol. Exp. Ther.* **150**, 469.

Endröczi, E. (1968). Unpublished data.

Endröczi, E. (1969). *In* "Recent Developments of Neurobiology in Hungary" (K. Lissak, ed.), Vol. 2, pp. 27-50. Akademia Kiado, Budapest.

Endröczi, E., and Lissák, K. (1962). *Acta Physiol.* **21**, 265.

Endröczi, E., Telegdy, Gy., and Lissák, K. (1958). *Acta Physiol.* **14**, 353.

Endröczi, E., Telegdy, Gy., and Lissák, K. (1959). *Acta Physiol.* **11**, 393.

Endröczi, E., Hartmann, G., Korányi, L., and Nyakas, Cs. (1968). *Acta Phsyiol.* **33**, 375.

Endröczi, E., Fekete, T., Lissák, K., and de Wied, D. (1970). *Progr. Brain Res.*, **32**, 254.

Feldman, S. (1970). *UCLA Workshop Conf.* (In press).

Feldman, S., Todt, J. C., and Porter, R. W., (1961). *Neurology* **11**, 109.

Fortier, C., a23, Labrie, F., Pelletier, G., Raynaud, J. P., Ducommun, P., Delgado, A., Labrie, R., and Ho-Kim, M. A. (1970). *In* "Ciba Foundation Collection" (G. E. W. Wolstenholme, and J. Knight, eds.), pp. 178-209. Churchill, London.

Fuxe, K. (1965). *Acta Physiol. Scand. Suppl.* **247**, 39.

Giurgea, C. (1953). "Elaborarea reflexului conditionat prin excitarea directa a scoartei cerebrale." Edit. Acad. Roman. Rep., Bucharest.

Grossman, S. P. (1969). *Ann. N. Y. Acad. Sci.* **157**, 902.

Guillery, R. W. (1957). *J. Anat.* **91**, 91.

Guthrie, E. R. (1942). "Conditioning: A Theory of Learning in Terms of Stimulus, Response and Associations." A forty-first yearbook. Nat. Soc. for the Study of Education, Bloomington, Ill.

Harris, G. W. (1964). *Endocrinology* **75**, 627.

Havelane, J., and Paul, C. (1963). Maze learning and open-field behavior of adrenalectomized rats. *Midwest. Psychol. Meeting, May, 1963* Abstract.

Hernandez-Peon, R. (1963). *Electroencephalog. Clin. Neurophysiol.* **24**, 188.

Hilgard, E. R. (1936). *Psychol. Rev.* **43**, 366.

Hilgard, E. R. (1948). "Theories of Learning." Appleton, New York.

Hilgard, E. R., and Marquis, D. G. (1940). "Conditioning and Learning." Appleton, New York.

Hollenberg, C. H., Raben, M. S. and Astwood, E. B. (1961). *Endocrinology* **68**, 589.

Hull, C. L. (1943). "Principles of Behavior. An Introduction to Behavior Study." Appleton, New York.

Jasper, H. (1949). *Electroencephalog. Clin. Neurophysiol.* **1**, 405.

Jouvet, M. (1961). *In* "The Nature of Sleep" (G. E. W. Wolstenholme, and M. O. O'Connor, eds.), pp. 188-261. Churchill, London.

Kato, J., and Villee, C. A. (1967). *Endocrinology* **80**, 567.

Kellogg, W. N., Scott, B. V., and Davis, R. C. (1940). *J. Comp. Physiol. Psychol.* **29**, 43.

Kesner, R. P., Fiedler, P., and Thomas, G. J. (1967). *J. Comp. Physiol. Psychol.* **63**, 452.

Koffka, K. (1935). "The Principles of Gestalt Psychology." Harcourt, New York.

Kohler, W. (1929). "Gestalt-Psychology." Liveright, New York.

Korányi, L., and Endröczi, E. (1965). *Acta Physiol.* **26**, 377.

Korányi, L., and Endröczi, E. (1967). *Neuroendocrinology* **2**, 65.

Korányi, L., Endröczi, E., and Lissák, K. (1963). *J. Psychosom. Med.* **11**, 159.

Korányi, L., Endröczi, E., and Tamásy, V. (1969). *Acta Physiol.* **36**, 73.

Korn, J. H. (1967). *J. Genet. Psychol.* **110**, 169.

Krivoy, W. A., Lane M., and Kroeger, D. D. (1963). *Ann. N. Y. Acad. Sci.* **104**, 312.

Kuo, Z. Y. (1921). *J. Phil.* **18**, 645.

Labrie, F., Pelletier, G., Labrie, R., Ho-Kim, M. A., Delgado, A., Macintosh, B., and Fortier, C. (1968). *Ann. Endocrinol.* **29**, 29.

Lashley, K. S. (1950). *Symp. Soc. Exp. Biol.* **4**, 454.

Levine, S., and Jones, L. E. (1965). *J. Comp. Physiol. Psychol.* **59**, 357.

Lewin, K. (1936). "Principles of Topological Psychology." McGraw-Hill, New York.

Li, C. H. (1956). *Advan. Protein Chem.* **11**, 101.

Li, C. H., and Oelofsen, W. (1967). *In* "Adrenal Cortex" (A. B. Eisenstein, ed.), pp. 185-201. Little, Brown, Boston, Massachusetts.

Li, C. H., Fønss-Bech, P., Geschwind, I. I., Hayashida, T., Hungerford, G. F., Lostroh, A. J., Lyons, W. R., Moon, H. D., Reinhardt, W. O., and Sideman, M. (1957). *J. Exp. Med.* **105**, 335.

Li, C. H., Ramachandran, J., Chung, D., and Gorup, B. (1964). *J. Amer. Chem. Soc.* **86**, 2703.

Liddell, H. S., Kotyuka, O., Anderson, O., and Hartman, F. A. (1935). *Arch. Neurol. Psychiat.* **34**, 973.

Light, J. S., and Gantt, W. H. (1936). *J. Comp. Psychol.* **21**, 19.

Lindsley, D. B., Bowden, J. W., and Magoun, H. W. (1949). *Electroencephalogr. Clin. Neurophysiol.* **1**, 475.

Lissák, K. (1969). *In* "Recent Developments of Neurobiology in Hungary" (K. Lissák, ed.), Vol. 2, pp. 1-26. Akademia Kiado, Budapest.

Lissák, K., and Endröczi, E. (1960) "Die Neuroendokrine Steuerung der Adaptationstatifkeit." Akademia Kiado, Budapest.

Lissák, K., and Endröczi, E. (1965)' "The Neuroendocrine Control of Adaptation." Pergamon, Oxford.

Lissák, K., and Endröczi, E., and Medgyesi, P. (1957). *Pfluegers Arch. Gesamte Physiol.* **117**, 265.

Loucks, R. B. (1935). *J. Psychol.* **1**, 5.

Loucks, R. B., and Gantt, W. H. (1938). *J. Comp. Psychol.* **25**, 415.

Maier, N. R. R., and Schneirla, T. C. (1942). *Psychol. Rev.* **49**, 117.

Markel, E., and Adam, G. (1969). *Acta Physiol.* **36**, 265.

McEwen, B. S., Weiss, J. M., and Schwartz, L. S. (1970). *Brain Res.* **17**, 471.

Miller, N. E. (1948). *J. Exp. Psychol.* **38**, 89.

Miller, N E. (1959). *In* "Psychology: A Study of a Science" (S. Koch, ed.), Vol. 2, pp. 196-292. McGraw-Hill, New York.

Miller, N. E. (1966). *Science* **148**, 328.

Miller, N. E., and Dollard, J. (1941). "Social Learning and Imitation." Yale Univ. Press, New Haven, Connecticut.

Miller, R. E., and Ogawa, N. (1962). *J. Comp. Physiol. Psychol.* **55** 211.

Mirsky, I., Miller, R., and Stein, M. (1953). *Psychosom. Med.* **15**, 574.

Morgane, P. J. (1961) *J. Comp. Neurol.* **117**, 1.

Morgane, P. J. (1969). *Ann. N. Y. Acad. Sci.* **157**, 806.

Morrison G. W., and Cunningham, B. (1941). *J. Comp. Physiol. Psychol.* **31**,413.

Moruzzi, G., and Magoun, H. W. (1949). *Electroencephalogr. Clin. Neurophysiol.* **1** 455.

Moss, F. A. (1924). *J. Exp. Psychol.* **7** 165.

Mowrer, O. H. (1947). *Harvard Educ. Rev.* **17**, 102.

Mowrer, O. H. (1960). "Learning Theory and Behavior." Wiley, New York.

Moyer, K. E. (1958). *J. Genet. Psychol.* **92**, 11.

Moyer, K. E., and Moshein, P. (1963). *J. Comp. Physiol. Psychol.* **56**, 163.

Munn, N. L. (1939). *J. Genet. Psychol.* **21**, 119.

Murphy, J. V., and Miller, R. E. (1955). *J. Comp. Physiol. Psychol.* **48**, 47.

Nauta, W. J. H. (1963). *Advan. Neuroendocrinol. Proc. Symp. 1961,* 5-25.

Olds, J. (1962). *Physiol. Rev.* **42,** 554.

Ordzonikidze, T., and Nutsubidze, M. (1959). *Tr. Inst. Fiziol. Akad. Nauk Gruz. SSR* **12,** 85.

Pavlov, I. P. (1902). "The Work of the Digestive Glands," transl. by W. H. Thompson. Griffin, London.

Pavlov, I. P. (1927). "Conditioned Reflexes." Oxford Univ. Press, London and New York.

Perrin, F. A. C., and Klein, D. B. (1926). "Psychology." Holt, New York.

Peters, R. H., Rosvold, H. E., and Mirsky, A. F. (1956). *J. Comp. Physiol. Psychol.* **49,** 111.

Popov, N. (1950). *Byull. Eksp. Biol. Med.* **30,** 1.

Razra, G. H. S. (1939). *Psychol. Rev.* **46,** 264.

Reiss, M. (1958). "Psycho-neuroendocrinology." Grune & Stratton, New York.

Richards, W. J., and Stockburger, J. C. (1958). *J. Comp. Physiol. Psychol.* **51,** 445.

Rosenberg, I. N. (1953). *Proc. Soc. Exp. Biol. Med.* **82,** 701.

Routtenberg, A. (1968). *Psychol. Rev.* **75,** 51.

Sakata, T., Agari, S., Kawasaki, S., Kuwahara, H., and Ogawa, N. (1966). *Fukuoka-Igaku-Zasshi* **57,** 752.

Schlosberg, H. (1934). *J. Genet. Psychol.* **45,** 303.

Schlosberg, H. (1937). *Psychol. Rev.* **44,** 379.

Schneirla, T. C. (1946). *J. Abnorm. Soc. Psychol.* **41,** 385.

Sheffield, F. D. (1948). *J. Comp. Physiol. Psychol.* **41,** 165.

Skinner, B. F. (1935). *J. Genet. Psychol.* **12,** 66. (1935). *J. Genet. Psychol.* **12,** 66.

Skinner, B. F. (1938). "The Behavior of Organisms." Appleton, New York.

Stumpf, W. E. (1968). *Science* **162,** 1001.

Sutin, J., and Eager, R. P. (1969). *Ann. N. Y. Acad. Sci.* **157,** 610.

Ten Cate, J. (1934). *Arch. Neerl. Physiol.* **19,** 191.

Thompson, R., and Kenshalo, D. R. (1954). *J. Comp. Physiol. Psychol.* **47,** 36.

Thorndike, E. L. (1898). *Psychol. Monogr.* **2,** No. 8.

Thorndike, E. L., "Animal Intelligence." Macmillan, New York.

Tolman, E. C. (1934). *In* "Comparative Psychology" (F. A. Moss, ed.). Prentice-Hall, Englewood Cliffs, New Jersey.

Warren, J. M., and Akert, K. (1960). *J. Comp. Physiol. Psychol.* **53,** 207.

Wertheim, G. A., Conner, R. L., and Levine, S. (1967). *J. Exp. Anal. Behav.* **10,** 555.

Whatmore, G. B., Morgan, E. A., and Kleitman, N. (1946). *Amer. J. Physiol.* **145,** 432.

Woodworth, R. S. (1921). "Psychology. A Study of Mental Life." Holt, New York.

Woodworth, R. S. (1947). *Amer. J. Psychol.* **60,** 119.

Zeliony, G. (1911). *Trans. Soc. Russ. Phys.* 80-88.

Zeliony, G. (1930). *Exp. Biol. Med. (USSR).* **14,** 3-18.

7
Hormones, Biogenic Amines, and Aggression

R. L. Conner

I. INTRODUCTION

Numerous authors have emphasized that aggression is not a unitary concept, but rather refers to a broad class of complex behavior patterns. Moyer (1968) has described seven types of behavioral patterns usually included under the general heading of aggression: predatory aggression, inter-male spontaneous aggression, terror-induced aggression, irritable aggression, territorial defense, defense of the young, and instrumental aggression. In the present paper, three specific types of aggressive behavior will be considered: isolation-induced fighting in mice, shock-induced fighting in rats and mice, and mouse and/or frog killing behavior in rats. These three kinds of aggressive behavior represent particular examples under Moyer's categories of inter-male spontaneous aggression, irritable aggression, and predatory aggression, respectively. Insofar as is possible, the materials to be presented here will be grouped around specific chemical compounds under each specific type of aggressive behavior. Under a separate heading (Social Behavior, Section V), some data relating various chemical compounds to behavioral patterns which are directly or indirectly related to aggressive behavior will be discussed. The electrical stimulation and brain ablation data will not be covered except when such data elucidates a particular relationship between hormones or biogenic amines and aggressive behavior.

The organization of the materials in this chapter reflects a recognition that the various behavioral patterns termed aggressive may bear little relationship among one another. One should not, therefore, expect a common underlying physiological mechanism (Brown and Hunsperger, 1963; Karczmar and Scudder, 1969; Moyer, 1968). At the same time, however, it must be recognized that physiological systems do not function independently. It is generally recognized that the functioning of the endocrine system is under the control of higher nervous centers, especially the hypothalamus (cf. Chapter 2), and there are numerous interactions among the various endocrine systems. The monoamines play an important role in the sympathetic nervous system, and evidence is accumulating that these compounds may also serve as neurotransmitters in the central nervous system (CNS) (cf. Chapter 8). Some of the possible interactions between brain monoamines and endocrine function are discussed in Chapter 2. For further information and current evidence about these interactions, the reader is referred to the report of a workshop devoted to this topic (Wurtman, 1971). In the present chapter, the relations of the endocrine hormones and biogenic amines to aggressive behavior will be discussed under separate headings.

Since pharmacological procedures are frequently employed in laboratory studies of aggressive behavior, some comments are in order. It is often easy to show a behavioral effect of injecting a drug into an organism. But the determination of the biological mechanism mediating the drug effect on behavior is usually another matter. Parameters such as dose, method of administration, onset of action, duration of action, site of action, metabolism, interactions with other systems, and side effects are of paramount importance in the assessment of the behavioral effects of drugs. Further, there are intra- and interstrain and genus differences in response to exogenously administered drugs, and chronic administration may produce very different effects than acute treatment. Thus, while pharmacological techniques are valuable tools in the analysis of behavior, one must exercise caution in the interpretation of the behavioral effects of drugs (Dews, 1962; Tedeschi and Tedeschi, 1968).

During the past decade, there has been an increasing effort to experimentally isolate and analyze the biological mechanisms underlying the expression of aggressive behavior. There are some excellent reviews available (Boelkins and Heiser, 1970; Carthy and Ebling, 1964; Clemente and Lindsley, 1967; Davis, 1964; Moyer, 1968; Scott, 1966) as well as a volume containing the proceedings of an international symposium on aggressive behavior (Garattini and Sigg, 1969). The older literature has been reviewed by Collias (1944).

II. ISOLATION-INDUCED FIGHTING

Most of the systematic evidence relating biochemical events to aggressive behavior has been derived from studies of isolation-induced fighting among male mice. Following a period of social isolation, male mice will engage in a characteristic behavioral sequence with one another which usually culminates in an attack. The behavioral characteristics and the experimental parameters of this phenomenon have been described by Scott (1966) and others (cf. Garattini and Sigg, 1969). Only male mice generally show the phenomenon, although there are several reports that female mice of some strains may also fight following isolation (Ginsburg and Allee, 1942; Weltman et al., 1968). The isolation usually consists of confinement of individual animals in small cages for periods ranging from several days to several weeks. There are marked differences among strains of mice in their readiness to fight following this treatment (Southwick and Clark, 1968). Rats generally do not exhibit the phenomenon. Following the period of isolation, the mice are usually tested in pairs, but in some studies the mice have been tested in groups of three or more. If the pairings remain constant, one mouse is likely to emerge as dominant after repeated tests; if each mouse is successively paired with every other mouse in the sample (the "round-robin" technique) dominance relations take much longer to develop. Mice can also be trained to fight ("trained fighters") by repeated exposure to a nonisolated mouse, usually done by dangling the nonisolate by the tail in the immediate vicinity of the isolate.

A. Pituitary-Gonadal System

There are hardly any data relating pituitary gonadotropic hormones [luteinizing hormone (LH) and follicle-stimulating hormone (FSH)] to the expression of isolation-induced fighting. Eleftheriou and Church (1967) exposed mice to trained fighting mice and studied the effects of such exposure on pituitary and plasma levels of LH. They found that plasma LH was significantly elevated in defeated mice. Most of the studies relating pituitary-gonadal hormones to isolation-induced fighting have examined the role of androgens on this kind of aggressive behavior.

1. Androgens

Beeman (1947) used the round-robin testing technique in an early demonstration of the important role that androgens play in isolation-induced fighting. She reported that castration virtually abolished fighting behavior, and subcutaneous implants of pellets of testosterone propionate (TP) reinstated the behavior. (TP is frequently used in such studies because it is longer-acting than testosterone.) There are several lines of evidence for the involvement of androgens in the expression of isolation-induced fighting. First is the observation that the first appearance of fighting following isolation generally coincides with puberty, when there occurs a marked increase in the amount of circulating androgen (Fredericson, 1950; Levy and King, 1953). Second, administration of TP to sexually immature mice results in the appearance of fighting at a much earlier age than seen in untreated mice (Levy and King, 1953). While these findings have been generally confirmed, subsequent data indicate that numerous other variables may be as important as androgen in mediating fighting behavior. The effect of castration and/or androgen treatment on aggressive behavior following isolation has also been shown to be a function of strain and genetic factors (Fredericson et al., 1955; Ginsburg and Allee, 1942; Marie Antonita et al., 1968), past experience (Uhrich, 1938), learning and conditioning (Ginsburg and Allee, 1942; Scott, 1958), age (Uhrich, 1938), time and duration of castration (J. M. Bevan et al., 1958), testing procedure (Moyer, 1968), biological potency of replacement androgen (W. Bevan et al., 1957), and dosage and frequency of hormone replacement (J. H. Bevan et al., 1958). Other variables could also be included on this list. In discussing the inconsistent effects of castration on aggressive behavior, both within and between species, Guhl (1961) concludes that "... the experimenter's connotation of aggressive behavior and the method of its measurement may result in variations in the interpretation of the effects of castration."

To elaborate on just one of the variables in the above list, consider how the effects of castration may be modulated by past experience. With respect to sex behavior, it often has been observed that castration of males does not usually lead to an immediate cessation of copulation, in fact, in some instances among sexually experienced higher mammals, such as cats and dogs, castration of the male does not seem to markedly impair coital behavior for some time (Beach, 1970; Rosenblatt and Aronson, 1958). However, if a sexually inexperienced animal (or a prepuberal animal) is castrated, the results indicate that androgens *and experience* are necessary for the full expression of sex behavior. Similar data have been obtained with respect to aggressive behavior. Uhrich (1938) and others (Yen et al., 1962) have shown that prepuberal castration more effectively decreases adult fighting in mice than postpuberal castration. Further, mice isolated at weaning subsequently fight more reliably than those isolated at a later age (Uhrich, 1938). Finally, J. M. Bevan *et al.* (1958) have noted that castration does not completely abolish isolation-induced fighting in all mice. These observations emphasize the role of past experience in the expression of aggressive behavior. The role of past experience in mediating the effects of rearing mice in isolation as opposed to group rearing has been discussed by Scott (1958, 1966). He has postulated a passive inhibition process, i.e., "a habit of not-fighting built up simply by not-fighting" in grouped conditions, and, according to Scott, this habit may become associated with certain environmental conditions.

2. Estrogens

In most mammalian species the males typically exhibit more aggressive behavior than the females. This observation is possibly the basis for the hypothesis that estrogens are inhibitors of aggressive behavior (cf. Rothballer, 1967). In studies with male mice, estrogen administered at weanling age did not affect the development of isolation-induced fighting, but estrogen was found to inhibit fighting in mature males (Suchowsky *et al.*, 1969; Terdiman and Levy, 1954). Mugford and Nowell (1970a) have shown that the tendency for male mice to attack females was significantly increased if the females were given a course of testosterone treatments. According to Mugford and Nowell (1970a,b), the female releases a pheromone in her urine which normally inhibits attack, and the treatment with androgen appears to suppress this urinary substance, thus changing her stimulus properties. Other data relating the hormones of the female reproductive system to aggressive behavior will be discussed later (see Section V, B).

3. Early Hormones

It has been suggested (Harris, 1964; Young, 1961) that one of the major differences between genetic males and females lies in the differential organization of the CNS. The role of the gonadal hormones in promoting this differential organization during the perinatal period is discussed in Chapter 3. Several studies have been reported which describe the effects of gonadal hormones present during the neonatal period on male and female behavioral patterns other than sex behavior. Since the expression of aggressive behavior is sexually dimorphic in most mammalian species, this behavior provides an excellent opportunity to determine if the effects of neonatal hormone treatments extend to sexually dimorphic behavior patterns other than sex behavior. Edwards (1968) administered TP to female mice on the day of birth and tested the animals in adulthood using the isolation-induced fighting paradigm. Before TP was administered in adulthood, none of the mice fought. After TP administration, however, more than 90% of the female mice showed fighting during at least one test. These findings are particularly striking since female mice do not normally exhibit fighting in response to isolation, even after TP administration (Levy, 1954; Tollman and King, 1956). Data reported by Bronson and Desjardins (1968) are in agreement with the Edwards findings, and further, suggest that estrogen administered to female mice neonatally may mimic some of the effects of neonatal androgen. These data indicate that gonadal hormones play a dual role in mediating aggressive behavior as well as sex behavior. Early in development hormones promote differentiation of the physiological mechanisms underlying the expression of male-like patterns of behavior. In the absence of androgens, as in genetic females or neonatally castrated males, the physiological substrate mediating female-like patterns of behavior develop. The hormones are also involved in the expression of behavior in adulthood when the sexually differentiated brain is more susceptible to the action of specific gonadal hormones.

B. Pituitary-Adrenal System

We turn now to a consideration of the data relating the hormones of the pituitary-adrenal system to isolation-induced fighting behavior. The pituitary-adrenal system is sometimes referred to as the hypothalamo-hypophyseal-adrenocortical axis in order to emphasize the role of the hypothalamus in this negative feedback neuroendocrine system. The system is activated by sensory stimuli or affective states which cause the release of a neurochemical factor from the hypothalamus known as corticotropin-releasing factor (CRF). This neurohumor is transmitted by the blood circulating in the hypothalamic-hypophyseal portal vessels to the anterior pituitary where it causes release of adrenocorticotropic hormone (ACTH). The action of ACTH on the adrenal cortex leads to synthesis and release of glucocorticoids which play a characteristic role in peripheral reactions to stressful stimuli. The glucocorticoids also reach the hormone-sensitive areas in the brain which are responsible for regulating the release of CRF and exert an inhibitory action on these areas.

It is of interest to note that the technique most often used to evoke aggressive behavior among male mice itself has an influence on pituitary-adrenal function. Isolation of male mice produces adrenal atrophy and a lowered level of adrenal activity in the absence of "stress," and possibly accentuates the magnitude of the adrenocorticoid response to stress (Welch and Welch, 1969a). This observation has been interpreted as evidence that isolated mice are more easily aroused, and are hyperresponsive to changes in level of stimulation (Welch, 1965).

Almost any change, especially abrupt ones, in the quantitative or qualitative properties of the stimuli impinging upon an organism will evoke an increase in the activity of the pituitary-adrenal system. It is not surprising, therefore, that high levels of plasma adrenocorticoids have frequently been reported after fighting episodes in mice (e.g., Bronson and Eleftheriou, 1965a,b; Yen *et al.,* 1962). Fighting behavior thus takes its place alongside innumerable other conditions, as well as various chemical and physical agents which are "stressful." The data derived from gland ablation studies do not go very far in suggesting a strong relationship between the pituitary-adrenal system and isolation-induced fighting behavior. Removal of the adrenal glands in male mice does not influence the development of expression of isolation-induced aggression (Yen *et al.,* 1962). While hypophysectomy does inhibit the development and expression of isolation-induced aggression in male mice (Sigg, 1969; Yen *et al.,* 1962), this effect is most likely accounted for on the basis of the absence of pituitary gonadotropins (and therefore androgen), or on the basis of gross skeletomotor debilitation, and is probably independent of the pituitary-adrenal system.

Kostowski *et al.* (1970) studied the effects of adrenal steroids in male mice isolated for 14 or 28 days and tested for fighting in groups of three. Hydrocortisone (15 mg/kg) increased fighting in this situation, but this finding is compromised by the high dose used and the observation that the treated mice also exhibited increased sensitivity to handling and increased general motor activity. Hydroxydione (20 mg/kg) suppressed fighting behavior and deoxycorticosterone (DOC) was without effect.

C. Biogenic Amines

Chemical compounds to be discussed under this heading include acetylcholine (ACh) and the indoleamine, serotonin (5-hydroxytryptamine, 5-HT). These compounds are generally thought to serve as synaptic neurotransmitter agents in the CNS, but the evidence is still equivocal on this point. Along with 5-HT and ACh, the catecholamines (CA) dopamine (DA), norepinephrine (NE), and epinephrine (E) belong to a class of compounds referred to as biogenic amines. Biogenic amines are synthesized both peripherally and in the brain and are characterized by the presence of an amino group. Since endogenous concentrations of the biogenic amines normally remain constant, estimates of the utilization rates of these compounds are the best indicators of possible biochemical-behavioral relationships in the intact animal. The importance of some estimate of the dynamic aspects of synthesis, release, and inactivation of biogenic amines is underscored by the observation that changes in utilization rates of biogenic amines may not be reflected by measures of static levels (Garattini *et al.,* 1967). Barchas *et al.* have discussed the concept of utilization rate and have described some of the techniques used to estimate it (see Chapter 8). The changes in the utilization rates of 5-HT and NE accompanying isolation will be discussed below, but no such data for ACh are presently available since methods for measuring ACh utilization rates are new and technically difficult.

1. *Serotonin*

Because of some unique aspects of the isolation-induced fighting phenomenon, several distinct experimental questions have been examined. Since pairs of mice will generally exhibit spontaneous fighting behavior only after a period of isolation, several investigators have examined the effects of isolation on 5-HT levels and utilization rates in the brain. Results from these studies indicate that levels are not changed but utilization of brain 5-HT is lower in individually housed than in group-housed male mice (Garattini *et al.*, 1967, 1969). Female mice, on the other hand, do not generally exhibit spontaneous fighting following isolation, nor do they show decreased rates of 5-HT utilization following isolation (Garattini *et al.*, 1969). Furthermore, there is some evidence that this decrement in utilization of brain 5-HT following isolation is most pronounced in the male mice of those strains which readily exhibit aggression following isolation (Garattini *et al.*, 1969). Finally, rats do not show changes in either brain 5-HT metabolism or fighting behavior following isolation. Taken together, these observations suggest a relation between brain 5-HT metabolism and isolation in mice.

The critical question, however, is to what extent are changes in brain 5-HT following isolation necessary for, and specific to, the occurrence of aggressive behavior. The available evidence on this point does not permit an unequivocal answer. Some observations that may indirectly bear on the question would indicate that reduced 5-HT metabolism is not a direct cause of the fighting behavior seen after isolation. First, there are independent reports of the effects of isolation on fighting and on brain 5-HT utilization rates. Following isolation, there are marked strain differences among mice in fighting behavior, and probably in brain 5-HT utilization rates as well. But there are no reports in the literature describing a relationship between 5-HT utilization rates and fighting behavior among various strains of mice. Second, Garattini *et al.* (1969) found that changes in brain 5-HT metabolism may be seen on the first day of isolation, but that the emergence of aggressive behavior generally requires more than 1 day of isolation. Finally, Essman (1969) has found that biochemical changes persist even following prolonged isolation or increasing age, but there is a trend toward decreasing behavioral differences with either prolonged isolation or increasing age.

Turning now to a consideration of the relation between brain 5-HT and the fighting episode itself, it has been reported that mice show an abrupt increase in brain 5-HT levels when they are brought together and fought (Welch and Welch, 1969b). But increases in brain 5-HT levels are hardly unique to fighting. For example, restraint stress, acute exposure to cold, and *d*-amphetamine may also effect an elevation of brain 5-HT content (B. L. Welch and A. S. Welch, 1968). The interpretation of the relevance of elevated brain 5-HT levels with respect to fighting is further complicated by the observation that changes in 5-HT utilization rates may not be reflected by changes in 5-HT levels (Garattini *et al.*, 1967).

When whole brain 5-HT levels were lowered pharmacologically by treatment with *p*-chlorophenylalanine (PCPA), a compound which inhibits the enzymic action of tryptophan hydroxylase, a decrement in the fighting behavior of previously isolated mice was observed (A. S. Welch and B. L. Welch, 1968). However, isolated mice also fought less if whole brain 5-HT levels were elevated by administration of the 5-HT precursor, 5-hydroxytryptophan (5-HTP) (Welch and Welch, 1969a). In fact, according to Welch and Welch, almost any pharmacological manipulation of the isolated mouse will decrease its tendency to engage in fighting behavior. Thus, while there might be a link between brain 5-HT metabolism and isolation-induced fighting behavior, the evidence of a strong relationship is not very compelling.

2. Catecholamines

Isolation of male mice also effects changes in levels and utilization rates of brain CA. As a function of isolation, whole brain levels of NE but not DA are lowered, and utilization rates for both of these amines are decreased. Peripherally, both levels and utilization rates of adrenal medullary NE and E are decreased following isolation (Welch and Welch, 1969b). Following fighting, adrenal medullary levels of E fall, but NE levels are unchanged. Similarly, there are no changes in NE levels in diencephalon-midbrain region following fighting. NE levels in the brain stem, however, tend to fall after fighting, while there is an increase in telencephalic NE levels. Again the question of the specificity of these changes in brain neurochemistry to fighting behavior must be raised. Restraint causes a different spectrum of changes in NE content than does fighting. Whereas NE levels in the brain stem were decreased after fighting, they increased following restraint. NE content in telencephalic areas was not changed as a function of restraint. Isolated mice also show greater utilization rates of both DA and NE in brain than grouped mice as a function of restraint. These results suggest that isolation-induced fighting may evoke a biochemical response different from that seen after restraint stress. But it has not been possible to determine utilization rates of brain CA as a function of fighting, since administration of α-methyltyrosine (α-MT), a compound which inhibits the enzymic action of tyrosine hydroxylase, to isolated mice markedly decreases fighting behavior (Welch and Welch, 1969a). This effect of α-MT suggests that the brain CA biosynthetic mechanisms must at least be intact for the expression of isolation-induced fighting, but it does not demonstrate that altered CA function is uniquely associated with fighting in an antecedent fashion.

3. Cholinergic Mechanisms

The levels of ACh in three mouse brain parts were determined by Karczmar and Scudder (1969) as a function of various treatments. Isolation effected modest changes in brain ACh levels that appeared to be quantitatively or directionally different from changes seen after avoidance training or inescapable shock. But Karczmar and Scudder were unable to find a consistent relationship between any kind of fighting behavior and brain ACh levels in mice. Pharmacological manipulation of cholinergic function by the blockade of cholinergic postsynaptic receptors with the drug scopolamine inhibits fighting in mice previously trained to fight (DaVanzo et al., 1966) and in mouse fighting seen following isolation (Janssen et al., 1960).

D. Conclusions

According to one theory of the effects of isolation (Welch, 1965), an overall lower level of physiological and behavioral activity is effected by the reduced stimulus input associated with isolation. When exposed to a novel testing situation, however, the isolate exhibits a greater response than the previously grouped control animal. Results from several studies employing various physiological and behavioral measures have generally provided support for this view. For example, isolated mice have been reported to exhibit more locomotor activity in a novel testing chamber than grouped animals and they show an enhanced adrenocortical response to stress (cf. Welch and Welch, 1969a).

Taken together, the most obvious conclusion that can be derived from the materials summarized in the foregoing paragraphs is that there are critical questions for which we do not yet have answers. Isolation of mice effects changes in biogenic amine and endocrine activity, but we do not know if these physiological changes are uniquely associated with fighting behavior. We need to know how isolation compares with other treatments with regard to effecting similar or different physiological changes. In addition, we need to know how the physiological changes seen after isolation are related to various kinds of behavior as well as fighting. It is tempting to speculate that isolation of male mice effects a unique spectrum of physiological activity, and that this spectrum of activity is uniquely associated with fighting behavior. Obviously a number of experiments remain to be done to assess this hypothesis empirically. In future experimentation it will be necessary to measure concurrently several parameters of biochemical activity. Thus, while androgens are frequently ascribed the role of potentiating aggressive behavior, we have seen that numerous other factors must also be considered in assessing the "well-known" effects of androgen on either aggressive or sex behavior. Androgens are thus only one facet of the physiological spectrum underlying behavior. Further, the various systems contributing to the whole physiological spectrum are constantly interacting. For example, removal of the gonads effects changes in pituitary-adrenal activity (Sigg, 1969) and also effects changes in the levels of NE in the brain (Wurtman, 1971). The temporal parameters of the activity of these interacting physiological systems must also be considered in any attempts to establish a link between biochemical events and behavior. There may be a lag between the occurrence of biochemical events in the brain and the emergence of a behavior pattern. As an example, it is known that estrogen reaches the brain very quickly after peripheral injection, but the reappearance of sex behavior in the ovariectomized female takes much longer. It appears unlikely, therefore, that any parameter of a single chemical compound will ever be found that can be uniquely associated with the occurrence of isolation-induced fighting in mice. Since the available evidence has implicated various hormones and biogenic amines in the modulation of isolation-induced fighting, it appears that either there is a redundancy of physiological mechanisms underlying the behavior or more likely that a complex pattern of activity among various physiological systems mediates the behavior.

III. SHOCK-INDUCED FIGHTING

Data relating brain neurochemistry to still another kind of aggressive behavior have been provided by Stolk et al. (1970) and others (Lal et al., 1968, 1970). The shock-elicited fighting phenomenon has been studied in various species, and the procedure has been standardized for rats by Ulrich (1966) and his colleagues. Animals exposed to electric shock through the grid floor of a small enclosure typically assume a stereotyped posture and begin to attack one another. This behavior has also been referred to as "shock-elicited aggression," and "pain-elicited aggression." The method has the advantage of permitting close experimental control over the occurrence of fighting by manipulation of various stimulus variables.

A. Pituitary-Gonadal System

The effects of castration on shock-induced fighting behavior have been studied in several laboratories. Hutchinson et al. (1965) reported a gradual decline in the frequency of fighting in castrated male rats after extended testing. Powell et al. (1971) found that rats castrated at 35 days of age tended to show a decrement in fighting during adulthood if the castrates had previous fighting or shock experience, but this effect tended to diminish with time. Castrates with no prior fighting or shock experience, on the other hand, showed a decrement in fighting only after repeated testing. Hutchinson et al. (1965) also reported that male rats showed a marked increase in shock-induced fighting behavior at 35 days of age, suggesting that levels of circulating androgens may underlie the expression of the behavior. Powell *et al.* (1971), however, administered TP to rats for 14 consecutive days, beginning at 17 days of age, and did not observe any effect on fighting behavior. As was true for isolation-induced fighting in mice, the effects of postweaning castration or androgen treatment on shock-induced fighting in rats appear to be somewhat inconsistent. Neonatal treatment, on the other hand, produces a more consistent effect. Powell *et al.* found that TP administered neonatally to rats effected increased levels of fighting during adulthood. Conner and Levine (1969) reported that neonatally castrated male rats exhibited female-like patterns of shock-induced fighting behavior in adulthood, and did not show typical male patterns of fighting even when treated with TP, while TP injections completely replaced decrements in the fighting behavior of weanling age castrates. These effects of hormone manipulations done early in development on shock-induced fighting in rats are consistent with the results of similar experiments done with mice in the isolation-induced fighting situation (see Section II, A, 3).

B. Pituitary-Adrenal System

Kostowski (1967) reported that corticosterone increased fighting among mice in the shock-induced fighting paradigm, but there are no other reports of significant effects on shock-induced fighting following administration of hormones of the pituitary-adrenal system. On the other hand, there is evidence that shock-induced fighting produces marked effects on pituitary-adrenal activity in rats. In a series of experiments reported by Conner *et al.* (1971), there were three major groups of rats: a Fight, Shock and Control group. Animals in the Fight group were shocked in pairs, thus evoking fighting behavior. Animals in the Shock group were exposed to the same electric shock stimulation individually, while the animals in the Control group were never shocked. Immediately after the testing session, and at various times thereafter, animals from each group were sacrificed and blood samples were collected for determination of plasma ACTH and corticosterone concentrations. Both Shock and Fight treatments produced elevations in plasma ACTH levels, but the Shock animals showed faster and significantly higher elevations than the Fight animals. Shock-induced fighting thus evokes less pituitary ACTH secretion than exposure of a single animal to the same shock. While measures of ACTH clearly reflected such differences, measures of plasma corticosterone were more variable and only suggestive of possible differences in hypothalamohypophyseal activity. These findings suggest that direct measures of ACTH and other pituitary hormones might provide more reliable data in studies designed to elucidate neuroendo-crine-behavior relationships.

Conner *et al.* (1971) interpreted the difference in plasma ACTH shown by the Shock and Fight animals as support for the view that the opportunity to engage in fighting behavior represents a coping response. Miller (1969) and his colleagues have presented evidence showing that the magnitude of the behavioral and/or physiological response to aversive stimulation is attenuated if a coping response (such as an avoidance or escape response) is made available to the animal. It is virtually impossible for animals in the shock-induced fighting situation to escape or avoid the electric shock, and it does not appear that simply engaging in fighting behavior would reduce the physical intensity of the electric shock stimuli. According to the coping behavior interpretation, therefore, the act of engaging in an organized pattern of behavior is itself a coping response, even though the actual execution or persistence in that behavior pattern does nothing to alleviate the intensity or duration of the aversive stimulation.

C. Biogenic Amines

There is no evidence that serotonergic mechanisms are involved in the regulation of shock-induced fighting in rats (Conner *et al.*, 1970). Current experiments being conducted by the author in collaboration with Stolk indicate that pharmacological manipulation of cholinergic mechanisms by injection of scopolamine inhibits the fighting behavior of rats in this situation. The finding that methylscopolamine, a compound which has all the peripheral but not the central effects of scopolamine, did not affect fighting, suggests that the effects of scopolamine on the inhibition of fighting may be mediated by the blockade of ACh receptors within the brain.

Brain CA metabolism has been studied in some detail following exposure of rats to the shock-induced fighting situation by Stolk *et al.* (1970). These investigators employed three groups of animals as referred to above, a Fight, Shock, and Control group, and utilized the technique of intracerebral administration of tracer amounts of a precursor of NE in order to study metabolism. Four hours following an intracisternal injection of a small amount of DA, the animals in each group were tested. Immediately after the testing sesssion, and at various times thereafter, animals from each group were sacrificed and CA metabolism in three brain parts was studied.

At the end of the testing session the Fight animals did not show any significant changes in CA metabolism in any brain part. Shock alone, however, evoked an increase in the rate of NE utilization in the brain stem. Other investigators have also found changes in brain NE levels and utilization rates as a function of exposure to electric shock or other "stressful" stimuli (cf. Bliss and Zwanziger, 1966). It is of interest, therefore, that paired exposure of rats to the same stimulus, thereby evoking fighting behavior, did not produce a change in brain CA metabolism. One interpretation of this finding is that the shock stimulation was not very "stressful" if administered under conditions where the animals could engage in fighting behavior. During the hour subsequent to the termination of the testing session, however, the Fight animals showed a marked increase in NE metabolism in both brain stem and the diencephalon. The Shock animals, on the other hand, showed a marked decrease in the rate of NE utilization and release in the brainstem, with no changes in the diencephalon or telencephalon during this same interval. At intervals still longer after the testing session, the Fight animals showed decreases in NE metabolism in the diencephalon while the Shock animals showed increased NE metabolism in this area. Further, in the Fight group, there was a good relation between brainstem NE levels 1 hour after the session and the frequency of fighting responses recorded during the session. Thus, following exposure to the same electric shock stimulation, the Shock and Fight animals showed patterns of brain NE metabolism which were directionally and temporally different, as well as being specific to gross but different brain areas. Thus, not only are shocked and fought animals different with respect to neuroendocrine function, but they are also different neurochemically.

A more definitive interpretation of these neurochemical and neuroendocrine data must await the results of further experimentation directed toward determining the specificity of the behavior which produces such physiological changes. Others (Paré and Livingston, 1970; Weiss *et al.,* 1970) have reported differential changes in brain NE levels in avoidance ("coping") and yoked control animals. While it does not appear that the animals in the shock-induced fighting situation can escape or avoid the electric shock, it is still unclear whether or not the findings described above are uniquely associated with shock-induced fighting behavior.

IV. MURICIDE

Karli (1956) has described the mouse-killing phenomenon (muricide) seen in both laboratory and wild strains of rats. Some rats will spontaneously attack and kill mice, usually by a bite through the spinal cord. Other rats, termed "spontaneously inhibited," do not exhibit killing behavior. Subsequent investigation has revealed that laboratory rats may be more likely to attack and kill frogs than mice. The mouse/frog killing phenomenon has also been referred to as predatory aggression (Bandler, 1970).

A. Hormones

Sex hormones do not appear to play an important role in killing behavior since rats of both sexes may exhibit the behavior and Karli found that both castration and TP were without effect. Leaf *et al.* (1969), however, have presented data suggesting that both testosterone and estrogens may play a slight inhibitory role in mouse-killing behavior.

There are no reports of acute treatment with ACTH producing marked or consistent effects on muricide behavior. The positive evidence that adrenocorticoids are directly involved in the modulation of this behavior is very sparse. Leaf *et al.* (1969) reported that extremely high nonphysiological doses (10 mg/kg) of cortisone acetate, corticosterone, or hydrocortisone were necessary to produce an unreliable inhibition of mouse-killing behavior in rats. Kostowski *et al.* (1970) found that even higher doses of hydrocortisone (20 mg/kg) facilitated the killing behavior of killer rats while DOC and the pregnanedione derivative, hydroxydione, in 20 mg/kg doses inhibited mouse-killing behavior.

B. Biogenic Amines

1. Serotonin

A surgical procedure which may convert "spontaneously inhibited" rats to mouse-killer rats is that of olfactory deafferentation. Two or three days following olfactory deafferentation of nonkiller rats, it was found that they often began to engage in killing behavior. Karli *et al.* (1969) examined the 5-HT content of the amygdala following removal of the olfactory bulbs. 5-HT content of the amygdala showed a modest decline 4-8 weeks following the operation, but 2 months later the content had returned to preoperative levels. The killing response, however, appeared much earlier than the drop in 5-HT content in the amygdala, and persisted beyond the time when 5-HT levels recovered. 5-HT levels in the fore and hind half of the brain were determined in killer and nonkiller rats by Goldberg and Salama (1969). These determinations were made in the killer rats 24 hours after the last mouse killing test. They found no significant difference between killer and nonkiller rats in the levels of 5-HT in forebrain or hindbrain. These findings provide little evidence of a relation between brain 5-HT levels and muricidal activity. Depletion of brain 5-HT levels by the pharmacological procedure of injections with PCPA, on the other hand, has been reported to promote mouse-killing behavior in previously nonkiller rats (Karli *et al.*, 1969; Sheard, 1969). Sheard also found that administration of the 5-HT precursor 5-HTP produced a suppression of muricidal activity.

2. Catecholamines

The available data relating catecholaminergic mechanisms to mouse-killing behavior are inconsistent. Sofia (1969) studied the effects of various drug compounds, and found that those agents causing increased levels of brain NE were most strongly associated with the suppression of mouse-killing behavior. Leaf et al. (1969) found that direct placement of NE into the medial amygdala via bilateral cannulae also produced some inhibition of mouse-killing. However, virtually complete depletion of brain catechols by peripheral injections of α-MT produced only a modest increment in mouse-killing behavior (Leaf et al., 1969). Moreover, the data reported by Goldberg and Salama (1969) appear to be inconsistent with the Leaf et al. findings. They found that killer rats have a higher level and increased turnover rate of NE in the forebrain, compared with nonkillers.

3. Cholinergic Mechanisms

There is good evidence for a relation between brain cholinergic mechanisms and killing behavior. This relationship has been studied by examining the effect of manipulating brain cholinergic mechanisms on the inhibition or facilitation of killing in spontaneous killers, or on the elicitation of killing in "spontaneously inhibited" animals. Bilateral stimulation of the lateral hypothalamus (Lt H) with carbachol evokes mouse killing in rats that do not ordinarily kill (Smith et al., 1970), and unilateral stimulation facilitates frog killing in natural frog killers (Bandler, 1970). The specificity of this effect is indicated by the finding that placement of related compounds (NE, d-amphetamine, 5-HT, 5-HTP) into the same site did not elicit killing. Further, carbachol placed in regions near the effective Lt H site did not evoke killing. Brain cholinergic mechanisms may also be manipulated by the administration of compounds which inhibit the action of acetylcholinesterase, the enzyme involved in the deactivation of ACh. Administration of the cholinesterase inhibitor, neostigmine, to the Lt H also elicits the killing response in ordinarily nonkiller rats, and the administration of the cholinergic blocker methyl atropine inhibits killing in killer rats (Smith et al., 1970). Bandler (1970), however, found that atropine produced only a very modest suppression of attack and kill behavior when applied to the Lt H of killer rats. On the other hand, either atropine sulfate or atropine methyl nitrate administered peripherally before placing carbachol in the Lt H resulted in significantly longer attack and kill latencies. Atropine methyl nitrate was less effective in this regard and since it does not readily pass the blood-brain barrier in any appreciable amounts, the differential suppression of killing behavior was attributed to the central action of the atropine sulfate and was viewed as support for the hypothesis that killing behavior is under central cholinergic regulation. Bandler (1970) also applied ACh, physostigmine, neostigmine, or a combination of ACh and physostigmine to the Lt H of natural frog killing rats. Based on the hypothesis that a cholinergic mechanism in the Lt H facilitates killing, it would be expected that all four treatments would shorten kill latencies. While the data generally supported this hypothesis, only the combined drug treatment condition produced a statistically significant facilitation. According to Bandler, the positive result obtained with the drug mixture suggests that the failure of ACh alone was due to the rapid rate of destruction of ACh by cholinesterase.

The Lt H has been further implicated in muricide behavior by the finding that electrical stimulation of this site elicits killing in rats that do not spontaneously kill mice (King and Hoebel, 1968; Panksepp and Trowill, 1969). Electrical stimulation studies of attack behavior of cats also implicate the Lt H, and further, indicate the involvement of the amygdala (Egger and Flynn, 1962). The administration of a cholinergic blocking agent (methylscopolamine) directly to amygdaloid sites inhibits mouse killing (Leaf *et al.,* 1969) and the cholinesterase inhibitor amitone caused an increase in mouse-killing behavior (Igić *et al.,* 1970).

Besides the Lt H and amygdala, still another brain area has been implicated in the neurochemical modulation of killing behavior. Bandler (1971), again working with rats that spontaneously killed mice or frogs, found that carbachol stimulation of medial and midline thalamic nuclei facilitated killing, while the application of atropine to the same sites inhibited killing. Bandler also examined the effects of concurrent chemostimulation of thalamic and hypothalamic sites on killing behavior. Both unilateral and bilateral atropine administration at the hypothalamic sites at which carbachol facilitated killing failed to block the carbachol-induced facilitation of killing at thalamic sites. Atropine applied at positive thalamic sites, on the other hand, blocked the killing usually induced by administering carbachol at positive hypothalamic sites.

By the placement of chemical compounds which modulate cholinergic mechanisms directly into specific sites in the brain, it is relatively easy to facilitate or inhibit killing behavior which some rats show in the absence of the drug. But even with brain chemostimulation, the facilitation of mouse killing in "natural frog-killers" is not so easily demonstrated, and apparently it is necessary to place relatively large amounts of carbachol into the brain to evoke killing in rats that are not "natural killers." These observations suggest that in a rat which exhibits "spontaneous" killing behavior, whether this is due to inhibition of CA mechanisms or stimulation of cholinergic mechanisms, exogenously administered compounds may facilitate or inhibit the response, but they may not be important determinants for the elicitation of the response in "spontaneously inhibited" rats. This may mean that these brain mechanisms are involved in the regulation of the behavior, and other factors (such as past experience) are the important determinants of whether or not the behavior occurs at all.

V. SOCIAL BEHAVIOR

The maintenance and expression of other kinds of social behavior patterns besides aggression have also been shown to be modulated by endogenously occurring hormones. Several examples of social behaviors which are directly or indirectly related to the topic of aggression will be considered under this heading.

A. Social Order

Dominant-submissive relationships and hierarchical orders among individual animals in social groups have been described among various species. The role of overt and ritualized aggressive behavior in the establishment and maintenance of social orders among animals has been described elsewhere (cf. Guhl, 1961) and . will not be elaborated here.

1. Pituitary-Gonadal System

Davis (1957) observed that castration of male starlings produced no decrement in aggressive behavior, and testosterone injections did not affect the social rank of individual birds in the group. A discrepancy between the annual behavioral and gonadal cycles in the male starling has also been observed: Aggressive behavior is frequently observed in the spring breeding season when the testis weight is greatest, but aggressive behavior also frequently occurs in the fall even though the gonadal weights remain at their minimum summer level (cf. Mathewson, 1961). These observations suggested that gonadal hormones (androgens) were not involved in aggression in this species. Mathewson therefore studied the effects of the pituitary gonadotropic hormone LH, on fighting and dominance in male starlings. Using a paired bird situation, dominance was determined by possession of the single perch, for which the birds fought vigorously. In one experiment it was found that LH injections administered to the subordinate bird effected dominance reversals in 6 out of 8 pairs studied. In another experiment one of the birds was treated with LH before initial pairing. It was found that the hormone-injected bird achieved dominance in 13 out of the 16 pairs studied. In pairs comprised of one castrate and one intact bird, it was noted that the castrated bird most frequently dominated in the absence of any hormone treatment. These observations suggest that elevated LH levels, whether effected by exogenous administration or by castration, are involved in aggressive behaviors and dominance in starlings.

2. Pituitary-Adrenal System

The gradual emergence of a relationship between pituitary-adrenal function and social order has been traced by Davis (1964). The background for this relationship is the observation that adrenal size increases as a function of population density (Christian and Davis, 1964; Davis and Christian, 1957). With respect to adrenal weights, there is an inverse relation between adrenal gland size and social rank in a hierarchically organized group. With respect to pituitary-adrenal activity, the most dominant animals exhibit less adrenocortical responsiveness than do the submissive animals. Thus, Flickinger (1961) reported a significant inverse correlation between adrenal weights and social rank in groups of sexually mature White Leghorn male chickens. There was no relation between social rank and adrenal weights among grouped hens or sexually immature cocks. The dominant males also tended to have the largest testes and the development of spermatogenic mechanisms was retarded in subordinate grouped birds. These observations suggest that the social position of a cock in a group, the maintenance of which involves overt or ritualized patterns of behavior, may be a factor in regulating gonadotropin output and hence fertility. There is also evidence from several other species which indicates a relationship between the social rank of an individual animal in an organized group and the pituitary-adrenal activity of that animal.

In an experiment using CFW male mice, Louch and Higginbotham (1967) placed the animals in groups of four following prolonged isolation and observed the occurrence of fighting behavior. They also ascertained, for each group, which mouse dominated the other three. After 24 hours, the animals were killed and plasma corticosterone levels were determined for the dominant, subordinate, and isolated control animals. The mean corticosterone level for the controls was 9.3 μg% and was not significantly different from that of the dominant animals (11.9 μg%). The subordinate animals, on the other hand, showed significantly elevated plasma corticosterone levels of 19.9 μg%. It is unlikely that these differences in steroid levels can be attributed to injury, since dominant and submissive animals presumably fought equally hard and both sustained injuries around the head and flanks. According to the investigators, these data indicate that an important stimulus acting on mice to produce adrenal response after fighting is associated with defeat. These data are consistent with the results of several other mouse studies in which an inverse relation between position in a social hierarchy and adrenal weight was found (e.g., Davis and Christian, 1957). More importantly, the Louch and Higginbotham data described above suggest that the enlarged adrenals observed in previous studies are also functioning at a higher level and secreting greater amounts of adrenocorticoids. The increased adrenal size has been shown to be primarily due to hypertrophy of the adrenal cortex, specifically the zona fasciculata. An interesting corollary to these data is the observation (Welch and Welch, 1969a) that prolonged grouping among mice is accompanied by an increased intragroup variability in indices of pituitary-adrenal function, an effect presumably mediated by the marked differences which develop between the dominant and subordinate group members.

A recent paper (Sassenrath, 1970) describes the attack and escape behavioral interactions and the adrenal responsiveness in two caged groups of five subadult rhesus monkeys over a 2-year period during which several changes in the social environment occurred. The groups described were each comprised of three males and two females. Under conditions of a stable dominance structure, the dominant male exhibited a lower adrenal response to exogenously administered ACTH than the subordinate animals, as revealed by urinary 17-hydrocorticosteroid (17-OHCS). There was a good inverse rank-order correlation between social rank and magnitude of ACTH response among the animals. Removal of the most subordinate female cagemate for an 8-week period resulted in a significant decrease in her ACTH response. Removal of the dominant male for a 4-week period effected marked decreases in the ACTH-response levels of the female cagemates, but no apparent change in the two subordinate males. When consort pair formation occurred between the α male and the No. 3 female, the social rank of the consort female rose to the No. 2 rank, accompanied by a decrease in ACTH response levels. While these shifts in the dominance status and changes in adrenal responsiveness were occurring with the consort female, the ACTH response levels of the other female (the most subordinate in the group) were rising.

The social behavior patterns of individual members of organized groups are known to vary as a function of the status of the individual in the social structure of the group. Given an organized group, it should therefore be possible to predict the status and probable behavior patterns of individuals in the group from measures of pituitary-adrenal function, and predictions in the opposite direction should also be possible. However, while experimentally induced changes in the social order of a group are reflected by changes in pituitary-adrenal function, the opposite may not be true. For example, ablation of the adrenal glands or injections of ACTH have not been observed to effect marked changes in the social order. These considerations suggest that the observed changes in pituitary-adrenal function are an effect of the behavior that organisms engage in as a function of their position in the social organization of the group. Other factors, such as learning and possibly genetics, are apparently the important determinants of whether or not an individual organism assumes a dominant or submissive role.

B. Sex Behavior and Fighting

Evidence was previously cited indicating that estrogen may play an inhibitory role in isolation-induced fighting among mice (see Section II,A,2). Other evidence indicates that estrogen may suppress fighting in domestic fowl (Davis and Domm, 1943) and lizards (Evans, 1936), but data obtained from golden hamsters (Kislak and Beach, 1955) and chimpanzees (Birch and Clark, 1946) suggest just the opposite. In an experiment reported by Mirsky (1955), implants of estrogen into rhesus monkeys produced no changes in the group hierarchical status. Results from golden hamsters (Kislak and Beach, 1955) and rhesus monkeys (Michael, 1969) indicate that changes in the frequency of patterns of aggressive behavior are associated with changes in sexual activity. Kislak and Beach did not observe any decrement in the number of attacks that an ovariectomized female hamster directed toward the male after estrogen treatment; if anything, there was a tendency for estrogen to increase her aggressiveness. But when she was made sexually receptive by the combined treatment of estrogen and progesterone, her aggressive behavior was virtually abolished. The picture that emerges from the rhesus monkey data reported by Michael (1969) is quite different, however. He noted a marked increase in aggressive exchanges (apparently threats) when the female of a male-female pair was ovariectomized, but no change was seen in this form of heightened aggressive behavior when she was administered estrogen. However, when she was made sexually receptive by treatment with estrogen and progesterone, the number of aggressive episodes by the female more than doubled. In an intact bisexual pair, Michael noted a striking increase in the number of times that the male attempted to mount the female *after* she became pregnant. The number of direct attacks (biting and hitting) that the female directed toward the male also increased dramatically. He reports that the male remained extraordinarily tolerant until finally he began to fight back. Then almost 3½ months after conception, the female had to be separated from the male to avoid possible injury.

C. Maternal Aggression

Hormones are generally assumed to play a role in the aggression exhibited by females in protecting their young, but there is hardly any systematic or consistent data. Scudder *et al.* (1967) have reported marked strain differences among mice in the aggression exhibited against an extraneous object by mothers in defense of their pups. A report that only lactating female rats will spontaneously kill frogs placed into their cage (Endroczi *et al.* 1958) has not been confirmed (Revlis and Moyer, 1969). Thoman *et al.* (1970) found that lactating rats exhibited less shock-induced fighting than females that were not lactating.

VI. CONCLUSION

The foregoing materials have provided several examples of how behavior may affect the physiological functioning of the organism. More particularly, a start has been made toward describing the effects of specific kinds of aggressive behavior on patterns of physiological function. For example, the evidence indicates that following shock-induced fighting there are very different effects on patterns of neuroendocrine and biogenic amine activity than those seen after exposing animals to shock individually.

It is clear from the present survey that specific details of the behavioral paradigm being employed should be clearly specified. We have seen that while hormones of the pituitary-gonadal system, especially androgens, potentiate the expression of isolation-induced fighting behavior in mice, and, to a lesser degree, also shock-induced fighting among male rats, these hormones do not appear to be involved in any important way in the modulation of the mouse/frog killing exhibited by some rats. The antecedent conditions, the expression of the behavior and the physiological consequences of inter-male spontaneous aggression, irritable aggression, and predatory aggression are thus different. It is meaningless, therefore, to refer to the effects of androgens on aggressive behavior without further elaboration of the behavior pattern and its antecedent conditions.

To what extent can we further characterize the physiological substrates underlying the expression of the laboratory models of aggressive behavior surveyed in this paper? The evidence that estrogen suppresses the expression of aggressive behavior is sparse and is derived primarily from studies of isolation-induced fighting. The role of the hormones of the pituitary-adrenal system appears to be indirect, and it is presently difficult to separate the causes from the effects. With the possible exception of cholinergic mechanisms and muricide, it is even more difficult to characterize the role of brain monoamines in the expression of aggressive behavior. In some cases it may be possible to describe a particular conjectured mechanism as inhibitory or facilitatory, but this may be premature at the present time since numerous possible interactions have not been examined yet. In a few cases, endogenous neurochemical events as a function of behavior have been described for specific brain areas, but more often the brain has been only grossly sectioned before biochemical analysis. The precise localization of chemical effects, the identification of neurotransmitter substances, and mechanisms of action still remain to be determined. Thus, only a vague and incomplete picture emerges from the present survey of the relation of brain monoamines and endocrine function to aggressive behavior. This state of affairs reemphasizes the necessity for investigators seeking behavioral-biochemical relations to specify precisely the procedures used to evoke a particular kind of aggressive behavior.

Even in the face of these gaps in our knowledge, there is a significant amount of empirical data documenting the behavioral effects of hormones and biogenic amines. The literature cited in the present survey indicates that our knowledge of the effects of biochemical events on aggressive behavior is accumulating at a rapid rate. As new and more refined measurement techniques are applied in this area of research, we may expect an even broader empirical basis for the conviction that biochemical events are involved in the modulation of behavior.

References

Bandler, R. J., Jr. (1970). *Brain Res.* **20**, 409.
Bandler, R. J., Jr. (1971). *Brain Res.* **26**, 81.
Beach, F. A. (1970). *J. Comp. Physiol. Psychol.* **70**, 1 (monograph).
Beeman, E. A. (1947). *Physiol. Zool.* **20**, 373.
Bevan, J. M., Bevan, W., and Williams, B. F. (1958). *Physiol. Zool.* **31**, 284.
Bevan, W., Levy, G. W., Whitehouse, J. M., and Bevan, J. M. (1957). *Physiol. Zool.* **30**, 341.
Birch, H. G., and Clark, G. (1946). *Psychosom. Med.* **8**, 320
Bliss, E. L., and Zwanziger, J. (1966). *J. Psychiat. Res.* **4**, 189.
Boelkins, R. C., and Heiser, J. F. (1970). *In* "Violence and the Struggle for Existence" (D. N. Daniels, M. F. Gilula, and F. M. Ochberg, eds.), pp. 15-52. Little, Brown, Boston, Massachusetts.
Bronson, F. H., and Desjardins, C. (1968). *Science* **161**, 705.
Bronson, F. H., and Eleftheriou, B. E. (1965a). *Science* **147**, 627.
Bronson, F. H., and Eleftheriou, B. E. (1965b). *Proc. Soc. Exp. Biol. Med.* **118**, 146.
Brown, J. L., and Hunsperger, R. W. (1963). *Anim. Behav.* **11**, 439.
Carthy, J. D., and Ebling, F. J., eds. (1964). "The Natural History of Aggression" (Inst. of Biol. Symp. No. 13). Academic Press, New York.
Christian, J. J., and Davis, D. E. (1964). *Science* **146**, 1550.
Clemente, C. D., and Lindsley, D. B., eds. (1967). Brain function, "Aggression and Defense. Neural Mechanisms and Social Patterns," Vol. V. Univ. of California Press, Berkeley.
Collias, N. E., (1944). *Physiol. Zool.* **17**, 83.
Conner, R. L., and Levine, S. (1969). *In* "Aggressive Behaviour" (S. Garattini and E. B. Sigg, eds.), pp. 150-163. Excerpta Medica Foundation, Amsterdam.
Conner, R. L., Stolk, J. M., Barchas, J. D., Dement, W. C., and Levine, S. (1970). *Physiol. Behav.* **5**, 1221.
Conner, R. L., Vernikos-Danellis, J., and Levine, S. (1971). *Nature (London)* **234**, 564.
DaVanzo, J. P., Daugherty, M., Ruckart, R., and Kang, L. (1966). *Psychopharmacologia* **9**, 210.
Davis, D. E. (1957). *Science* **126**,253.
Davis, D. E., (1964). *In* "Social Behavior and Organization Among Vertebrates" (W. Etkin, ed.), pp. 53-74. Univ. of Chicago Press, Chicago, Illinois.
Davis, D. E., and Christian, J. J. (1957). *Proc. Soc. Exp. Biol. Med.* **94**, 728.
Davis, D. E., and Domm, L. V. (1943). *In* "Essays in Biology," pp. 171-181. Univ. of California Press, Berkeley.
Dews, P. B. (1962). *In* "Experimental Foundations of Clinical Psychology" (A. J. Bachrach, ed.), pp. 423-441. Basic Books, New York.
Edwards, D. A. (1968). *Science* **161**, 1027.
Egger, M. D., and Flynn, J. P. (1962). *Science* **136**, 43.
Eleftheriou, B. E., and Church, R. L. (1967). *Gen. Comp. Endocrinol.* **9**, 263.
Endroczi, E., Lissak, K., and Telegdy, G. (1958). *Acta Physiol.* **14**, 353.
Essman, W. B. (1969). *In* "Aggressive Behaviour" (S. Garattini and E. B. Sigg, eds.), pp. 203-208. Excerpta Medica Foundation, Amsterdam.
Evans, L. T. (1936). *Science* **83**, 104.
Flickinger, G. L. (1961). *Gen. Comp. Endocrinol.* **1**, 332.
Fredericson, E. (1950). *J. Psychol.* **29**, 89.
Fredericson, E., Story, A. W., Gurney, N. L., and Butterworth, K. (1955). *J. Genet. Psychol.* **87**, 121.

Garattini, S., and Sigg, E. B., eds. (1969). "Aggressive Behaviour." Excerpta Medica Foundation, Amsterdam.

Garattini, S., Giacalone, E., and Valzelli, L. (1967). *J. Pharm. Pharmacol.* **19**, 338.

Garattini, S., Giacalone, E., and Valzelli, L. (1969). *In* "Aggressive Behaviour" (S. Garattini and E. B. Sigg, eds.), pp. 179-187. Excerpta Medica Foundation, Amsterdam.

Ginsburg, B., and Allee, W. C. (1942). *Physiol. Zool.* **15**, 485.

Goldberg, M. E., and Salama, A. I. (1969). *Biochem. Pharmacol.* **18**, 532.

Guhl, A. M. (1961). *In* "Sex and Internal Secretions" (W. C. Young, ed.), Vol. II, pp. 1240-1267. Williams & Wilkins, Baltimore, Maryland.

Harris, G. W. (1964). *Endocrinology* **75**, 627.

Hutchinson, R. R., Ulrich, R. E., and Azrin, N. H. (1965). *J. Comp. Physiol. Psychol.* **59**, 365.

Igić, R., Stern, P., and Basagić, E. (1970). *Neuropharmacology* **9**, 73.

Janssen, P. A. J., Jageneau, A. H., and Niemegeers, C. J. E. (1960). *J. Pharmacol. Exp. Ther.* **129**, 471.

Karczmar, A. G., and Scudder, C. L. (1969). *In* "Aggressive Behaviour" (S. Garattini and E. B. Sigg, eds.), pp. 209-227. Excerpta Medica Foundation, Amsterdam.

Karli, P. (1956). *Behaviour* **10**, 81.

Karli, P., Vergnes, M., and Didiergeorges, F. (1969). *In* "Aggressive Behaviour" (S. Garattini and E. B. Sigg, eds.), pp. 47-55. Excerpta Medica Foundation, Amsterdam.

King, M. B., and Hoebel, B. G. (1968). *Commun. Behav. Biol.* **2**, 173.

Kislak, J. W., and Beach, F. A. (1955). *Endocrinology* **56**, 684.

Kostowski, W. (1967). *Diss. Pharm. Pharmacol.* **19**, 619.

Kostowski, W., Rewerski, W., and Piechocki, T. (1970). *Neuroendocrinology* **6**, 311.

Lal, H., Defeo, J. J., and Thut, P. (1968). *Commun. Behav. Biol.* **1**, 333.

Lal, H., Nesson, B., and Smith, N. (1970). *Biol. Psychiat.* **2**, 299.

Leaf, R. C., Lerner, L., and Horovitz, Z. P. (1969). *In* "Aggressive Behaviour" (S. Garattini and E. B. Sigg, eds.), pp. 120-131. Excerpta Medica Foundation, Amsterdam.

Levy, J. V. (1954). *Proc. W. Va. Acad. Sci.* **26**, 14.

Levy, J. V., and King, J. A. (1953). *Anat. Rec.* **117**, 562.

Louch, C. D., and Higginbotham, M. (1967). *Gen. Comp. Endocrinol.* **8**, 441.

Marie Antonita, Sr., Scudder, C. L., and Karczmar, A. G. (1968). *Pharmacologist* **10**, 168.

Mathewson, S. F. (1961). *Science* **134**, 1522.

Michael, R. P. (1969). *In* "Aggressive Behaviour" (S. Garattini and E. B. Sigg, eds.), pp. 172-178. Excerpta Medica Foundation, Amsterdam.

Miller, N. E. (1969). *Ann. N. Y. Acad. Sci.* **159**, 1025.

Mirsky, A. F. (1955). *J. Comp. Physiol. Psychol.* **48**, 327.

Moyer, K. E. (1968). *Commun. Behav. Biol.* **2**, 65.

Mugford, R. A., and Nowell, N. W. (1970a). *Psychonom. Sci.* **20**, 191.

Mugford, R. A., and Nowell, N. W. (1970b). *Nature (London)* **226**, 967.

Panksepp. J., and Trowill, J. (1969). *Psychonom. Sci.* **16**, 118.

Paré, W. P., and Livingston, A., Jr. (1970). *Physiol. Behav.* **5**, 215.

Powell, D. A., Francis, J., and Schneiderman, N. (1971). *Commun. Behav. Biol.* **5**, 371.

Revlis, R., and Moyer, K. E. (1969). *Psychonom. Sci.* **16**, 135.

Rosenblatt, J., and Aronson, L. R. (1958). *Anim. Behav.* **6**, 171.

Rothballer, A. B. (1967). *In* Brain function "Aggression and Defense. Neural Mechanisms and Social Patterns" (C. D. Clemente and D. B. Lindsley, eds.), Vol. V, pp. 135-170. Univ. of California Press, Berkeley.

Sassenrath, E. N. (1970). *Horm. Behav.* **1**, 283.

Scott, J. P. (1958). "Aggression." Univ. of Chicago Press, Chicago, Illinois.

Scott, J. P. (1966). *Amer. Zool.* **6**, 683.

Scudder, C. L., Karczmar, A. G., and Lockett, L. (1967). *Anim. Behav.* **15**, 353.

Sheard, M. H. (1969). *Brain Res.* **15**, 524.

Sigg, E. B. (1969). *In* "Aggressive Behaviour" (S. Garattini and E. B. Sigg, eds.), pp. 143-149. Excerpta Medica Foundation, Amsterdam.

Smith, D. E., King, M. B., and Hoebel, B. G. (1970). *Science* **167**, 900.

Sofia, R. D. (1969). *Life Sci.* **8**, 1201.

Southwick, C. H., and Clark, L. H. (1968). *Commun. Behav. Biol.* **1**, 49.

Stolk, J. M., Conner, R. L., Levine, S., and Barchas, J. D. (1970). *Soc. Biol. Psychiat., San Francisco, May 1970.*

Suchowsky, G. K., Pegrassi, L., and Bonsignori, A. (1969). *In* "Aggressive Behaviour" (S. Garattini and E. B. Sigg, eds.), pp. 164-171. Excerpta Medica Foundation, Amsterdam.

Tedeschi, D. H., and Tedeschi, R. E., eds. (1968). "Importance of Fundamental Principles in Drug Evaluation." Raven Press, New York.

Terdiman, A. M., and Levy, J. V. (1954). *Proc. W. Va. Acad. Sci.* **26**, 15.

Thoman, E. B., Conner, R. L., and Levine, S. (1970). *J. Comp. Physiol. Psychol.* **70**, 364.

Tollman, J., and King, J. A. (1956). *Brit. J. Anim. Behav.* **4**, 147.

Uhrich, J. (1938). *J. Comp. Psychol.* **25**, 373.

Ulrich, R. E. (1966). *Amer. Zool.* **6**, 643.

Weiss, J. M., Stone, E. A., and Harrell, N. (1970). *J. Comp. Physiol. Psychol.* **72**, 153.

Welch, A. S., and Welch, B. L. (1968). *Biochem. Pharmacol.* **17**, 699.

Welch, B. L. (1965). *Symp. Med. Aspects Stress in Military Climate.* (Originally published as part of U. S. Govt. Printing Office Publ., pp. 778-714.)

Welch, B. L., and Welch. A. S. (1968). *Nature (London)* **218**, 575.

Welch, B. L., and Welch, A. S. (1969a). *In* "Aggressive Behaviour" (S. Garattini and E. B. Sigg, eds.), pp. 188-202. Excerpta Medica Foundation, Amsterdam.

Welch, B. L., and Welch, A. S. (1969b). *Commun. Behav. Biol.* **3**, 125.

Weltman, A. S., Sackler, A. M., Schwartz, R., and Owens, H. (1968). *Lab. Anim. Care* **18**, 426.

Wurtman, R. J. (1971). *Neurosci. Res. Program Bull.* **9**, 182.

Yen, H. C. Y., Day, C. A., and Sigg, E. B. (1962). *Pharmacologist* **4**, 173.

Young, W. C. (1961). *In* "Sex and Internal Secretions" (W. C. Young, ed.), Vol. II, pp. 1173-1239. Williams & Wilkins, Baltimore, Maryland.

8

Biogenic Amines and Behavior

Jack D. Barchas, Roland D. Ciaranello, Jon M. Stolk, H. Keith H. Brodie, and David A. Hamburg

I. INTRODUCTION

Biogenic amines are derivatives of amino acids. They include two groups of compounds which are the subject of this review. The first group, catecholamines, includes compounds such as epinephrine, norephinephrine, and dopamine. The second is the indoleamine group which includes serotonin (Fig. 1).

The catecholamines are involved in two completely different functional processes, both of which will be considered in this chapter. The first process involves catecholamines formed and released by the adrenal gland. Epinephrine (adrenaline) and norepinephrine (noradrenaline) are the two principal members of this class. Compounds released from the adrenal affect other areas of the body, although only small amounts can enter the brain due to a barrier (blood-brain barrier) which restricts their entry. Catecholamines are generally viewed to act as transmitter agents between adjacent nerve cells. Thus, catecholamines formed by the adrenal gland act as circulating hormones while those formed in the brain act as transmitter agents. The catecholamines and the indoleamines are concentrated in brain areas thought to modulate emotional behaviors, and are affected by many drugs which are known to alter the

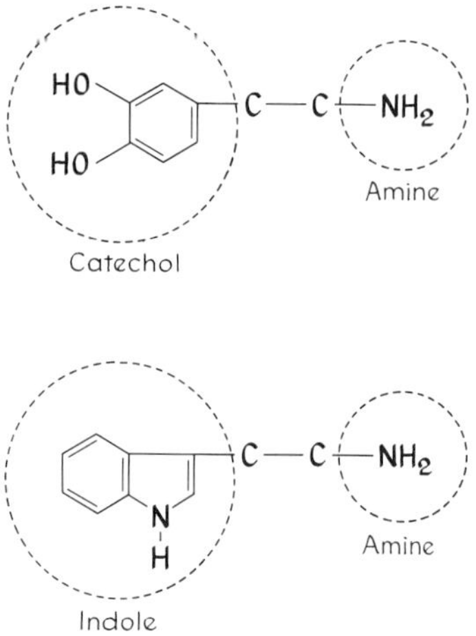

Fig. 1. Diagram of catecholamine and indoleamine structure. Portions of the material presented here are reprinted by permission of the publisher from *Advances in Psychological Assessment*, Volume Two, edited by Paul McReynolds, Palo Alto, Calif.: Science and Behavior Books, Inc., 1971, pp. 260-292.

behaviorial state of the organism. Derivatives of these compounds have powerful behavioral effects. Because the role of biogenic amines in brain may be either as transmitter agents or as modulators of neural function, we will frequently refer to the compounds as neuroregulators.

This review will emphasize the possible importance of: (1) catecholamines released from the adrenal gland functioning as hormones in terms of their effects on behavior and the behavioral states in which the compounds are released, (2) catecholamines synthesized in the brain acting as proposed neurotransmitters at synapses involved in the modulation of behavior, and (3) serotonin in the brain as a proposed neurotransmitter involved in the modulation of behavior.

Because of the quantity of information which has accumulated within the past decade relating to the biochemistry and pharmacology of biogenic amines, which is not generally available to those interested in behavior, this review will focus on biochemical and pharmacological studies. Such a choice has been made since many of the behavioral studies have utilized biochemical and pharmacological techniques and it appears clear that such a trend will become a dominant research strategy during the coming decade. Further, we have chosen to discuss a few topics in detail with the hope of giving a sense of the issues and type of research being conducted in fields related to biogenic amines. Various aspects of processes involving neuroregulators have been subject to major reviews including the following: neuroregulators and emotional illness (Eiduson *et al.*, 1964; Schildkraut and Kety, 1967; Mandell and Spooner, 1968; Mandell and Mandell, 1969; Schildkraut, 1970; Hamburg, 1970; Williams, 1970; Himwich,

TABLE I. Prerequisites for Identification of a Putative Chemical Transmitter as a neurotransmitter in the brain

Requirement	Serotonin	Dopamine	Norepinephrine
Present in brain tissue, accompanied by the necessary metabolic enzymes	Yes	Yes	Yes
Located intraneuronally in specific nerve tracts	Yes	Yes	Yes
Physiological effects identical to effect produced by electrical stimulation of the nerve tract in question	Probably	?	Probably
Drug effects on putative transmitter chemical cause expected effects in brain	Yes	Yes	Yes
Stimulation or activation of specific nerve tracts results in release of the putative transmitter	Yes	?	Yes

1971), catecholamines (Axelrod, 1959; Rothballer, 1959; Acheson, 1966; Malmejac, 1964; Wurtman, 1966 a,b,; von Euler, 1967; Mason, 1968; Melmon, 1968; Geffen and Livett, 1971), serotonin (Garattini and Valzelli, 1965; Erspamer, 1966; Garattini and Shore, 1968; Page, 1968; Sjoerdsma, 1970; Barchas and Usdin, in press), and psychopharmacology (Kety and Sampson, 1967; Bloom and Giarman, 1968a,b; Efron, 1968; Hollister, 1968; Klein and Davis, 1969; Clark and del Guidice, 1970; Usdin and Efron, 1967; Cooper *et al.*, 1970; Smythies, 1970; Rech and Moore, 1971).

II. BIOGENIC AMINES AS NEUROTRANSMITTERS

Neurohumoral transmission, regardless of the transmitter substance or the nervous tissue involved, requires several components for efficient functioning: Enzyme systems are necessary for the production and destruction of the chemical messengers; the transmitter must be released, either as a precursor or in an active form; specific target cells or organs must be able to receive and act upon the message of the transmitter to effect an appropriate action. The criteria required for acceptance of a chemical as a neurotransmitter, and evidence for norepinephrine (NE), dopamine (DA), and serotonin (5-hydroxytryptamine, 5-HT) fulfilling these requirements, are summarized in Table I (Bloom and Giarman, 1968a,b; Weight and Salmoiraghi, 1968).

The original studies of Vogt (1954) established the presence of NE in the brain. During the subsequent ten years, a considerable volume of information appeared regarding the regional distribution in brain of NE, as well as DA and 5-HT (e.g., Brodie and Shore, 1957; Carlsson et al., 1957a). These studies showed that DA was found in high concentrations only in the basal ganglia, whereas NE and 5-HT had a wider distribution with highest concentrations in the midbrain and diencephalon. A major contribution to the discrete study of these compounds in the brain was made by the development of a histochemical fluorescence method for visualization, which first demonstrated that these amines were (1) located within nerve cells, as opposed to vascular or glial tissue, (2) highly concentrated in synaptic regions of neurons, and (3) localized within specific fiber tracts in the brain (Carlsson et al., 1962; Falck, 1962). Subsequent investigations documented the precise distribution of the amine-containing neurons (Fig. 2). Briefly stated, DA-containing nerve pathways are established in only two regions of the brain: (1) the nigroneostriatal fibers running from the substantial nigra to the caudate nucleus, putamen, and, to a lesser extent, the globus pallidus, and (2) the tuberoinfundibular tract originating in the arcuate nucleus of the ventral hypothalamus and terminating on the capillaries of the hypophyseal portal system in the median eminence. The distribution of NE- and 5-HT-containing tracts is much more extensive when compared to dopaminergic tracts. For 5-HT, the cell bodies of origin are located primarily in the raphe nuclei of the brain stem and midbrain (Fuxe et al., 1968). The most prominent tract distributing the 5-HT neurons to other brain regions is the median forebrain bundle in the medial hypothalamus. 5-HT-containing nerve terminals also have been observed in a number of regions in the telencephalon, basal ganglia, and limbic system. This distribution of fibers is somewhat comparable to those of the noradrenergic system. Most of the cell bodies of NE-producing neurons lie in the ventrolateral tegmental area. The median forebrain bundle contains the majority of the noradrenergic outflow from the brain stem, but the cerebellum, neocortex, and amygdala also possess appreciable quantities of NE-containing nerve endings. It has been pointed out that the distribution of these three amines is predominantly within the phylogenetically older portions of the central nervous system (CNS) which adds credence to their participation in the variously described emotional and drive behaviors.

A.   Adrenergic System

1.   Biochemistry of the Catecholamines

A schematic representation of the synthetic pathway of catecholamines (CA) is shown in Fig. 3. The initial enzyme in CA biosynthesis is tyrosine hydroxylase (TH). High levels of TH activity have been found in particulate fractions isolated from adrenal medulla and from other peripheral sympathetically innervated

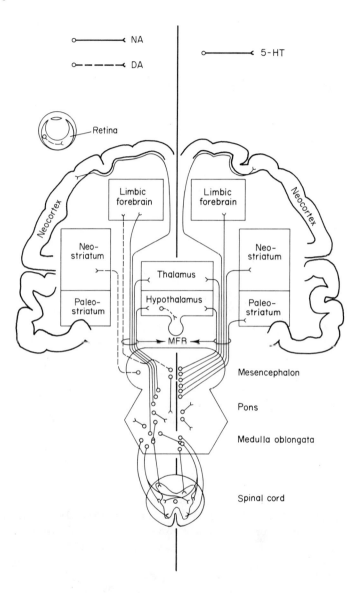

Fig. 2. Schematic representation of the distribution of norepinephrine (NE), dopamine (DA), and serotonin containing (5-HT) fiber tracts in the brain. MFB refers to the median forebrain bundle of the hypothalamus. This figure is taken from Andén *et al.* (1966).

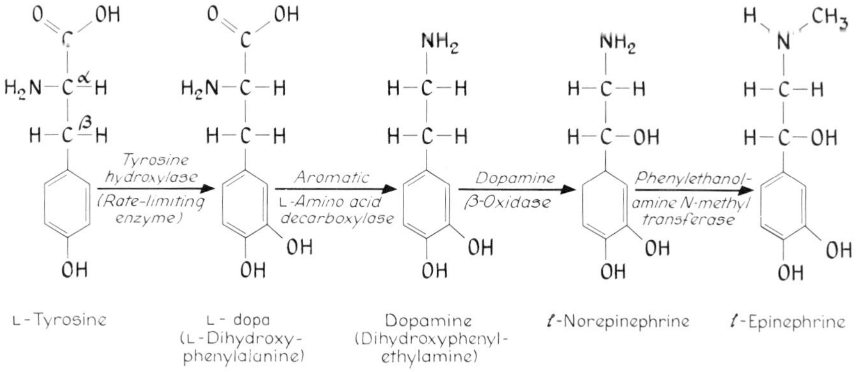

Fig. 3. Metabolic pathway of catecholamine synthesis. Portions of the material presented here are reprinted by permission of the publisher from *Advances in Psychological Assessment,* Volume Two, edited by Paul McReynolds, Palo Alto, Calif.: Science and Behavior Books, Inc., 1971, pp. 260-292.

tissues. Enzyme activity in the brain is greatest in those areas known to have high concentrations of CA-containing nerve endings (McGeer et al., 1967). As will be discussed in detail below, TH appears to be the rate-limiting step in CA formation and, thus, assumes an important role in regulating the levels and activity of CA in various tissues as shown in the elegant studies of Udenfriend and his group who discovered the enzyme (Nagatsu et al., 1964; Gordon et al., 1966a).

The product of tyrosine hydroxylation, dihydroxyphenylalanine (DOPA), is rapidly decarboxylated to DA by the enzyme DOPA decarboxylase. The latter enzyme appears predominantly in soluble fractions isolated from cell tissue and is widely distributed throughout the organism. Due to its high activity, relatively little DOPA is found in any tissue in the body. The product of the decarboxylation step, DA, by virtue of its structure, is the first of the CA formed in the synthetic pathway from tyrosine. Normally DA is found in high concentrations only in the basal ganglia of the brain where enzymes for further modifying DA are absent or in very low concentrations. DA has definite and important roles in motor function and also has been related to other behaviors.

Conversion of DA to NE is accomplished by the enzyme dopamine β-oxidase (DβO). This enzyme appears to be located within specific submicroscopic granules which are known to store NE. To effect conversion to NE, DA must first be transported into the granule by an energy-requiring enzyme system. As will be described in detail below, this transport step and the conversion of DA to NE are susceptible to drug action. The conversion of DA to NE represents the final step in the CA synthetic pathway in most neural tissues. After its synthesis, NE may be disposed of in various ways. As mentioned above, the bulk of the NE in the cell is stored within granular structures in close proximity to the neuroeffector junction (in nerve cells) or to the cell surface (in the adrenal medulla). The NE which is released, either physiologically or pharmacologically, may be handled in different ways; it may (1) react with an appropriate receptor, thereby resulting in the transmission of an effect; (2) undergo reuptake, which involves active transport back into a CA-containing cell, a mechanism which probably is the most important means for terminating the action of CA and is an important step with regard to the action of many drugs; or (3) be metabolized extraneuronally.

The final synthetic enzyme, phenylethanolamine N-methyltransferase, converts NE to epinephrine (E) (Axelrod, 1962a). Enzyme activity is high only in the adrenal medulla, although low levels of enzyme activity resulting in formation of E have been found in mammalian brain.

The most important intracellular enzyme responsible for the degradation of CA is monoamine oxidase (MAO). Most MAO activity is found in mitochondrial and microsomal cell fractions (Schnaitman et al., 1967). Multiple forms of mitochondrial MAO have been described (Ragland, 1968; Squires, 1968). The other major enzyme-catabolizing CA, catechol O-methyltransferase (COMT), is located extraneuronally (Axelrod, 1959). As will become evident from further discussion, a great deal of important information has been inferred from the pattern of CA catabolism in various conditions. A summary of the possible pathways of CA metabolism is presented in Figs. 4, 5, and 6.

2. Distribution of Enzymes Required for Synthesis and Degradation of the Catecholamines

The regional distribution in brain of the enzymes required for synthesizing DA and NE is related to the regional differences in CA content. For purposes of comparison, endogenous NE and DA levels, together with the activity of various enzymes associated with the metabolism of these agents in rats, are listed in Table II. In comparing data from other species with that for the rat, there are no gross differences in distribution of these amines. Thus the highest NE levels in all

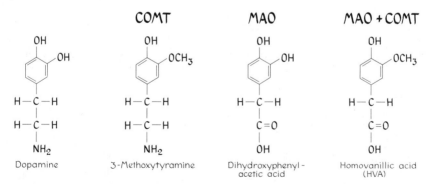

Fig. 4. Metabolic pathway of dopamine. Portions of the material presented here are reprinted by permission of the publisher from *Advances in Psychological Assessment*, Volume Two, edited by Paul McReynolds, Palo Alto, Calif.: Science and Behavior Books, Inc., 1971, pp. 260-292.

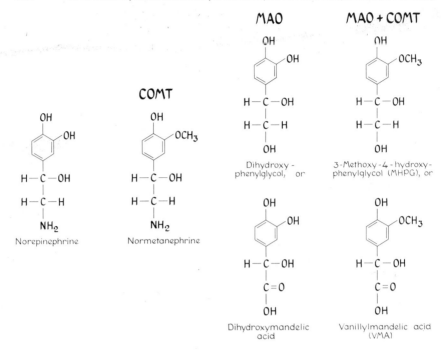

Fig. 5. Metabolic pathway of norepinephrine. Portions of the material presented here are reprinted by permission of the publisher from *Advances in Psychological Assessment,* Volume Two, edited by Paul McReynolds, Palo Alto, Calif.: Science and Behavior Books, Inc., 1971, pp. 260-292.

species studied are found in the hypothalamus, with the midbrain, medulla-pons, and striatum at intermediate levels, and the other brain structures containing low concentrations of NE. DA is present in appreciable amounts only in the striatum.

Regional differences in brain TH activity in the rat, rabbit, and cat were compared by McGeer, *et al.* (1967). Although TH activity generally parallels NE and DA levels, it is of note that all three species had very high TH activity localized in the septal area (about five times the TH activity measured in the hypothalamus). In the only study examining TH activity in human brain, postmortem analysis revealed little or no activity in any area except the basal ganglia (Vogel *et al.,* 1969). The data presented in the latter study were quite variable, and it is possible that the elapsed time between death and enzyme assay (about 16 hours) grossly interfered with accurate measures of enzyme activity. Such studies obviously are important with regard to brain CA metabolism in man and need to be repeated.

Activity of DβO has been detected in the hypothalamus, substantia nigra, and globus pallidus in man (Vogel *et al.,* 1969). However, there have been many difficulties encountered specifically in brain with the *in vitro* assay procedures used for measuring DβO (Molinoff *et al.,* 1969); thus, the data published for

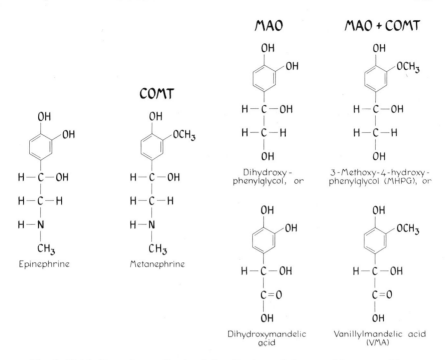

Fig. 6. Metabolic pathway of epinephrine. Portions of the material presented here are reprinted by permission of the publisher from *Advances in Psychological Assessment*, Volume Two, edited by Paul McReynolds, Palo Alto, Calif.: Science and Behavior Books, Inc., 1971, pp. 260-292.

this enzyme in brain may not reflect the true disposition of the enzyme. Perhaps the best assay currently available for estimating brain DβO activity *in vivo* is that used by Iversen and Glowinski (1966) and Glowinski and Iversen (1966b). They measured the amount of ^{3}H-NE formed in areas of rat brain following the intraventricular injection of ^{3}H-DA. Their data indicate DβO activity is high in the medulla oblongata, hypothalamus, and hippocampus, with the striatum (basal ganglia) and cortex having the lowest activity. Similar data in monkeys was presented by Goldstein *et al.* (1967). Since intraventricular injection limits the number of brain structures capable of being studied, these data must be cautiously interpreted. They do, however, illustrate the differences obtained between various groups of investigators with regard to measuring DβO activity in brain.

The work of Vogt (1954) demonstrated E in the dog hypothalamus. Further investigations by Gunne (1962) using biochemical and bioassay techniques established that E was present in hypothalamic tissue from a number of species. Data from the present authors' laboratory confirm the presence of E in the hypothalamus of perfused cat brains. Several investigators have reported the presence of a brain enzyme which synthesizes E, although its activity is quite low and there are problems with interfering reactions in the assay procedure (McGeer and McGeer, 1964; Pohorecky *et al.*, 1968; Barchas *et al.*, 1969;

TABLE II. Comparison of Norepinephrine (NE) and Dopamine (DA) levels with Tyrosine Hydroxylase (TH) and Monoamine Oxidase (MAO) Activities in Various Regions of the Rat Brain

| Brain area | Levels[a] | | TH activity[b] | MAO activity[c] |
	NE	DA		
Striatum	0.25	7.50	56.0	1.1
Hypothalamus	1.79	—	3.8	1.8
Midbrain	0.37	—	2.8	1.2
Hippocampus	0.20	—	1.4	1.2
Medulla oblongata	0.72	—	2.2	—
Cortex	0.24	—	2.4	1.0
Cerebellum	0.17	—	1.0	—

[a]Data listed in $\mu g/gm$ wet weight; from Glowinski and Iversen (1966a).
[b]TH activity relative to activity found in the cerebellum; from McGeer et al. (1967).
[c]MAO activity relative to the activity found in the cortex, DA used as substrate; from La Motte et al. (1969).

Ciaranello et al., 1969b; Deguchi and Barchas, 1971).

The data summarized in Table II for MAO are in general agreement with other reports for rats as well as other species (cf. Vogel et al., 1969). COMT activity, like MAO, shows only minor regional differences in brain.

3. *Physiology of Noradrenergic Function* (Figure 7)

a. Storage of Catecholamines. The physiologically active CA, E and NE, were shown by Blaschko and Welch (1953) and by Hillarp et al. (1953) to be stored in submicroscopic granules within the adrenal medulla. The fully developed medulla of most mammals contains two types of granule-containing chromaffin cells—one type selectively storing E and the other NE. The predominance of E-containing cells correlates with the relative amounts of E in the mature gland (Elfvin, 1965). Analysis of the pre- and postnatal development of chromaffin cells within the medulla of the rat indicates that the NE-containing granules are the first to appear, apparently formed in the Golgi region of the cell. Further differentiation of a population of NE granules to E-type organelles in the rat is associated with an increasing ratio of E to NE during postnatal development (Roffi, 1964; Elfvin, 1967). The mechanisms controlling morphological and biochemical differentiation of the granules is not known.

von Euler and co-workers proved that NE was the active substance concentrated in peripheral sympathetic nerves and sympathetically innervated organs, such as the heart, spleen, etc. Electron-dense organelles in these tissues have been found to be morphologically similar to the NE-containing granules of the adrenal medulla (von Euler and Hillarp, 1956). Although organ and tissue differences are known, the neuronal granules appear to be functionally and chemically related to the medullary structures. The presence of NE in the CNS suggested that CA-containing granules also might be present within the brain. Indeed, axons in brain areas known to accumulate NE also contain numerous granular and agranular vesicles. Such studies are undertaken using CA labeled with a radioactive atom; thus, CA radiolabeled with carbon-14 (^{14}C) or tritium (^{3}H) are used. Pellegrino de Iraldi and co-workers (1963) were the first to suggest that NE within the CNS is stored in large electron-dense structures similar to those previously described in peripheral sympathetic nerve and adrenal medulla. Although other pharmacological studies appeared to substantiate this, Fuxe et al. (1966) and Hökfelt (1967) challenged the view that CA in the brain were stored in large electron-dense granules. Although the large granular vesicles did appear to be the site at which exogenous radiolabeled NE introduced via the cerebrospinal fluid (CSF) was bound intracellularly, changes in the electron opacity of these organelles did not correlate well with the magnitude of CA depletion produced by various drugs (Bloom and Aghajanian, 1968). Thus, the relationship between specific granules and the storage of brain CA is not clear, although it is apparent that microanatomical structures for the storage of amines are present in all nerve cells where these amines have a documented or postulated role as neurotransmitters.

Recent work by Swedish investigators indicates that the storage granules in adrenergic neurons are made in the region of the cell body and are transported down the axon to the nerve terminals. Evidence for this comes from work in which ligatures are made on the spinal cord or the splenic nerve. Above the ligation there is an accumulation of NE and storage granules, whereas below the tied portion of the nerves there is a steady decrease in NE and storage granule population (Dahlström, 1967). A crucial test of these data, at least within the CNS, would be whether synaptosomes (pinched-off nerve endings, known to contain all the enzymes for making NE) (Udenfriend, 1969; Levitt et al., to be published) can synthesize the storage protein. If so, it is conceivable that the nerve endings could produce their own storage granules, or a portion of them, thereby being able to function somewhat autonomously from the cell body in certain circumstances of increased need. The relative importance of amines formed in the nerve cell body and those formed at the synapse in neuronal function remains unclear. It is possible that the CA implicated in neural transmission are synthesized by a specialized synthesizing granule at the synapse.

Apart from being the site at which NE is synthesized from DA, the storage granules also possess mechanisms for sequestering amines from the cytoplasm. Carlsson et al. (1963) and Kirschner (1962) have described an uptake mechanism in adrenal medullary granules which is specific for CA. This uptake system is temperature-dependent, and is stimulated in vitro by adenosine triphosphate (ATP) and magnesium ion, all of which constitute presumptive evidence for an enzymic process. A similar uptake system also appears to be present in granules isolated from brain. In all cases, active uptake of CA into the storage granules can be blocked pharmacologically with reserpine (see below). Another uptake process occurring in the granules may be important pharmacologically. This process is not energy-dependent; it is also not specific for CA, and is not blocked by reserpine (Hamberger, 1967).

b. Release of Catecholamines. The fate of the CA-containing granule, or chromaffin granule, during release of CA from the adrenal medulla has been studied intensively. Much of the published data indicate that the granular contents of medullary cells are discharged upon stimulation of the gland. Thus, CA secretion from the adrenal gland is accompanied by the release of DβO, ATP and specific proteins, as well as NE and E, all of which enter the blood draining the adrenal (Banks, 1966; Poisner *et al.*, 1967; Viveros *et al.*, 1968). In addition, both electron microscopic and biochemical evidence suggest that the storage granule membranes remain within the medullary cells, indicating that amines may be secreted by a process of exocytosis (Malamed *et al.*, 1968). Factors involved in the release of catechols from the adrenal medulla have been summarized by Poisner and Trifaró (1967).

The release mechanism for NE in brain neurons is less clear than that in the medulla although certain parallels do exist. Electrical stimulation *in vitro* of brain slices is accompanied by the release of endogenous or radiolabeled NE into the perfusate (Kirpekar and Misu, 1967; Baldessarini and Kopin, 1966, 1967) with metabolic requirements similar to those in the adrenal. To date, however, the fate of the CA-containing granules in nerve is unknown although at present various laboratories are examining this problem. In addition, *in vivo* release of radio-labeled NE within the brain recently was described by Stein and Wise (1969).

c. Uptake of Catecholamines by the Cellular Membrane. Although enzymic destruction is one factor involved in terminating the actions of CA, an equally important mechanism is the uptake process which is a specific membrane "pump" possessed by medullary and adrenergic nerve cells. The membrane mechanism for sequestering extracellular CA is known to be an energy-requiring system which obeys the generally accepted rules of enzyme kinetics. The membrane systems use an Na^+-K^+-dependent adenosinetriphosphatase "pump" mechanism (Berti and Shore, 1967; Kopin *et al.*, 1965). The uptake system on the cell surface appears to be distinct from the previously described uptake processes of the CA storage granules within the cell, both by biochemical and pharmacological criteria. As will be apparent from subsequent sections, pharmacological alteration of the membrane uptake system is an effective means of altering the behavioral state of the organism, both clinically and experimentally.

4. Regulation of Catecholamine Biosynthesis

The factors regulating CA biosynthesis in adrenergically innervated tissues and in sympathetic neurons have been under intensive investigation in the past few years. Although earlier investigators proposed that increased neuronal activity might cause acceleration in the rate of CA synthesis, confirmation of these ideas awaited discovery and characterization of the enzymes involved in synthesis.

a. Tyrosine Hydroxylase.   Hökfelt and McLean (1950) observed that stimulation of the splanchnic nerves to the adrenal gland resulted in a marked rise in the CA content of the adrenal venous effluent, yet intramedullary amine content was unchanged. Numerous other investigators confirmed these findings. von Euler (1962) proposed a model of sympathetically innervated organs which assumed a relatively constant level of neurotransmitter based on adjustments of the CA biosynthetic rate in response to nervous activity. By 1966, a number of laboratories were engaged in the study of this problem. Using the isolated guinea pig vas deferens-hypogastric nerve preparation, several groups (Alousi and Weiner, 1966; Roth *et al.*, 1967) independently demonstrated an increase in the amount of ^{3}H-NE synthesized from ^{3}H-tyrosine during nerve stimulation. By pharmacological means Alousi and Weiner were able to correlate alterations in the NE synthetic rate with changes in intracellular amine levels. They offered the suggestion that intracellular NE might regulate its own synthesis, possibly by feedback inhibition of TH. Nagatsu *et al.* (1964) had previously shown that purified beef adrenal TH could be inhibited by NE, the end-product of the CA biosynthetic pathway.

Although the above studies showed an acceleration of NE biosynthesis by nerve stimulation, it was not clear at which enzymic step in the pathway stimulation occurred. Although speculation pointed to TH, it was not until the work of Sedvall and Kopin (1967b) and Sedvall *et al.* (1968) that convincing evidence on this point emerged. Using a double-label technique, these investigators were able to show a dramatic increase in *in vivo* TH activity in the rat submaxillary gland following stimulation of the cervical sympathetic chain. They infused ^{14}C-tyrosine and ^{3}H-DOPA which were converted to ^{14}C-NE and ^{3}H-NE, respectively. The amount of ^{14}C-NE synthesized represents the overall activity of the entire CA biosynthetic pathway, while the ^{3}H-NE represents the activity of the last two steps (Fig. 3). Thus, the CA pathway is divided into two separately measurable parts. Sedvall showed that, following stimulation of the nerves to the submaxillary gland, the amount of ^{3}H-NE synthesized from ^{3}H-DOPA in the stimulated animals was not different from that in the unstimulated controls. However, the amount of ^{14}C-NE in the stimulated rats was increased fivefold. Since the conversion of ^{3}H-DOPA to ^{3}H-NE was not altered, but the overall pathway from ^{14}C-tyrosine to ^{14}C-NE was elevated, this

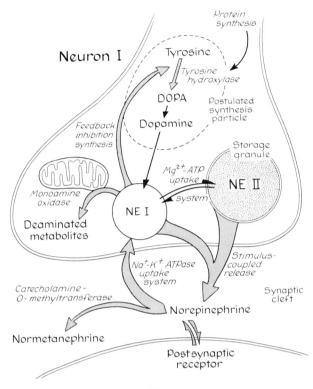

Fig. 7. Functional model of a noradrenergic neuron. The presynaptic neuron (Neuron I) contains all the synthetic enzymes for producing norepinephrine (NE). The synthetic pathway in this figure is shown to enter a labile cytoplasmic compartment (NE I) rather than the storage granule (NE II) because of certain theoretical reasons discussed in the text. Monoamine oxidase, located on the mitochondrion, also is an intracellular enzyme that catabolizes NE. NE released from Neuron I into the synaptic cleft by a nerve impulse may react with the receptor on the postsynaptic neuron (Neuron II), thereby propagating the response that released the neurotransmitter. Other fates of released NE include conversion to the metabolite normetanephrine by the extracellular enzyme catecholamine O-methyl-transferase, or uptake by a transport system located on the presynaptic nerve terminal membrane. The latter uptake system is considered to be quantitatively the most important fate of NE released into the synaptic cleft. Refer to text for full details.

could only mean that TH was activated. This method has also been used to study NE synthesis and TH activity in brain.

Gordon *et al.* (1966a) had earlier used slightly different techniques to arrive at the same conclusion. Studying CA synthesis in a number of organs, this group measured the amount of ^{14}C-NE synthesized from ^{14}C-tyrosine and found it to be elevated two- to threefold when animals were subjected either to cold or exercise. In most tissues studied, NE levels were not lower than control values, suggesting that accelerated synthesis was compensating for the increased release of NE. However, when a TH inhibitor (α-methyl-*para*-tyrosine, α MT) was administered, NE levels fell markedly in heart and brain. These data were taken as evidence that cold or exercise results in a massive utilization of NE in brain, but that under these conditions an accelerated synthesis rate is able to keep pace with demand and maintain normal NE levels. The role of TH as prime mediator of this increase in CA biosynthesis is demonstrated by the fall in NE levels when the enzyme is blocked.

Several hypotheses have emerged to explain the mechanisms whereby neural activity might regulate the activity of TH (Fig. 8). One possibility was that the nerve impulses were in some way stimulating the synthesis of more TH. This

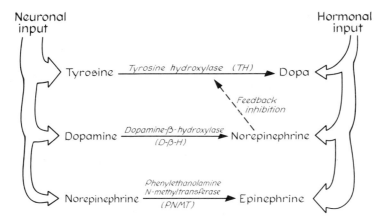

Fig. 8. Role of neuronal and hormonal stimuli on the regulation and induction of tyrosine hydroxylase, dopamine β-hydroxylase, and phenylethanolamine N-methyltransferase. This diagram shows, in a highly schematic way, the qualitative importance of neuronal and hormonal stimuli in the induction of the three enzymes. TH appears to be regulated principally by neuronal stimuli, although ACTH appears to be essential to the maintenance of basal levels of the enzyme (Axelrod *et al.*, 1970b). Neuronal (Molinoff *et al.*, 1970) and hormonal (Weinshilboum and Axelrod, 1970) stimuli seem to be equally important in the regulation of DβH activity. ACTH may be essential in the maintenance of basal DβH activity (Weinshilboum and Axelrod, 1970). PNMT is regulated primarily by corticosteroids, although neuronal stimuli play a role in enzyme activity as well (Axelrod *et al.*, 1970b; Molinoff *et al.*, 1970; Ciaranello and Black, 1971). Both neuronal and hormonal stimuli are essential in regulation of tissue content of these enzymes by stimulating synthesis of enzyme protein. In addition, short-term neural stimuli activate TH without increasing the absolute tissue content of the enzyme by releasing norepinephrine, thus removing the feedback-inhibition of this compound on TH (dashed lines in the diagram). The conversion of DOPA to dopamine, the second step in the catecholamine pathway, is not shown here, since little is known about the regulation of this enzymic conversion.

would increase the number of enzyme molecules, thus increasing the amount of NE formed from tyrosine. The possibility of *de novo* induction of TH was considered by Sedvall and Kopin (1967b), who repeated their earlier experiments on the salivary gland and also measured the activity of submaxillary gland *in vitro*. Although they confirmed *in vivo* activation, they were not able to detect any change in the *in vitro* content of TH. Protein synthesis inhibitors do not alter the *in vivo* rise in TH seen following short-term cold exposure or exercise (Gordon *et al.,* 1966b), but do inhibit the rise seen following prolonged stimulation (Weiner and Rabadjija, 1968).

A second hypothesis to account for the neuronal activation of TH suggested that more tyrosine might be made available to the enzyme during periods of stimulation, either by increased transport of the amino acid into the cell, by decreased metabolism of tyrosine, or by altered cell permeability. This does not appear to be a tenable notion, however, since most investigators have reported that neither the endogenous tyrosine levels nor the amount of radioactive tyrosine in the cell is appreciably altered during nerve stimulation.

By far the most popular hypothesis is that *in vivo* activity of TH is controlled by the level of CA and that CA inhibit the enzyme through feedback inhibition. Thus, nerve stimulation results in utilization and thereby some degree of depletion of NE. This would, it is argued, diminish the NE available to inhibit TH activity and, hence, TH would be more active. Evidence for this notion has been brought forth by Spector *et al.* (1967) who studied the effect of altering tissue NE levels on TH activity. When NE degradation was blocked by MAO inhibitors, the levels of NE in the brain stem rose; but there was a simultaneous decrease in the conversion of ^{14}C-tyrosine to ^{14}C-NE, with TH activity being reduced by about 50%. Since the MAO inhibitor did not alter either tissue tyrosine or the uptake of ^{14}C-tyrosine, and since conversion of ^{3}H-DOPA to ^{3}H-NE was not reduced, inhibition of TH is believed to be due to the increase in intracellular NE.

Weiner and Rabadjija (1968) have proposed an additional and distinct mechanism in situations involving prolonged stimulation. In such situations, TH activity may remain elevated after the stimulus is terminated. This poststimulation increase in TH activity differs markedly from that seen during stimulation in that the poststimulation activity is blocked by puromycin, whereas the rise in TH activity during stimulation is not affected by this drug. Further, the presence of exogenous NE abolishes the rise in TH activity seen during the stimulation period but has no effect on the increased NE synthesis seen during the poststimulation period. As a result of these data, Weiner and Rabadjija proposed that there might be two distinct mechanisms for the regulation of NE biosynthesis by neuronal activity: (1) increased TH activity due to removal of feedback inhibition by NE, and (2) an increase in NE synthesis secondary to induced synthesis or decreased degradation of TH itself.

More recently, studies from Axelrod's laboratory have emphasized that there is a neuronally mediated induction of TH in the adrenal gland. Using pharmacological agents which cause a reflex activation of the nerve supply to the adrenal medulla, Mueller *et al.* (1969), and Thoenen *et al.* (1969) have shown that TH activity rises after drug exposure. The increase in TH can be blocked by cycloheximide, an inhibitor of protein synthesis, suggesting that neuronal stimulation is inducing TH, possibly by increasing synthesis of the enzyme protein (Mueller *et al.*, 1969). These results tend to substantiate the notion that TH activity is under two types of neuronal control: (1) a short-term increase in enzyme activity but not content, mediated via relief of feedback inhibition, and (2) a longer-acting induction of the enzyme with a net increase in tissue content of the enzyme mediated via chronic stimulation.

The role of the pituitary-adrenal axis in TH regulation has been probed by Mueller *et al.* (1970). Enzyme activity falls following hypophysectomy, but does not respond to glucocorticoid administration. Only adrenocorticotropic hormone (ACTH) is effective in restoring enzyme levels to near-normal. This effect of ACTH is not blocked by inhibitors of glucocorticoid synthesis, suggesting that ACTH is acting directly to stimulate TH. This proposal, if substantiated, would prove to be an extremely novel and interesting refinement of the role of ACTH in enzyme regulation. Weinshilboum and Axelrod (1970) have proposed that a similar mechanism may be operant in the maintenance of DβO activity.

b. Dopamine β-Oxidase.   The third enzymic step in the production of the CA involves the addition of an hydroxyl (OH) group to the β-carbon of DA, thereby forming NE (Fig. 3). The regulation of this enzymic process, a key step in NE formation in adrenergic nervous tissue, is being investigated at present in many laboratories (Friedman and Kaufman, 1965). There are inhibitors of the enzyme present in tissues where the enzyme is found. One could postulate that DβO, in certain circumstances, acts as the rate-limiting step in NE biosynthesis rather than TH. Recent studies of the regulation of this enzyme have emerged from the laboratory of Axelrod and his co-workers. Molinoff *et al.* (1970) demonstrated that neural activity plays a role in the maintenance of enzyme activity in sympathetic ganglia. Weinshilboum and Axelrod (1970) have demonstrated that the adrenal enzyme is reduced markedly in the hypophysectomized rat; activity can be restored by ACTH but not by glucocorticoids. These investigators have interpreted their results to mean that the enzyme is under complex endocrine control with ACTH possibly being the primary regulator of enzyme activity.

C. Phenylethanolamine N-methyltransferase.   The last step in the biosynthesis of E is the *N*-methylation of NE. This reaction was described by Axelrod (1962a), who purified and characterized the enzyme from monkey adrenal glands. Because of its ability to catalyze the transfer of a methyl group to the amino nitrogen of a variety of phenylethanolamine derivatives, Axelrod named the enzyme phenylethanolamine N-methyltransferase (PNMT). Methyla tion is accomplished by energy derived from ATP, and the methyl donor for this reaction is known to be S-adenosylmethionine.

The majority of PNMT activity in the body is located in the adrenal medulla. There, Axelrod (1962a) and others have shown that the enzyme resides almost exclusively in the supernatant fraction of the cell homogenates. This would suggest that, following the intragranular conversion of DA to NE, NE is released from the storage granules and N-methylated in the cytoplasm. The E formed then returns to the granule where it is stored until released into the blood. However, Ciaranello et al. (1969b) have obtained evidence that in brain PNMT activity is associated with particulate fractions in the neurons.

The adrenal enzyme N-methylates a number of phenylethanolamine deriva- tives, among them phenylethanolamine itself, normetanephrine, and NE (Axel- rod, 1962a; Molinoff et al., 1969). The β-OH group appears to be of paramount importance in determining whether a compound will be a substrate for this enzyme, since phenylethylamine derivatives are not N-methylated. Krakoff and Axelrod (1967) have shown that a number of MAO inhibitors block PNMT activity in vitro although this has not yet been demonstrated in vivo. The in vivo effects of PNMT inhibitors must be tested over prolonged periods of time to take into account the slow turnover of adrenal E.

Fuller and Hunt (1967) have shown that E, the natural product of PNMT activity in vivo, markedly inhibits its own formation from NE. This might be expected purely on structural grounds, i.e., NE and E are structurally similar. Hence, one might expect that epinephrine would compete with NE for sites on the enzyme and, in sufficient concentrations, E would inhibit its own formation. Axelrod (1962a) has shown that N-methylepinephrine, the methyl derivative of E, exists in adrenal medullary tissue. He demonstrated that E itself is a substrate for PNMT, but is methylated (to N-methylepinephrine) by the enzyme only to about one-fifth the extent of NE. All of these data constitute circumstantial evidence for competitive inhibition of NE methylation by E. However, Fuller and Hunt (1967) suggested that the inhibition of E methylation by E is noncompetitive. This finding was substantiated by Kitabchi and Williams (1968), who showed that human adrenal PNMT is inhibited by E in a noncompetitive fashion. It appears, therefore, that more than simple structural similarity is involved in E inhibition. These data raise the question whether E might fit onto some noncatalytic binding site of the enzyme that may alter enzyme activity. Evidence for the existence of such a site is not yet available.

Perhaps the most exciting aspects of the control of PNMT activity deal with the regulation of the enzyme within the adrenal gland. Coupland (1953) observed that marked species differences exist with respect to the E content of the adrenal gland. Those species whose adrenal medulla was enveloped by a glucocorticoid-producing cortex had high concentrations of E and NE, whereas those species whose adrenal medulla was separate from the cortex contained only NE. Furthermore, the presence of E in the extraadrenal chromaffin tissue was dependent on anatomical contact with some steroid-producing source, as in the rabbit where intra- and extraadrenal chromaffin tissue are contiguous. Jost and Roffi (1958) showed that the pressor activity from the adrenal gland of decapitated rat fetuses decreased markedly, but could be restored with cortisol treatment. These data suggested that the adrenal medulla might be a target organ for glucocorticoids (Fig. 8).

The work of Wurtman and Axelrod (1966) ultimately confirmed Coupland's hypothesis. They demonstrated that hypophysectomy causes a decrease of PNMT activity in adrenal tissue to about 10% of normal. Activity could be restored by administering cortisol, ACTH, or dexamethasone. Only glucocorticoids or ACTH were effective in restoring enzyme activity. When a variety of other pituitary hormones were tested, only ACTH caused this effect on PNMT activity (Wurtman, 1966a).

The stimulation of PNMT in the hypophysectomized animal was shown to proceed by an increase in enzyme synthesis (Wurtman and Axelrod, 1966). When protein synthesis inhibitors were administered with the glucocorticoid, there was no detectable rise in enzyme activity. Neither did the addition of glucocorticoids or ACTH to the enzyme *in vitro* increase activity. *In vivo*, however, it was found initially that the enzyme could not be stimulated in the intact animal using ACTH, dexamethasone, or a variety of short-term stresses (cf. Fuller and Hunt, 1967). It now appears that enzyme activity can be elevated in the intact animal, but that its rate of rise proceeds much more slowly than in the hypophysectomized animal. Thus, in the hypophysectomized rat, PNMT activity doubles after 3-4 days of dexamethasone or ACTH treatment. Using prolonged physiological stresses, Vernikos-Danellis *et al.* (1968) and Ciaranello *et al.* (1969a) demonstrated that PNMT activity doubled in the intact animal over a 20-50-day period.

These results suggest that control mechanisms operating in the intact rat subjected to physiological stress are different from the mechanisms which regulate PNMT activity in the hypophysectomized animal treated with ACTH or glucocorticoids. The effects of the relatively slow turnover of PNMT and E in the intact animal might be to ensure adequate supplies of E in times of stress and to limit the amount of E released at any given time, which could have detrimental effects on the organism. The increase in PNMT activity with long-term stress could have special significance in terms of physiological, biochemical, and behavioral aspects of chronic stress.

Recent studies have demonstrated that PNMT also is under partial neuronal control (Fig. 8). When the splanchnic nerves to the adrenal are stimulated by administration of the drug 6-hydroxydopamine, PNMT activity rises slowly (Mueller *et al.*, 1969). This rise can be blocked by denervation, suggesting that the response is neuronally triggered. Hypophysectomy has no effect on the enzyme response to 6-hydroxydopamine, indicating that the pituitary-adreno-cortical axis is not involved in this aspect of PNMT regulation (Thoenen *et al.,* 1970). Similarly, these same investigators demonstrated that denervation has no effect on the response of the enzyme to dexamethasone in hypophysectomized animals. These results are interpreted to mean that the neuronal and hormonal controls on the enzyme are mediated via different routes.

5. *Selected Aspects of the Pharmacology of Adrenergic Neurons*

An understanding of the relationship between the CA (or the indoleamines (IA)) and behavior depends, in large measure, upon comprehension of the basic pharmacological actions of various drugs on the nervous system. This is especially important with regard to the functions of amines in the CNS, since many of the standard methods of studying CA physiology are inadequate for analyzing their central function. This section will summarize briefly the basic actions of drugs widely used in studying CA and behavior. A more detailed consideration of particular drugs is presented where appropriate in succeeding sections of this chapter.

a. Reserpine and Other Amine-Depleting Agents. Reserpine, an alkaloid extracted from *Rauwolfia serpentina,* was being investigated as a potential antihypertensive agent by Bein (1953), who noted that the drug caused behavioral depression in several patients. This accidental finding led Kline (1954) to evaluate the effects of reserpine in psychotic patients, where the drug met with limited therapeutic success. Subsequently, Carlsson *et al.* (1957a) and Paasonen and Krayer (1957, 1958) found that reserpine depleted peripheral organs of their endogenous CA and also affect 5-HT stores. Possibly more than any other drug, subsequent studies with reserpine served to focus attention on the relationship of brain CA and 5-HT to behavior (Brodie and Shore, 1957). It is now recognized that reserpine has multiple effects on the organism, many unrelated to the drug's action on aminergic systems; nevertheless, although more specific pharmacological agents are available, reserpine maintains a relatively prominent position in the experimental arsenal for studying aminergic processes in the brain.

Treatment with reserpine causes a long-lasting depletion of brain and peripheral NE and inhibits uptake of NE by the granular transport mechanism (von Euler and Lishajko, 1963). Subsequent investigations on the mechanism of action of reserpine, summaraized by Alpers and Shore (1969), demonstrate that specific intracellular binding of reserpine, probably to adrenergic nerve granules, is associated with NE depletion. Reserpine-induced depletion of tissue NE is known to be accompanied by changes in the electron microscopic appearance of the granules. Only the granule NE-sequestering system, and not the cell

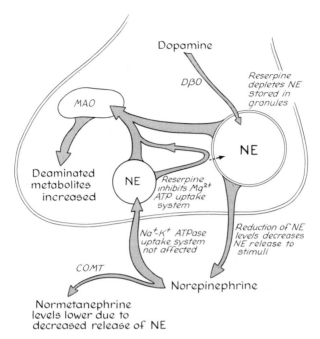

Fig. 9. Effect of reserpine on a functional model of a noradrenergic neuron. The action of reserpine on different components of the model neuron depicted in Fig. 7 is illustrated. Refer to text for further details.

membrane uptake system (Fig. 7), is inhibited by the drug (Glowinski *et al.*, 1966). Further, release of stored NE is accompanied by a large increase in the intracellular metabolism of amines due to mitochondrial MAO, with little or no alteration in COMT-derived metabolism. These changes are summarized in Fig. 9. The temporal duration of these effects is similar to the behavioral depressant effects of reserpine (cf. Stein, 1964; Rech *et al.*, 1968).

Another series of drugs, benzoquinolizine and its derivatives, have actions on adrenergic storage granules similar to those of reserpine but lasting for a shorter period of time (Quinn *et al.*, 1959). Tetrabenazine, the most widely used benzoquinolizine drug, is able to block the biochemical actions of reserpine on CA stores and metabolism, but unlike reserpine, does not cause the prolonged behavioral depression or overt side effects of the *Rauwolfia* alkaloid. There is reason to believe that tetrabenazine has a prominent effect on "free" NE within adrenergic neurons—an action not shared by reserpine.

There are other classes of drugs which effect brain CA depletion but are not related to reserpine or tetrabenazine. Perhaps the most important of these are the compounds which inhibit the various enzymes responsible for synthesizing CA. One such drug, α MT, has been discussed previously. This important

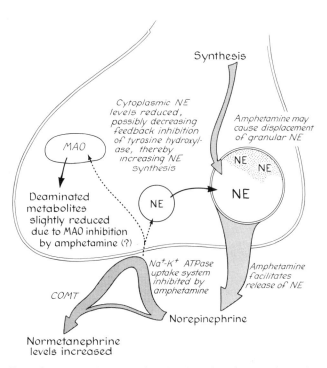

Fig. 10. Effect of amphetamine on a functional model of a noradrenergic neuron. The action of amphetamine on different components of the model neuron depicted in Fig . 7 is illustrated. Refer to text for further details.

category of CA-depleting agents is summarized in Table III. Other classes of drugs which modify tissue amine levels by methods other than enzyme inhibition are listed in Table IV.

b. Amphetamine and Related Sympathomimetic Amines.   The classical work on the active principle of the adrenal medulla conducted by Oliver and Schäfer (1895) and by Abel and Crawford (1897) led quickly to the elucidation of the chemical structure of "sympathin," or epinephrine (E). In 1910, Barger and Dale published their comprehensive structure-activity study of E-like compounds, called sympathomimetic amines. Although their usage goes back at least five centuries to the native Chinese and Indian cultures (Chen and Schmidt, 1930), the behavioral properties of sympathomimetic amines were first elegantly and completely defined by Nathanson in 1937. In current terminology, sympathomimetic amines are classified on the basis of their innate ability to stimulate adrenergic receptors. Using this criterion, the concept of direct- and indirect-acting sympathomimetic amines has evolved (Trendelenburg, 1963). Direct-acting compounds are those which directly excite adrenergic receptors, i.e., NE and E. Indirect-acting amines are relatively inactive by themselves in

TABLE III. Drugs Which Deplete Tissue Catecholamines by Inhibiting the Enzymes which Synthesize the Endogenous Amines

Enzyme	Drug	Mechanism of action
Tyrosine hydroxylase	α-Methyl-*para*-tyrosine (αMT) (and its congeners)	Possibly competes with enzyme cofactor; can also be converted to α-methyl-DOPA to a limited extent
DOPA decarboxylase	α-Methyl-DOPA	Although inhibits enzyme, main effect is to be converted by DOPA decarboxylase and dopamine β-oxidase to α-methyl-NE, which displaces endogenous NE from the granule
Dopamine β-oxidase	Disulfiram Diethyldithiocarbamate (metabolite of disulfiram)	Complexes with copper ion necessary for enzyme activity
	p-Hydroxyamphetamine (a major metabolite of amphetamine in many species)	Direct competition with dopamine for active site of enzyme
Phenylethanolamine N-methyltransferase	Pargyline (a mono-amine oxidase in-hibitor)	*In vitro* only?
	S-Adenosylhomocysteine	

stimulating adrenergic receptors and require, as we shall see, the presence of NE (or E) for their action. The most representative indirect-acting sympathomimetic amine with regard to its behavioral effects is amphetamine. The following discussion, therefore, will concentrate on the general mechanism of action of this drug.

One fundamental characteristic of an indirect-acting sympathomimetic amine is its decreasing ability to evoke a maximal response during successive administrations of the drug over relatively short periods of time. Thus, amphetamine causes a large increase in blood pressure or heart rate upon initial injection, but an identical dose of the compound given shortly thereafter will be less effective than the previous response, and so on for succeeding doses. This phenomenon is called tachyphylaxis. Tachyphylaxis to indirect-acting sympatho-mimetic amines has been demonstrated in many different peripheral test systems. Using CA release from the adrenal medulla as a case in point, amphetamine was found to cause a hundredfold increase in the secretion rate of

TABLE IV. Drugs Which Decrease Tissue Catecholamine Levels by Mechanisms Other Than Inhibiting the Enzymes Responsible for Amine Synthesis

Drug	Mechanism of depletion
Benzoquinolizine derivatives Benzquinamide Tetrabenazine	Mechanism similar to reserpine.[a] block granular uptake system; release NE stored in granule
Sympathomimetic amines Tyramine Amphetamine	Converted by $D\beta O$ to NE-like amines which displace NE in granules
α-Methyl-*meta*-tyrosine	Depletes NE stored in granule
Guanethidine	Causes inhibition of adrenergic transmission by unknown mechanism, and results in a slow reduction of NE content in the cell, also by unknown mechanism
6-Hydroxydopamine	Destroys NE-containing neurons and cells by an unknown mechanism; this effect is reversible in the peripheral nervous system, since cells can regenerate, but is permanent in central NE-containing neurons

[a]See text.

CA in the venous effluent of the perfused gland (Harvey *et al.*, 1968). Following development of tachyphylaxis by repeated doses of amphetamine, a subsequent dose of the stimulant did not cause any significant alteration in the "resting" CA concentration in plasma. When NE was infused after the development of tachyphylaxis, amphetamine once again caused a hundredfold increase in amine secretion from the adrenal medulla. These data suggest that reduction of adrenal CA content by amphetamine was one aspect in the development of tachyphylaxis.

It is apparent, however, that the tachyphylaxis observed to amphetamine is not simply a manifestation of reduced tissue CA stores, since tachyphylaxis to amphetamine developed when CA levels were nearly normal (Bhagat, 1965). In addition, tolerance to the central behavioral effects of the drug has not been demonstrated (Brown and Searle, 1938). These and other results prompted the formation of a number of hypotheses regarding the mechanism of action of amphetamine; among these have been postulates concerning (1) the heterogeneity of endogenous CA stores and (2) the effects of amphetamine on endogenous CA metabolism. The current view is that one of the major effects of amphetamine is the preferential release of a relatively small pool of intraneuronal NE (e.g., see Fig. 7).

Amphetamine also has documented effects on CA catabolism. Several laboratories have shown that amphetamine decreases the uptake of NE into adrenergic neurons. This effect appears to be localized in the cell membrane uptake system. On the basis of this action, one would predict that metabolism of NE released by the drug would be shifted toward COMT metabolites, which has been shown to occur (Glowinski et al., 1966). Although early workers suggested that part of amphetamine's stimulant effects on behavior were due to inhibition of MAO (Mann and Quastel, 1940), discrete evidence does not reveal a significant degree of *in vivo* MAO antagonism. Additionally, since amphetamine simultaneously releases NE and blocks its recapture, one would expect that the drug has a stimulant action, which it has. The combined effects of increasing CA release, presumably of the small pool of NE, and decreasing the recapture of NE from the synaptic cleft has been postulated to result in a decrease in feedback inhibition by NE on TH, thus causing an increase in CA synthesis. Although this mechanism is hypothetical, amphetamine does cause a prominent increase in NE synthesis (Javoy et al., 1968). The various effects of amphetamine on the adrenergic neuron are illustrated in Fig. 10.

c. *Drugs Inhibiting the Uptake of Catecholamines.* Early work on cocaine revealed that administration of this drug prior to giving NE or E potentiated the responses of various tissues to these CA. Subsequent work has shown that cocaine blocks the cell membrane CA-uptake mechanism, thereby increasing the concentration of NE (or E) at the receptor and accounting for the potentiated response. The alterations in metabolism of ^{3}H-NE, in brain, (i.e., decreased intraneuronal ^{3}H-NE, increased COMT-derived metabolites and decreased MAO-derived products) reflect the postulated site of action of cocaine (Glowinski and Axelrod, 1965).

Another group of drugs, the tricyclic antidepressants, also inhibit the membrane "pump" system which accumulates extraneuronal CA. The best known compounds in this category, desmethylimipramine (DMI) and imipramine, have effects on brain ^{3}H-NE metabolism somewhat comparable to those described for cocaine (Schanberg et al., 1967a; Sulser et al., 1969). Recent evidence, however, also indicates that DMI may have an additional intraneuronal effect of blocking the granular uptake system and stabilizing the granular stores of NE (Reid et al., 1969). The relationship of these intraneuronal effects to the behavioral and clinical effects of DMI is not known. A summary of drugs which block the nerve cell membrane uptake system appears in Table V.

d. *Drugs Affecting the Catabolism of Catecholamines.* The major class of drugs affecting the enzymes responsible for the degradation of CA that have found extensive use, either experimentally or clinically, are the MAO inhibitors. As expected from the model proposed in Fig. 7 and the catabolic pathways illustrated in Fig. 3, the main alteration in NE metabolism following MAO inhibitors is an increase in NE as well as in normetanephrine and other COMT-derived metabolites (Schanberg et al., 1967a,b). Comparable effects are observed on E and DA metabolism. Although one might postulate a concurrent

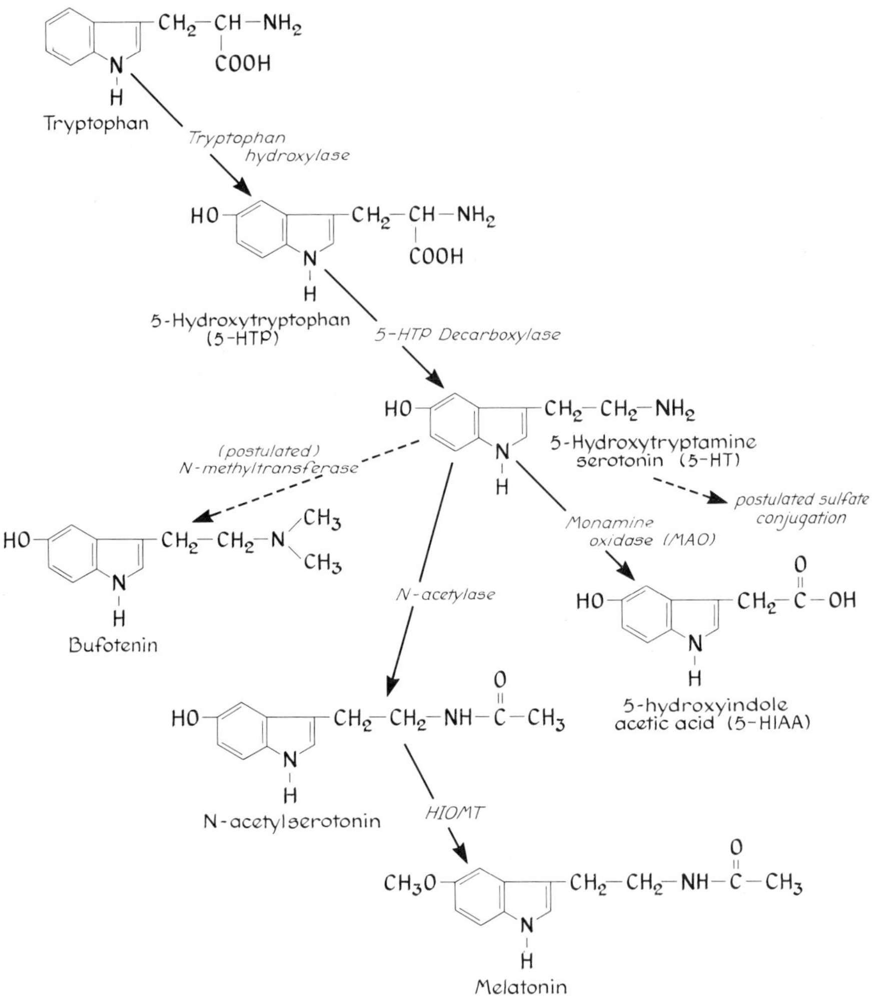

Fig. 11. Metabolic pathway of indoleamine formation and metabolism. Portions of the material presented here are reprinted by permission of the publisher from *Advances in Psychological Assessment*, Volume Two, edited by Paul McReynolds, Palo Alto, Calif.: Science and Behavior Books, Inc., 1971, pp. 260-292.

increase in the levels of NE at the receptor level, turnover studies reveal that there is a reduction in the utilization rate of NE under such conditions (Neff and Costa, 1966). The accepted mechanism for the latter effect is that the increased intraneuronal NE levels result in the end-product inhibition of TH, thereby decreasing the synthesis rate of the amine. Pyrogallol, an inhibitor of COMT, has found limited use due to its high toxicity.

TABLE V. Drugs Which Inhibit the Na⁺—K⁺ ATPase Catecholamine Transport System on the Adrenergic Cell or Neuronal Membrane

Ouabain, a member of the digitalis
  family of drugs
Cocaine
Imipramine
Desmethylimipramine
Phenoxybenzamine, and other receptor—
  blocking drugs
Sympathomimetic amines, such as
  amphetamine, tyramine, etc.

e. Drugs Affecting Adrenergic Receptors. Both the metabolic effects of E and NE secreted by the adrenal medulla and the NE or DA released into synapses by nerve stimulation cause their physiological effects by reacting with hypothetical molecules or structures called receptors. Although the mechanisms involved in receptor activation have not yet been defined, specific inhibitor chemicals are able to block the activity of CA selectively on postsynaptic receptors, at least in the peripheral adrenergic system. The principle durg used to block the effects of NE on the postsynaptic membrane of peripheral sympathetic nerves is phenoxybenzamine, a so-called α-adrenergic blocking agent. Although this agent is effective in almost completely antagonizing the peripheral actions of NE, attempts to block the actions of central NE with phenoxybenzamine have not been universally successful. With respect to the central stimulant effects of amphetamine, however, various reports have demonstrated that phenoxybenzamine is partially able to antagonize amphetamine's action (e.g., see Rech and Stolk, 1970).

In addition to blocking NE's effects in the periphery, phenoxybenzamine also causes alterations in the turnover of CA. These changes entail a relatively large increase in the turnover of NE in spinal cord ceurons (Andén *et al.*, 1967). The mechanism of this action is not clearly understood, but Andén and his associates have postulated that the increased turnover is attributable to a reflex increase in neuronal impulse activity with the possible concomitant activation of TH.

Another group of drugs, the phenothiazines, also are thought to have prominent antiadrenergic activity in the brain (Sulser and Dingell, 1968). Phenothiazines are universally accepted as the drug of choice in the treatment of schizophrenia, and widespread use of these compounds significantly decreased the number of hospital beds required for schizophrenic in-patients in the U.S. since 1955. Chlorpromazine, the most widely used phenothiazine, shares the same activity as described above for phenoxybenzamine. In addition, chlorpromazine was found to increase by threefold the accumulation of ^{14}C-DA from

[14]C-tyrosine, indicating a prominent increase in TH activity (Nybäck and Sedvall, 1968).

B. Serotonergic Neurotransmission

1. Biochemistry of the Indolealkylamines and Serotonin

Serotonin was first investigated in the 1950's (see Erspamer, 1966; Page, 1968). This compound has a wide distribution throughout the body. The metabolic pathway responsible for synthesis of the indolealkylamines is diagramed in Fig. 11. Tryptophan hydroxylase is the initial enzyme in the synthesis of 5-HT and was recently characterized by Ichiyama et al. (1970). Levels of tryptophan hydroxylase appear to correlate with the regional distribution of 5-HT in brain (see below).

5-Hydroxytryptophan (5-HTP), the product of tryptophan hydroxylation, is decarboxylated rapidly by the enzyme 5-HTP-decarboxylase to form 5-HT. This decarboxylase enzyme is similar, if not identical, to DOPA decarboxylase. Some investigators propose the use of the name aromatic l-amino acid decarboxylase for these enzyme activities since the current belief is that both decarboxylations are performed by the same enzyme.

A further series of synthetic enzymes for producing melatonin (5-methoxy-N-acetyltryptamine) is present in the pineal gland. The overall synthetic pathway has been shown to progress as follows: 5-HT ⇒ N-acetylserotonin ⇒ melatonin (Axelrod and Weissbach, 1961).

The last enzyme in melatonin synthesis, hydroxyindole O-methyltransferase (HIOMT), was discovered by Axelrod and Weissbach in 1961. The only mammalian tissue known to contain HIOMT activity is the pineal parenchyma. Axelrod, Wurtman and other collaborators have elegantly demonstrated the many complex and intriguing mechanisms controlling the activity of this enzyme. Melatonin may function as a hormone secreted from the pineal (Barchas et al., 1967). The body of literature pertinent to the pineal gland and melatonin has been summarized by Wurtman et al. (1968).

MAO was believed to be the major intracellular catabolic enzyme for 5-HT as well as for the CA (Fig. 11). The enzyme converts the amine to an aldehyde and most of the aldehyde is then transformed to 5-hydroxylindoleacetic acid (5-HIAA). The latter compound is found in the CSF of many species, including man (Gottfries et al., 1969), and has been used to measure the rate of 5-HT turnover in brain. Recently, two other potentially important enzymes metabolizing 5-HT have been studied. The first, indole(ethyl)amine N-methyltransferase, has generated considerable interest. Axelrod (1962b) originally described a nonspecific N-methyltransferase in various peripheral organs of the rabbit, but not in the brain. Morgan and Mandell (1969; Mandell and Morgan, 1971) have also investigated such an enzyme in brain. This enzyme appeared in the supernatant and synaptosomal fractions of pituitary and pineal homogenates. The discovery of this enzyme in brain raises the possibility of endogenous production of N-methylated indolealkylamines, which are potent psychotomimetic agents, thus linking the enzyme in a tenuous way to psychoses and psychotic reactions to various drugs (e.g., MAO inhibitors). The possibility that N-methylated derivatives of indoles could be produced and have behavioral effects has stimulated considerable interest (Himwich, 1971).

Another IA enzyme, 5-HT sulfotransferase, (Goldberg and Delbruck, 1959; Hidaka et al., 1969b), is present in the high speed supernatant fraction of brain and has a variable regional distribution (Hidaka et al., 1969a). Korf and Sebens (1970) report that serotonin O-sulfate, the product of the sulfotransferase, constitutes about 33% of the 5-HT metabolites excreted in the urine.

2. Distribution of Enzymes Required for the Synthesis and Degradation of Indolealkylamines

As is true for the CA, there appears to be a consistent distribution of 5-HT in the brain of various species (Table VI). Thus, hypothalamus and midbrain areas consistently have the greatest concentration of the amine, while cerebellum has a low 5-HT concentration. Melatonin formation has been demonstrated only in the pineal gland in mammals; theoretically it may be transported elsewhere via either the third ventricle of the brain or the blood supply from the pineal. A summary of the localization of 5-HT in the brains of non-mammalian species has

TABLE VI. Distribution of Serotonin (5-HT) and Tryptophan Hydroxylase in the Brain of the Rat, Cat, and Dog

Brain area	5-HT (µg/gm brain)			Tryptophan hydroxylase[a]		
	Rat[b]	Cat[c]	Dog[d]	Rat[b]	Cat[c]	Dog[d]
Caudate nucleus	0.39	2.44	—	4.70	31.0	—
Hypothalamus	0.81	2.44	1.72	20.0	20.0	2.00
Midbrain	0.61	2.34	—	13.9	17.6	—
Pons	0.50	1.20	0.41	11.8	5.40	1.00
Neocortex	0.31	0.14	—	3.70	1.30	—
Cerebellum	0.06	0.19	0.05	0.30	1.00	—

[a]Tryptophan hydroxylase activity relative to activity found in hypothalamus.
[b]From Deguchi and Barchas (1971).
[c]From Peters et al. (1968). Tryptophan hydroxylase activity relative to activity found in cerebellum.
[d]From Grahame-Smith (1967). Tryptophan hydroxylase activity relative to activity found in the pons.

been presented by J. H. Welsh (1968). A comparison of 5-HT concentrations and tryptophan hydroxylase activity in various brain regions of the rat, dog, and cat are compiled in Table VI. Other regional distribution studies are in general agreement with the values reported in the table. MAO activity shows little, if any, regional specificity (Table II). The remaining catabolic enzymes have not been studied in any detail.

3. Physiology of Serotonergic Function

a. *Serotonin Storage Granules.* Early work by Giarman and Schanberg (1958) and by Schanberg and Giarman (1962) revealed that approximately 70% of the 5-HT in brain is particulate-bound as opposed to being "free" in the supernatant of brain homogenates. These results strongly suggested that 5-HT, like NE, is stored within morphologically distinct granular structures similar to those sequestering the CA. However, the lack of a peripheral nervous system model has hindered the detailed study of specific 5-HT binding organelles.

Aghajanian and Bloom (1967) studied the localization of ^{3}H-5-HT after intraventricular injection. As is true for labeled CA, the labeled IA is concentrated in periventricular areas known to contain large amounts of dense-core vesicles. Further elaboration of the bound radioactivity was not possible using the techniques employed by those workers. Subsequent investigation by Wesemann (1969) revealed that 5-HT may be bound in a specific type of vesicular fraction isolated from rat brain. Snipes *et al.* (1968) have demonstrated that exogenous 5-HT is capable of being incorporated into granules usually storing NE.

b. *Release of Serotonin.* Chase *et al.* (1967, 1969) have studied the *in vitro* release of ^{3}H-5-HT from brain slices subjected to pharmacological and electrical challenge. Whether the labeled indole was given *in vivo* or *in vitro* prior to the start of the experiment, electrical stimulation was found to cause a marked increase in the amount of ^{3}H released into the superfusing medium. The radioactivity consisted of both ^{3}H-5-HT and labeled degradation products. Unlike NE release, release of ^{3}H-5-HT did not appear to be calcium dependent, but was somewhat specific in that (1) the efflux of radiolabeled urea which distributes homogeneously in most tissue media is unaffected by stimulation, and (2) the amount of 5-HT released is related to the density of 5-HT-containing nerve terminals in each of the brain regions analyzed.

Another means of demonstrating the release of 5-HT from brain neurons has been employed by several investigators. In these studies, changes in the levels of 5-HIAA, the principal metabolite of 5-HT, are measured and assumed to bear some functional relationship to altered release of 5-HT from nerve endings. Aghajanian *et al.* (1967) and Sheard and Aghajanian (1968) found that electrical stimulation of the midbrain raphe caused an elevation in forebrain 5-HIAA levels in the rat. There also was a concomitant decrease in forebrain 5-HT concentration. These changes were observed only when 5-HT-containing fiber tracts were stimulated. Similar experiments have been reported recently by Eccleston *et al.* (1970), and are interpreted as strong evidence favoring electrically coupled release of 5-HT from brain neurons.

   c. Uptake of Serotonin by the Cellular Membrane.   Numerous studies have demonstrated both metabolic and temperature requirements for 5-HT uptake by brain tissue which are similar to those described for NE uptake (Blackburn *et al.*, 1967; Ross and Renyi, 1967) and for 5-HT accumulation in nonneural peripheral tissues (Green, 1966). Uptake of labeled 5-HT injected intraventricularly followed a regional pattern which was dissimilar to that of NE (Aghajanian and Bloom, 1967), indicating at least some differentiation of transport sites and amine-containing cell population.

   The metabolic requirement for the 5-HT system is also different from the NE-concentrating mechanism at the nerve cell membrane. Ouabain, a relatively specific inhibitor of the Na^+-K^+ ATPase system thought to mediate CA transport (Berti and Shore, 1967), has only a minor inhibitory action on 5-HT accumulation (Ross and Renyi, 1967; Blackburn *et al.*, 1967). The latter investigators also reported that neither NE nor DA affected 5-HT uptake, thus further minimizing the possibility that 5-HT was being concentrated by the CA membrane transport system.

4. Regulation of Serotonin Biosynthesis

   In contrast to the wealth of data compiled on the regulation of CA synthesis, relatively little work has been done on the control of 5-HT metabolism. The decarboxylase step does not seem to be rate-limiting in the formation of 5-HT.

   Shein *et al.* (1967) measured 5-HT production in organ cultures of pineal gland and concluded that the hydroxylation of tryptophan was rate-limiting. The latter study was substantiated by Moir and Eccleston (1968), who examined 5-hydroxyindole metabolism in rats and dogs using both tryptophan and 5-HTP injections. They concluded that there were regional differences in the metabolism of 5-HT and that turnover through the system normally was controlled by the enzyme tryptophan hydroxylase. In the same report, Moir and Eccleston also postulated an interesting model of the functional relationships extant in 5-HT neurons. They proposed that 5-HT formed from exogenous 5-HTP was handled in a manner considerably different from that formed from endogenous or exogenous tryptophan. In their model, 5-HT formed from 5-HTP is rapidly deaminated by MAO rather than stored within the neuron as 5-HT. These data are consistent with a two-pool model of 5-HT metabolism in brain serotonergic neurons. This is similar to hypotheses of NE distribution within adrenergic neurons. However, a recent publication indicates that 5-HT production following 5-HTP administration is markedly different from that after tryptophan administration. Aghajanian and Asher (1971) using an histochemical method, demonstrated that the increase in whole brain 5-HT levels after tryptophan administration is accounted for by an increase in the fluorescence of cells that normally synthesize 5-HT. There was no qualitative difference in the distribution of 5-HT in brain, although absolute levels increased. Following 5-HTP administration, however, all cells in the brain showed fluorescence, especially those that normally were nonfluorescent. Thus, distribution of 5-HT in brain is altered both qualitatively and quantitatively after 5-HTP, in contrast to the changes observed after tryptophan.

5. Selected Aspects of the Pharmacology of Serotonin-Containing Neurons

There are relatively few drugs which specifically affect either the 5-HT- or the NE-containing neuronal systems without affecting both amines. For this reason much of the pharmacology of NE is applicable to 5-HT and will not be discussed in detail here. Similarities in drug action on the two systems emphasize the many parallels seen in their biochemistry and physiology.

a. Serotonin-Depleting Drugs. As previously mentioned, reserpine and related drugs cause a profound decrease in the levels of 5-HT and CA in the brain. In the case of 5-HT, however, recovery of normal functional mechanisms occurs more rapidly than for NE (Brodie *et al.,* 1966a), and similar differences are seen in the rate of repletion of brain amine stores after the drug. Although reserpine causes alterations in 5-HT metabolism comparable to those for NE (Fig. 9), the extent of the biochemical effects on 5-HT are quantitatively less prominent. For instance, following the intracisternal injection of ^{3}H-5-HT, rats pretreated with reserpine had 30% less ^{3}H-5-HT remaining in brain than did controls 1 hour after the injection of the radioactive amine (Schildkraut *et al.,* 1969). The reduction in the case of NE was much greater (about 80%; Glowinski and Axelrod, 1965). Deaminated metabolites of ^{3}H-5-HT were increased (relative to 5-HT content), but to a smaller extent than for NE. Reserpine appeared to increase the turnover of 5-HT in brain (Tozer *et al.,* 1966). As was true for CA-containing neurons, reserpine does not appear to affect *in vitro* uptake of 5-HT by the nerve cell membrane (Blackburn *et al.,* 1967). Even though the transport systems are not the same for each amine; available data suggest that storage granules are the main site of action of reserpine on brain content and metabolism of both 5-HT and NE.

One candidate for a relatively specific brain 5-HT-depleting agent appears to be *p*-chloroamphetamine and its derivatives. These compounds have been shown to cause prolonged (i.e., several weeks) reduction in brain 5-HT and 5-HIAA levels, but no change in brain CA concentration. Since synthesis from trypto-phan does not appear to be affected, the most widely accepted mechanism of action for *p*-chloroamphetamine is depletion of 5-HT from storage sites combined with an inhibition of MAO.

In 1966, Koe and Weissman introduced a chlorinated amino acid, *p*-chloro-phenylalanine (PCPA), which caused profound and relatively long-lasting reductions in brain 5-HT concentrations. The originally postulated mechanism of this effect was an inhibition of tryptophan hydroxylase. Subsequent work by Jequier *et al.* (1967) revealed that inhibition of the enzyme was reversible in an *in vitro* assay system, but was not reversible when PCPA was injected into the animals prior to isolating the enzyme, indicating that PCPA causes a structural or chemical alteration in the enzyme itself and recovery from the drug effect requires synthesis of new enzyme protein. Deguchi and Barchas (in press) have also studied the mechanism of inhibition. Much work has indicated that PCPA's effects are not confined solely to 5-HT-containing cells. Phenylalanine hydroxylase also is inhibited by PCPA (Koe and Weissman, 1966), presumably in a manner similar to tryptophan hydroxylase (Lipton *et al.*, 1967; Jequier *et al.*, 1967). Other alterations include effects on brain CA levels (Koe and Weissman, 1966) and metabolism (Stolk *et al.*, 1969) and must be taken into account when interpreting the effects of this drug.

A summary of 5-HT-depleting drugs is listed in Table VII.

b. Serotonin-Releasing Drugs and Serotonergic Stimulants. With the exception of PCPA, all the 5-HT-depleting drugs listed in Table VII have been postulated to cause an increase in the levels of "free" 5-HT at the receptor level, thus resulting in an increased transmission across serotonergic synapses (see Vogt, 1968). Other classes of compounds which do not fall into the above category are classified as 5-HT stimulants. Many of the sympathomimetic

TABLE VII. Drugs Causing a Depletion of Brain Serotonin

Drug	Mechanism of action
Reserpine and the *Rauwolfia* alkaloids	Disruption of 5-HT storage sites by an action similar to that on NE (postulated)
Benzoquinolizine derivatives Benzquinamide Tetrabenazine	Same as above
p-Chloroamphetamine	Displacement of stored 5-HT and inhibition of MAO. Inhibits tryptophen hydroxylese
α-Methyl-5-hydroxytryptophan	Inhibits *l*-amino acid decarboxylase; it is also converted by the same enzyme to α-methyl-5-HT which displaces 5-HT and NE from storage sites
Oxypertin and related piperazine derivatives	Disruption of storage sites for DA, NE, and 5-HT. Affects 5-HT only in high doses (Bak *et al.*, 1969)
p-Chlorophenylalanine	Inhibits tryptophan hydroxylase

amines, particularly amphetamine, have been postulated to have direct effects on 5-HT receptors (Vane, 1960), as is true of the tryptamine derivatives (Winter, 1969); indeed, 5-HT receptors have been termed "tryptaminergic" receptors by Vane. Sabelli and his associates have studied the deaminated metabolites of 5-HT and find that certain compounds (i.e., 5-HIAA and its aldehyde intermediate, 5-hydroxy-indoleacetaldehyde) are able to mimic certain effects of 5-HT on behavior and in neurophysiological tests (Sabelli et al., 1969; Sabelli, 1970).

   c. Drugs Affecting the Uptake of Serotonin into Neurons.   Various investigators have reported that the tricyclic antidepressants, like imipramine and desmethylimipramine (desipramine), inhibit the in vitro uptake of 5-HT into brain slices (Blackburn et al., 1967; Ross and Renyi, 1967, 1969) and into synaptosome preparations (Segawa et al., 1968). However, in vivo studies reveal no alterations in amine uptake (Fuxe and Ungerstedt, 1967; Schildkraut et al., 1969). Some members of this series of compounds cause a decrease in 5-HT turnover in brain, while others have little or no effect (Corrodi and Fuxe, 1969). Of possible interest in this regard is the finding of Schildkraut et al., (1969) that desipramine is ineffective in retarding ^{3}H-5-HT turnover, whereas imipgramine has a marked effect.

   In light of current clinical interest, lithium treatment is known to stimulate the uptake of 5-HT into platelets (Murphy et al., 1969); an identical action is seen on NE transport (Colburn et al., 1967). Lithium also increases the deamination of both 5-HT and NE (Schildkraut et al., 1969; Schanberg et al., 1967a), but has opposite effects on amine turnover, slowing down 5-HT and increasing NE utilization (Stern et al., 1969).

   Other drugs affecting uptake of 5-HT into cells include cocaine, tryptamine, N-alkylated tryptamine derivatives and bufotenin (some of which may be metabolites of 5-HT; see Fig. 11). Ouabain, a potent inhibitor of CA uptake, has but a small effect on 5-HT-containing nerve cells.

   d. Drugs Affecting Receptors Stimulated by Serotonin.   Gaddum (1954) originally proposed that the hallucinogenic potency of lysergic acid diethylamine (LSD) is related to the blockade of 5-HT receptors in the brain. Although other works have vacillated between interpreting LSD's effects as being attributable to receptor stimulation or to receptor blockade, the prevailing bulk of neurophysiological and neuropharmacological data appears to sustain Gaddum's original thesis (Aghajanian et al., 1968; Clineschmidt and Anderson, 1969). The proposed decrease in 5-HT turnover after administration of LSD (Diaz et al., 1968; Schildkraut et al., 1969) is supported by the findings that endogenous 5-HT levels are increased and 5-HIAA concentrations reduced by the drug (Rosecrans et al., 1967). Lin et al. (1969c) have reported that conversion of ^{14}C-tryptophan to ^{14}C-serotonin is reduced. It would appear that hallucinogenic potency bears some relationship to these effects since brom-LSD, which inhibits peripheral

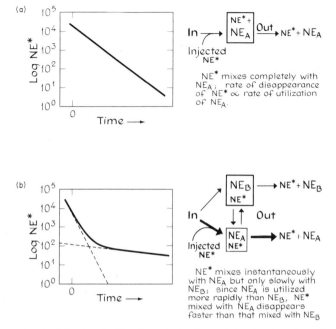

Fig. 12. Basic principles for the kinetic analysis of catecholamine function using radioactive norepinephrine (NE*) for illustrative purposes.

5-HT receptors but has no hallucinatory effects, has no effect on brain 5-HT synthesis or metabolism (Lin *et al.,* 1969c).

Another antiserotonin compound postulated to block the effects of 5-HT on brain receptors is methysergide (Dewhurst and Marley, 1965a,b), a drug which has been tried in the treatment of mania with variable success (Dewhurst, 1968; Haskovek and Soucek, 1968; Fieve *et al.,* 1969).

C. Methods of Studying Metabolism of Neuroregulatory Agents in Brain

1. *General Concepts*

The issues involved in measurement of levels of brain amines and determination of their metabolic pathways have come to be of major importance in behavioral and psychoactive drug-oriented research. In this section of the chapter, the first portion will be a general survey of the techniques followed by more detailed sections on CA, 5-HT, and human investigation.

Two general approaches have been used to study amines in brain. The first has been to measure levels of the compounds in tissues to determine whether the levels are altered. There are certain types of information which can be obtained from static measurement studies, if the information deviates sufficiently from the norm. For instance, in Parkinson's disease, levels in the brain of DA and of homovanillic acid (HVA), the main metabolite of DA (Fig. 4), are markedly reduced in the spinal fluid. Despite the value of measuring the levels of compounds, there are serious drawbacks to such methods, the most formidable being the interpretation of the data. The levels of the compound do not provide information on fluctuations in the synthesis, degradation, or utilization rate of the compound. Indeed, there is now considerable evidence that there may be a marked increase or decrease in the rate of utilization of an amine due to drug treatment, stress, or behavioral states, and, yet, the measured level of the compound may be normal. An analogy may be drawn to measuring the level of water in a dam: the levels can shift somewhat, but we learn little of the rate of the inflow or outflow from a single static measure of the level of the water. Measures of the dynamic state are referred to as kinetics.

The second approach involves measurement of rates of synthesis and utilization, and determination of metabolic pathways. Obtaining information about the kinetics of processes supplies data about the rates of synthesis and destruction, utilization, uptake, etc. In essence, information is obtained about the effects over time of a particular parameter. In coming years, it is expected that studies correlating behavior with biogenic amines will be concerned increasingly with the measurement of dynamic states. Presently, techniques for studying kinetic processes involving neuroregulatory agents in animals, in relation to behavioral states, are just beginning; there have been very few studies in humans.

One approach to analysis of dynamic states involves administration of a drug which inhibits synthesis of a particular amine (or prevents enzymic destruction or removal of a metabolite of the amine) and then monitors the rate of change in the level of the amine or metabolite. Samples of tissue are taken at different times after administering the drug and the levels of the amine are determined. The rate of change in the levels of the amine provides information about the utilization. Examples of such techniques include administration of αMT, an inhibitor of CA synthesis, and determination of the rate of decline of CA. An example which applies to the serotonergic system involves administration of an MAO inhibitor, such as pargyline, which prevents destruction of 5-HT and monitoring the rate of increase of 5-HT. Another example involves the administration of probenecid which blocks the exit of the acid metabolites from the spinal fluid. Levels of 5-HIAA or HVA can be monitored in the brain or spinal fluid allowing determination of the rate of utilization of either 5-HT or DA by observing the rate rise in the levels of the metabolites. Through these procedures, each of which involves measuring levels of the compound under conditions which enable assessment of kinetic processes, it is possible to learn a great deal about the rate of utilization of amines in brain in various behavioral states. Nevertheless, although techniques involving blockage of synthesis, metabolic breakdown, or removal of a compound can give information about rate of utilization, such methods do not provide information about metabolic pathways, a vital factor in the assessment of biochemical processes.

Another approach which enables one to determine information about metabolic pathways involves the use of radiolabeled compounds. With this approach, one can either administer a precursor compound or the actual amine. Studies of this type involve administration (intravenously or intraperitoneally) of biogenic amine precursors, such as tyrosine or tryptophan, and determination of the formation of the resultant CA or IA. For example, radiolabeled tryptophan crosses the blood-brain barrier and one can measure the rate of uptake of tryptophan, the degree of conversion to 5-HT that might serve as an indicator of the activity of tryptophan hydroxylase, and the amount of radioactivity present as the major metabolite of 5-HT, 5-HIAA, which could give an indication of the rate of release and utilization of 5-HT. A completely different approach involves the administration of the radiolabeled amine into the CSF via the intraventricular or intracisternal route (Glowinski et al., 1965; Nobel et al., 1967; Schanberg et al., 1967a,b; Maas and Landis, 1968). One then follows the rate of disappearance of the amine or the pattern of its metabolites. The procedure has been used extensively for NE and it has been demonstrated that most of the radiolabeled NE is taken up from the cerbrospinal fluid by the nerve endings in a pattern similar to the endogenous distribution of the amine. A disadvantage of this procedure is that some of the amine so administered is transferred from the CSF to the blood, or is taken up by cells which do not normally contain NE. A variation of this technique involves the use of push-pull cannulae which enable perfusion of a small area of brain following labeling of the amine stores.

2. Kinetic Measures of Biogenic Amine Metabolism in Animals

a. Catecholamines—Animal Studies. Since the subject of CA turnover and utilization rate will recur many times throughout the following sections of this chapter, the methods used to measure the dynamic state of these compounds will be described briefly. A more elaborate description of the methods and concepts outlined below is covered well by Costa and Neff (1966). There are two general techniques used to measure CA turnover—a nonisotopic and an isotopic method. The basic principles behind each of the methods are similar.

The isotopic techniques employ a radioactive CA (i.e., ^{3}H-NE will be used as a representative compound) that is injected into the organism. All tissues with specific cellular membrane uptake systems (Fig. 7) are able to accumulate and store a portion of the injected ^{3}H-NE. Assuming that the radioactive CA is indistinguishable physiologically from endogenously produced NE, the radioactive compound taken up into the cell may be used to trace the utilization of total cellular NE. The rate at which the ^{3}H NE disappears from the cell, then, will be identical to the rate at which endogenous NE is utilized.* This general approach has been extremely useful in studying brain NE metabolism. Since NE in the bloodstream has but limited passage into the brain due to the presence of the blood-brain barrier, peripheral injections of radioactive NE cannot be used to measure brain NE turnover. Many of the NE-containing cells in the brain, however, are distributed in close proximity to the brain ventricular system. Introduction of radioactive NE into the ventricular system, whether by intraventricular or intracisternal injection, results in the labeling of a portion of the CA-containing neurons in the brain. Assuming that the NE levels within the cell remain constant, the rate of ^{3}H-NE disappearance is exponential and reflects both the synthesis rate and the utilization rate of cellular NE.

If all the NE within the cell is homogeneous (i.e., if the cytoplasmic NE is in rapid equilibration with that stored in the granules), then the radioactivity in the cell disappears monophasically (Fig. 12a) and the slope of the line indicates the turnover rate. However, if the cellular NE is not homogeneous, a monophasic decline in ^{3}H-NE levels will not be seen except in one specific case (when the two pools are independent of one another and the radioactive NE enters but one of these pools). Let us assume for the moment that the NE within the cell is divided between two distinct compartments, one being bound in the granules and another being free within the cytoplasm of the cell. If neither compartment changes size with time, and if the outflow of one compartment is greater than the outflow from another, then the turnover of the NE within the more mobile pool is greater. (Conversely, since the amount of NE does not change, input via synthesis is faster in one compartment, too.) This is illustrated diagrammatically in Fig. 12b. Under these circumstances, when ^{3}H-NE is taken up by the cell, it will be distributed differentially between the two compartments within the cell as long as there is communication between the compartments. Likewise, the compartment with the greater turnover rate will lose its radioactivity faster than the pool with the slower rate of utilization, resulting in a biphasic disappearance of ^{3}H-NE. It is precisely this type of result which originally led many investigators to propose that NE was not stored homogeneously within adrenergic nerve cells. For instance, Axelrod et al. (1961) and Kopin et al. (1962) followed the time course of ^{3}H-NE disappearance from the rat heart after intravenous injection. They found that radioactivity in the heart declined rapidly at first, but thereafter decayed at a progressively slower rate. Similar findings with regard to the disappearance of ^{3}H-NE from rat brain have been presented (Glowinski and Iversen, 1966a).

----

*The kinetic measures are defined by the following equation (Brodie et al. 1966b): $C_t = C_0 e^{-kt}$, where C_t is the concentration of ^{3}H-NE at time t after injection, C_0 is the concentration of the radioactive amine at 0 time and k is the fractional rate constant (hr^{-1}), utilization rate of ^{3}H-NE is defined by the product of k and C_0, and the turnover time of the compartment in question is $1/k$.

Theoretical support for the existence of two compartments of NE in adrenergic neurons can be marshaled. End-product regulation of TH, which suggests participation of unbound NE, is one such example. Different uptake mechanisms in adrenergic neuronal and granular mechanisms is another. The data of Kopin *et al.* (1968), showing preferential release of newly synthesized NE from the spleen is also strongly suggestive, if not proof, of heterogeneous NE compartments. Similarly, recent experiments by Stolk and Barchas (to be published) demonstrate that NE formed from either DA or DOPA in the brain turns over more slowly and is metabolized by different pathways than NE introduced directly into the brain.

Despite these considerations, most of the previous work showing multiphasic decline of ^{3}H-NE in adrenergic nerves was challenged on methodological grounds. Costa *et al.* (1966) and Neff *et al.* (1968) demonstrated that true tracer doses of ^{3}H-NE disappear exponentially from the heart, signifying a single homogeneous pool of NE. On the other hand, nontracer doses of the labeled amine (i.e., doses causing an increase in the endogenous NE content of the heart) disappeared in a polyfunctional manner. As far as disappearance of labeled NE in brain is concerned, similar arguments have been voiced against interpreting such data as evidence for two or more functional compartments of NE.

In addition to the above criticisms, the nonisotopic method for measuring CA turnover consistently has shown that NE decline is monophasic (i.e., NE stores are homogeneous). This second method of measuring CA turnover utilizes the drug α MT, a specific inhibitor of TH (Weissman *et al.*, 1966; Spector *et al.*, 1967). As developed by Brodie and co-workers (1966b), inhibition of TH by α MT is accompanied by a single exponential decline of CA content in all adrenergic systems tested. Once again making the initial assumption that CA within adrenergic neurons exist in a steady state, this method stops input into the system and assumes that outflow continues at an unaltered rate (similar to the situation depicted in Fig. 12a, except that one measures the decline in endogenous NE levels rather than the fall in radioactive NE). The measurements of turnover rate constants for NE in various tissues obtained by the α MT method agree extremely well with those obtained using isotopic techniques. Although these findings argue strongly for homogeneous NE stores, a counter-argument for this interpretation of α MT turnover studies has been lodged (Van Orden *et al.*, 1969). The latter investigators used the histochemical fluorescence microscopy techniques developed by the Swedish workers (Andén *et al.*, 1966) which visualized the cellular localization of biogenic amines, in conjunction with electron microscopic analysis of adrenergic nerve granule density, to study the kinetics of NE depletion in the iris after α MT. They found that cytoplasmic NE, which they claim is preferentially measured by the histochemical techniques, disappears much more rapidly than does granular NE. These data, once again, were suggestive of multiple NE compartments within adrenergic neurons.

Although perhaps confusing, the data summarized above may not be inconsistent. It has been emphasized by many investigators that adrenergic nerve granules contain approximately 90% of cellular NE. Thus, in all chemical measurements of NE, even a large change in the remaining 10% of the NE in the cell (presumably cytoplasmic) would not greatly affect total NE content. With these considerations in mind, the present authors, like other investigators (Weissman *et al.*, 1966; Rech *et al.*, 1968; Sulser *et al.*, 1968), view the adrenergic neuron as a multicompartment system consisting of at least two NE pools: a "free" cytoplasmic store and a "bound" granular store (see Fig. 7). The "free" NE is the store that most likely regulates TH activity, and would appear to be the compartment which is preferentially released on nerve stimulation. The same pool is preferentially labeled by exogenous radiolabeled NE and has a greater turnover rate than does the "bound" granular store of NE. We feel that this model best fits the available data, although more sophisticated analytical procedures modifying our relatively ignorant present conceptualizations are needed. Eventually, it is hoped there will be information relevant to the problem of the relationship between the various stores of CA, the factors controlling entry and exit from the various compartments, and binding within the compartments.

The uptake of peripheral amines by brain is relevant to our discussion of brain processes. The classic studies in this area were performed by Axelrod *et al.* (1959) who found that, although brain has but a very limited ability to take up E and other amines from the blood, some brain areas—particularly the hypothalamus—have been shown to be relatively more permeable than others. Because of the limited transport of E from blood into brain, it is necessary to correct for the amounts of blood remaining in the brain after sacrificing the experimental animal. Using a saline perfusion technique to clear all blood from the brain, it has been shown (Barchas *et al.*, 1969; Steinman *et al.*, 1969) that E could be accumulated in small amounts by brain areas in the rat other than the hypothalamus. In comparing the metabolic pathway of E transported into brain from the blood (after intravenous injection) with that of intraventricularly injected E, it was found that the two routes of administration led to differences in E metabolism. In both situations, the half-life of E, which is a reflection of the turnover rate, was about 2.5 hours. These data show that normally E may be present in the hypothalamus and other brain areas of many species whether it is formed in the brain or sequestered from cerebral blood flow. Whether or not brain E levels or turnover can be altered by various stressors remains to be established, but the need for further investigation of the relation of peripheral amines to central amines is evident.

b. Serotonin—Animal Studies. There are, at present, three nonisotopic methods for determining the rate of 5-HT turnover in the brain, all of which

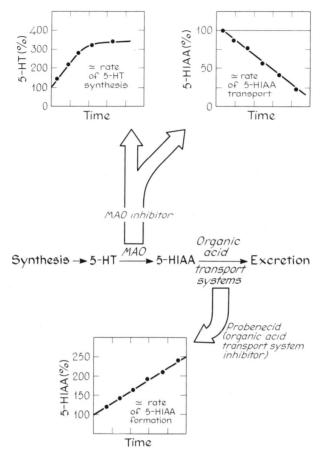

Fig. 13. Schematic diagram of the methods used to study serotonin (5-HT) turnover. 5-HIAA represents the major serotonin metabolite, 5-hydroxyindoleacetic acid.

have emanated from Brodie's laboratory (Tozer *et al.,* 1966; Neff *et al.,* 1967; Neff and Tozer, 1968). The first of these methods utilizes the measurement of the rate of rise of 5-HT following inhibition of MAO (Fig. 13). As illustrated by Neff and Tozer (1968), brain levels of 5-HT increase linearly for about an hour, then gradually approach a horizontal asymptote about three times the normal resting levels.

The second measure utilizes the procedure just described, but focuses instead on the 5-HIAA levels in brain. Following inhibition of MAO, the deamination product of 5-HT, 5-HIAA, is no longer formed. Since 5-HIAA is actively transported out of the brain (Roos *et al.,* 1964), the rate of 5-HIAA decrease after MAO inhibition is exponential with time, Assuming that 5-HIAA is the prime metabolite of consequence of 5-HT, the rate constant for 5-HIAA decline is proportional to the utilization rate of 5-HT, and, assuming a steady-state relationship in the unaltered 5-HT neuron, the rate of 5-HT synthesis (Fig. 13). The third method also involves the measurement of 5-HIAA levels and takes advantage of the active transport of this metabolite out of the brain. Probenecid, a drug which blocks organic acid transport systems, antagonizes the exit of 5-HIAA from the CNS; by measuring the rate of rise of 5-HIAA, one can arrive at the rate of utilization of 5-HT, once again assuming that 5-HIAA is the only important metabolite of the amine (Fig. 13).

These methods of measuring turnover demonstrate that at least one mechanism for regulating synthesis of NE is not available to 5-HT—that of end-product inhibition of the rate-limiting step in the synthetic pathway. Increasing the 5-HT levels by inhibiting MAO does not affect the rate of rise of 5-HT, at least not until amine levels are increased by threefold. This lack of feedback inhibition in serotonergic neurons has been verified using an isotopic procedure for measuring 5-HT synthesis (Lin *et al.*, 1969b; also, see below).

It should be pointed out that the assumption made in all of the above nonisotopic methods of measuring 5-HT turnover, namely, that all or most of the 5-HT is metabolized via MAO to 5-HIAA, may not be strictly valid. The possibility of alternate pathways of metabolism of 5-HT would invalidate the use of inhibitor methods unless this possibility had been excluded. Further studies are necessary to substantiate the use of MAO inhibitors and 5-HIAA level changes in calculating the turnover rate and, especially, the synthesis rate of 5-HT.

One isotopic method developed to measure 5-HT synthesis uses a constant-rate infusion of ^{14}C-tryptophan (Lin *et al.*, 1969a). This procedure utilizes the specific activity of plasma tryptophan and of brain 5-HT to calculate the synthetic rate. Although this is the purest measure of 5-HT synthesis rate available, the method has the drawbacks of high cost and the need for restraining the animal for the necessary infusion of precursor. All of the data thus far obtained using the isotopic techniques yield values comparable to those obtained using the nonisotopic methods; it is this consistency obtained using quite different methods that is cited as evidence substantiating the validity of the above procedures.

3. Studies on Brain Amine Metabolism in Humans

Many of the procedures just described are not applicable to human studies, since studies with synthesis inhibitors or metabolic blockers in tissues require removal of tissues and large number of samples. Apart from autopsy materials, the most important technique to date has been the measurement of metabolites of the neuroregulators in the CSF, although the neuroregulators themselves are not present in CSF (Table VIII).

The major metabolite of 5-HT is presumed to be 5-HIAA, and that compound is found in the CSF of humans. It is believed, from animal studies, that 5-HT is utilized and metabolized to 5-HIAA and that the metabolite then passes into the CSF from which it is then absorbed into the circulation. A spinal fluid has been found. This gradient is steep with considerably higher concentrations of 5-HIAA at higher levels. The issue of whether the 5-HIAA in lumbar spinal fluid can be taken as a measure of brain or spinal cord 5-HT utilization remains to be answered. In cats, some data have been presented that suggest the 5-HIAA in spinal fluid may not reflect the levels of the compound formed in the brain (Bulat and Zivković, 1971). On the other hand, an important study in humans suggests that the lumbar spinal fluid may give a valid measure of the metabolite produced by brain (Curzon et al., 1971). Clearly, further investigation will be necessary and it may be that investigators will be forced to conduct studies using CSF derived from the cisterna magna. However, at this time, lumbar spinal fluid has been used as an indicator of levels of 5-IIIAA derived from the brain.

In an attempt to obtain information beyond that possible from static measurements of the amine metabolite, probenecid has been used to block the exit from the spinal fluid of the acid metabolites of the biogenic amines (5-HIAA derived from 5-HT, or HVA derived from DA), by blocking the active transport system that removes the metabolites from the spinal fluid. In animal studies, high doses of the drug can be used and there is a rapid rise in the CSF level of 5-HIAA since the 5-HIAA is not being removed from the spinal fluid, and, as described earlier, from the rate of rise obtained, it is possible to gain information about the rate of utilization of 5-HT. However, such studies are not as easily performed in humans, since the doses of probenecid which would cause complete blockage of 5-HIAA transport have untoward side effects. To circum-

TABLE VIiI. Levels of Serotonin and Dopamine Metabolites in Spinal Fluid[a]

Neuroregulator	Metabolite	Level of metabolite	Reference
Serotonin	5-hydroxyindoleacetic acid (5-HIAA)	0.030 μg/ml	Gerbode and Bowers, 1968
		0.056 μg/ml	Dubowitz and Rogers, 1969
		0.04 μg/ml	Gottfries et al., 1969
		0.04 μg/ml	Olsson and Roos, 1968
Dopamine	Homovanillic acid (HVA)	0.06 μg/ml	Gottfries et al., 1969
		0.05 μg/ml	Olsson and Roos, 1968
		0.01 μg/ml	Curzon et al., 1970
		0.15 μg/ml	Weiner et al., 1969
Norepinephrine	3-Methoxy-4-hydroxy-phenylglycol (MHPG)	0.022 μg/ml	Wilk et al., 1971

[a]Portions of the material presented here are reprinted by permission of the publisher from *Advances in Psychological Assessment*, Volume Two, edited by Paul McReynolds, Palo Alto, Calif.: Science and Behavior Books, Inc., 1971, pp. 260-292.

vent this, the drug is given in multiple doses over a 24-hour period and the increase in metabolite levels is monitored. Using this technique, varying conditions may be employed or individuals with different illnesses may be studied. The procedure does not allow an exact calculation of the rate of utilization of 5-HT but does give a relative value. For example, with this technique it has been found that at least some depressed individuals utilize less 5-HT per unit of time than do control subjects (van Praag *et al.*, 1970). Among the questions to be investigated are: (1) Is there actually a decreased utilization of 5-HT in such patients? (2) Is 5-HT being metabolized by a different route in such patients? (3) Is probenecid, for some reason, less effective in blocking transport in such individuals? (4) Is the change indicative of a change in brain 5-HT? If the findings and interpretation of decreased 5-HT utilization are valid, some important questions arise: Why does decreased utilization occur? What does such a finding tell us of the etiology of depression and of potential therapy?

Much of the reasoning used in studies involving 5-HT and its metabolite, 5-HIAA, has also been applied to DA and its metabolite, HVA. In the case of NE, measurement of 3-methoxy-4-hydroxyphenylglycol (MHPG) has proved difficult. In addition, probenecid cannot be used to study NE kinetics. Thus far, there is no satisfactory means of studying NE utilization in humans, although Maas and Landis (1968) from studies in dogs have suggested a technique that may allow such studies in man by circumventing the problem of removal of tissues for assay.

In the Maas and Landis technique, radiolabeled NE is administered intracisternally, the goal being to measure the metabolites formed by the brain and excreted in the urine. The NE is metabolized in the brain; the metabolites are transported via the spinal fluid to the blood and ultimately appear in the urine. The investigators faced the problem that immediately after the intracisternal injection, some of the administered NE is transported unchanged into the blood, metabolized peripherally, and excreted in the urine. This raised the dilemma of differentiating the material metabolized by the brain from that metabolized peripherally. The investigators took advantage of the fact that there is no blood-brain barrier for the material *from* the brain, but there is a blood-brain barrier from the body *to* the brain. At the same time that ^{3}H-NE is injected into the cisterna magna, ^{14}C-NE is injected into a peripheral vein. The blood-brain barrier precludes passage of the ^{14}C material into brain; however, the ^{3}H material can pass from the brain into the body compartments. Thus, the ^{3}H metabolites appearing in the urine originate from both central and peripheral metabolic reactions, while the ^{14}C metabolites are only formed peripherally. By means of a set of equations, the contribution of extracerebral metabolism of the tritiated material can be determined and an estimate of CA metabolism by the brain obtained. This technique would allow experiments using the subject as his own control for repeated testing over time without sacrificing the subject.

Neurologists have expressed the opinion that this technique could be feasible in humans. With more basic research, the method might enable a direct test of the hypothesis that there is an alteration of NE metabolism in depression, or could allow investigation of the biochemical aspects of other conditions such as paranoid states.

We have discussed these measures using spinal fluid for brain amine metabolism in humans in considerable length, because of their potential use in psychological studies in the future, and because they represent one of the few ways of studying neuroregulators in the human brain. Studies which focus on metabolism of brain amines in brain or spinal fluid have a great advantage over those which measure compounds in urine. Studies emphasizing the latter are difficult to interpret because the amounts of various materials in the urine are a reflection of both brain and peripheral metabolism of the compounds. Thus, one can profitably study peripheral amines by studies utilizing urine, but one cannot draw many valid conclusions regarding central amines from simple urinary studies.

III. ADRENAL MEDULLARY CATECHOLAMINES AND HUMAN BEHAVIOR

A. Behavioral Effects of Infused Catecholamines—Human Studies

One method frequently used to evaluate the behavioral effects of biogenic amines has been to infuse the amines into humans and observe behavioral results. Such studies involve a number of difficulties: (1) Lack of double blind controls so that the experimenter was aware of the drug that was being administered. In some cases, this problem was compounded by the fact that the subject also knew which drug was being administered and what to "expect." (2) Drugs were given to an individual already in a strong emotional state so that the range of response was limited. In some instances, this has been done intentionally as part of the experimental design, but on other occasions, the subject has been "anxious" about the experiment such that that affective state has been part of an unintended underlying affective continuum in the subject. (3) The dose of the drug may be outside the range that might normally be considered as physiological.

One of the earliest studies of the psychological effects of E was performed by Wearn and Sturgis (1919). Their report begins with one of man's recurring dilemmas: "With the mobilization of our troops, and especially the drafted troops, at the entrance of this country into the war, the problem of sorting the fit from the unfit was one of the first to come up." With that problem in mind, the investigators gave 0.486 mg E intramuscularly to army subjects and observed subjective behavior as well as respiratory and vascular responses. They noted that there was a difference between normal individuals and individuals with "anxiety" sometimes called "irritable heart syndrome" or "neurasthenia." The normals had no reaction. The anxious subjects had no response to the control injections but responded dramatically to the E injections. All changes occurred within 1 hour of the initial injection with the marked effect occurring within 12 minutes. The peak of the response was at 32 minutes. The subjects manifested restlessness, complaints of nervousness, precardial pain, palpitation, and frequent apprehension. In reviewing the life style of the "irritable heart" subjects, the most striking characteristic of these individuals to Wearn and Sturgis was their intolerance to exercise as seen with general muscular fatigue and tiredness. In many of their subjects, there was a lifelong inability to handle stress and a tendency to be nervous and easily excited.

The authors concluded that the subjects with "irritable heart" had a hypersensitivity to E, and that these patients classed as neurotic and neurasthenic are " . . . not good material from which to make a soldier . . . They are not fit to fight. . . ." The paper raises several basic questions relating peripheral CA to behavior which have yet to be resolved. First, what is the relationship of E to behavior and what emotional tone is produced by E? Does it have a multitude of roles in activation of emotional tone? Further, are there individuals who are more sensitive than others to the effect of catechols, and if so, could such differences account for any forms of emotional distress or impairment?

Marañon (1924) first described the subjective perception in some persons who were given E as an "as if" or "cold emotion." He noted that some persons taking the compound (dose usually 0.5 mg) had no effect, while others experienced autonomic changes which they associated with strong emotional states; however they lacked the psychological component of the emotion. There was another factor seen in some of the patients, which was considered to be a secondary reaction in which the person felt invaded by an emotional flux, usually of an anxious nature. The whole phenomenon can be described as an emotional state. This second-degree reaction was seen in a more limited number of persons. In such persons, topics with an emotional overlay had no effect before the injections, but would elicit strong emotion after the injection. Marañon was dealing with three classes of individuals: (1) those who have no reaction to the drug, (2) those with autonomic changes and a "cold emotion," and (3) those with autonomic changes and evidence of a true emotional state. He found that he could elicit a positive reaction, including emotional changes from some nonresponders by treating them with thyroid hormone. This finding is consistent with many subsequent studies showing potentiation of E by thyroid hormone. This relationship between thyroid and E was not a constant one.

There was considerable variation and many exceptions. Marañon also noted that the likelihood of a positive emotional response was high in individuals with what he termed a high emotional index. This has been described by investigators in many endocrine disorders and psychiatric syndromes. Marañon emphasized the potential importance of the emotional reaction produced by E, stating that no other drug or hormone known had such an effect on on emotional status. The main thrust of Marañon's writing was in terms of the "cold emotion" component seen in most of his subjects. Following his work, there was some disagreement over the presence of an emotional component in his patients. Various investigators focused on the "cold emotion" aspect, entirely accepting that as the main effect. The various results and interpretations were summarized by Cantril and Hunt (1932) who also performed a series of investigations concerning the effects of E in 11 persons, including themselves. Their dose was not stated. In all of their subjects they noted physiological manifestations after drug administration, including muscular tremor lasting up to 2 hours and an increase in heart rate. Several of their subjects reported a "cold emotion" but others had a genuine emotion which varied considerably from subject to subject, and included feelings ranging from an experience similar to great positive excitement, to those of anxiety or foreboding, or intensive fear. Of interest was the repeated report of those experiencing the cold emotion of feeling as though they might be readily subject to any kind of emotional suggestion. Cantril and Hunt conclude that the interpretation that the subject puts on the physiological experience will vary from subject to subject and from time to time, and may vary with the same subject. Along the dimension of "pleasantness-unpleasantness," they found that the injections had no specific effect. They were also struck by the need for catharsis noted by some of the subjects. Thus, their results question, in several crucial ways, those of Maranon, for they showed that the situation must contain certain logical cognitive relationships for the experience to contain an element of genuine emotion.

An extremely thorough study was performed by Lindemann and Finesinger (1940) who studied a population of 40 neurotic individuals, all of whom had symptoms of anxiety attacks. In their study, the patients were given an injection of E (1 mg, administered intramuscularly) in a design that allowed for controls injected with saline or mecholyl, a parasympathomimetic drug. Patients were asked a series of questions, and a transcription was made of responses, thereby allowing for a detailed analysis of the data obtained. After the E injections, there was a gradual development of noncommunicativeness, and the patients spoke hesitantly, used few words, and seemed to have difficulty in describing their feelings. Remarks tended to be internal rather than external. Particularly striking was the occurrence of references to mood in the study, for 30% of the subjects reported feelings of depression after the E injections, a finding markedly in contrast with the mood after saline or mecholyl; indeed, the latter drug resulted in references to feeling happy in 60% of the patients. Saline produced no such emotional reports. A number of questions arise from the report which to this day have not been adequately answered. Perhaps the most important is whether there is a subpopulation of persons with psychiatric illness, particularly affective (referring to illnesses which relate to emotional tone such as depression or anxiety), who are more susceptible to the effects of CA. There would be a number of ways of testing such a statement, although the extent to which it has been tested, even in patients with anxiety, is very limited.

Of tremendous theoretical and experimental interest have been the studies of Schachter and Singer (1962) and Schachter and Wheeler (1962) who applied the tools of sophisticated social psychology to a problem that had been repeatedly investigated in a series of medical paradigm studies. First, in reviewing the literature they pointed out the observation made by a number of psychologists that cognitive situational factors influence the way in which a particular autonomic activation is perceived, and that this may be particularly true with the effects of E. Further, if individuals know *why* they are having a state of autonomic arousal, they would no longer need to label the feelings in terms of some alternate explanation. Finally, they pointed out that the physiological aspect of the response was important for the individual to know he was experiencing an emotion which was appropriate to his cognitions. In the Schachter-Singer study, these relationships were put to experimental test in an interesting design using 185 male college students. Subjects were told that they were being given a medication affecting vision and were given either a saline injection or ½ mg of E. By giving three types of explanations, the investigators manipulated an appropriate explanation for the subjects of what they would experience from the E injections, in no case telling the subjects that they were receiving E. A group labeled "epinephrine-informed," was given a correct description of what the subjects would feel as side effects of the drug; a second group labeled "epinephrine-ignorant" was not told about any of the autonomic effects the subjects would encounter, while the third group, "epinephrine-misinformed" was given a set of autonomic changes which do not occur with the drug. Subjects given saline injections were similarly divided. Subjects were put into a situation that would cause a cognitive state of anger or euphoria by the use of a confederate of the experimenter. Schachter's other work had demonstrated that people evaluate their feelings by comparing themselves with others around them. In this experiment, he took advantage of those findings by using confederates who went through a routine indicating either euphoria or anger. Subjects were observed during the interactions, and after the experience with the stooge were given questionnaires to fill out asking them to rate their moods in terms of euphoria or anger, and provide information on the various physiological effects of the drug, including whether they had experienced any effects which were not actually a part of the response to E. Subjects who clearly were suspicious of the setup (11 of the 185) were excluded from the data analysis.

In interpreting the data, it becomes clear that regardless of whether the behavior of the stooge was euphoria or anger, there was a greater tendency for the subject to follow the emotional lead of the stooge in the group that had not been preinformed of the physiological responses the subjects would experience. Hence, the authors state that on the basis of their experiment "providing the subject with an appropriate explanation of his bodily state greatly reduces his tendency to interpret his state in terms of the cognitions provided by the stooges' . . . behavior." Thus, the authors conclude that the emotional tone is not directly related to the degree of activation, but rather to the cognitive accompaniments of the activation, and that without any prior information, the subjects will attempt to fix a cognition to explain the physiological activation. Subjects who received the drug and were told what would happen did not "catch" the emotion of the confederate. The authors also discuss the placebo groups which in these experiments pose certain problems of interpretation, for the placebo itself may lead to self-arousal and, hence, general excitation of the sympathetic nervous system.

In an extension of the studies on the effect of E on emotional responses, Schachter with Wheeler performed an experiment in which subjects viewed a comedy movie after having been given E (dose same as in previous experiment), or saline. The subjects were observed by observers who did not know which drug had been given. They were rated according to the extent to which they showed evidence of finding the film humorous. After the film, the subjects were given a questionnaire to verify their emotional responses and to determine the degree of physiological change. The group treated with E clearly experienced the film as more humorous than did the saline group. The results are interpreted as consistent with the notion that emotional state is "a function of a state of physiological arousal and an appropriate cognition."

There have been a number of attempts to relate E to behavioral states in psychiatric populations or to anxiety *per se*. The experiments of Schachter, as powerful and convincing as they are, do not directly rule out such a relationship since, for a specific individual, there may be a psychological (conditioning) or a biochemical process which predisposes him to experience the arousal caused by E as a signal of anxiety or a situation which leads to anxiety. For example, what would be the results of the experiments if the same design were used in a population of various types of emotional disorders? Would the social cueing still be as important if the individual did not know what he would be experiencing? Further, even if he knew what he was experiencing, would that factor be as important, or would the hormone trigger some affective state? There have been no studies which specifically look at these issues, although there have been a number of studies concerned with psychiatric issues.

A study of the effects of E on certain motor behaviors as well as subjective psychological processes was performed by Basowitz et al., (1956). Their experiments were performed on 12 volunteer medical interns who were interviewed and then, on later occasions, given either saline or E. The hormone was administered in an intravenous dose of 0.005 mg/kg/hr. Thus, their conditions are not parallel to those used by most other investigators. The experiments lasted for a period of over an hour, and the subject continued to receive the drug throughout the experience. The most important finding, as the authors describe it, was the suggestion that the general lability of mood and differing ego defenses also affect the manner and extent to which E has an effect. Thus, subjects whose behavior revealed an openness for the experience and expression of affect readily perceived both the physical and psychological experiences they had with E, while those subjects who were evaluated as having personalities which would constrict emotional experience and suppress their awareness of it showed less appreciable subjective and objective signs. For some of the subjects, E was capable of precipitating a full-blown anxiety attack, yet with limited or no physical effects on the cardiovascular system. Indeed, the effects of the drug on the cardiovascular system were not only not directly related to the magnitude of the emotional response, but indeed, there may have been the opposite correlation. Thus, for example, the individual who had the greatest cardiovascular change apparently experienced almost no emotional change. In terms of the physical tests, E caused a decrease in performance of motor tasks, such as hand steadiness, but no effect on sensory threshold or intellectual tasks. The fact that the subjects clearly anticipated having an emotional experience of anxiety because they were asked about their experiences with that emotion is a problem in this study. The study can be partially explained by Schachter's finding that a situation in which there is autonomic arousal creates social and internal cues toward the affect of anxiety, thus causing the subjects to interpret the autonomic arousal as anxiety. However, the Basowitz study demonstrates that there is considerable variability in subjects and suggests that the personality structure in terms of openness to emotional response and tendencies toward expression or denial of affect may be extremely important factors. This clearly is very important from a psychiatric standpoint.

An unusual study investigating the subjective psychological effects of E and NE was undertaken by Hawkins et al. (1960), who used four psychiatrists as subjects. E was given intravenously at a rate of 12 μg/min, although other rates were also studied. A naturalistic approach was used except that a measure of blood pressure and pulse was taken every minute, a factor which clearly interrupted the experience and interfered with the naturalistic aspects of the experiment. The higher doses of E caused a difficulty in speech, felt to have a CNS component, with some disordering or thought and memory. Strikingly, the subjects were all aware of when they were receiving E and, as Schachter had predicted for such a situation, the affect of anxiety was rarely present. One subject described feelings of transitory moments when things felt disorganized and out of control, during which time there would be anxiety, but when he regained control, the anxiety would go away. At one point, due to an error, this subject was given a much higher but unstated level of the drug which caused temporary severe disorganization and near panic, although it is not clear to what extent that feeling was a result of what probably was a feeling of marked concern by the research team. In these investigations, the drug was given to the subjects on multiple occasions and it became increasingly clear that the psychological effect diminished, although the subjects still had a strong physical reaction. The impression of the investigators was that E was most likely to have an emotional effect if some association meaningful to the patient was made. They believed that the subjects treated with E were predisposed or prepared for anxiety and any appropriate association would permit the genuine affect.

NE was also studied by Hawkins and his group in two of their regular subjects, as well as in a group of 12 student volunteers. The drug was given intravenously at a dose level of 8-12 µg/min and, although there were clearcut physiological changes, there were no changes in affect. The subjects were aware of generalized cooling and very mild restlessness. The investigators were interested in whether there would be any statements suggestive of the affect of anger, and found no such effect. Hawkins and his co-workers conclude by suggesting that the usual assumption that E is associated with anxiety and NE with outward directed anger is incorrect. When persons are given E, they appear anxious to the observer even if they are not subjectively anxious, while those given NE demonstrate no clear-cut changes. Further E causes a change in terms of the readiness with which the individual will take on an affect which, in these instances, was anxiety. All of the subjects recognized the physiological effects, including a sensation like a "lump in the throat," etc., that they would feel in an anxiety situation.

Kety and his group have studied the effects of E in a group of schizophrenic patients in an attempt to validate or invalidate the beliefs that E is involved in the symptoms of the disease. As part of the broad scale observations which also included metabolic and physiological studies, Pollin and Goldin (1961) investigated the psychological aspects of E. They administered the compound to a group of 12 schizophrenics and 12 normals, although there were unavoidable discrepancies between the two groups. The compound was given at a rate of 0.15 µg/kg/min. A team of raters was present in the observation room at the time of the experiment. All subjects demonstrated a narrowing of their field of awareness and a shift of attention from the environment to themselves with the onset of the E infusion. Subjects varied as to whether they felt more or less alert and awake after the start of the infusion. Behaviors in a number of the subjects were exaggerated. Several subjects, both schizophrenics and controls, showed a decreased ability to cope in the situation, although this was most pronounced among the schizophrenic group. The schizophrenic patients did display changes in their behavior but not to such an extent that it would be considered an increase in psychotic behavior, for, although half of the patients became more psychotic, it was felt that this was in response to the overall test situation rather than due to the infused E. This untoward response to stress, a characteristic of schizophrenic patients, could have been in response to the purely psychological aspects of the stress or to the patients' hormonal output of CA or some other hormone which then affected an ongoing psychological state. Of interest is the finding that the schizophrenics may have shown less anxiety with E than the normals, although the interpretation of this may be difficult since the schizophrenics were more aroused by the baseline situation.

There are several ways the varying patterns with which persons respond to E might be of importance both theoretically and clinically. Assuming that there are variations in patterns of response, and that some individuals are "more sensitive" to the effects of the drug, one could imagine that the psychological effects could be due to a number of different causes, including (1) increased likelihood of associating the drug with a behavior normally experienced, such as anxiety, because the compound is excreted normally by the individual when experiencing such an emotional state—in this explanation, the effect would be the result of psychological conditioning; or (2) a difference in susceptibility of the CNS effects due to such changes as an altered permeability of the blood-brain barrier or to an alteration in the pattern of uptake, utilization, or metabolism of the compound by the brain.

A major difficulty in giving the subject a drug such as E and asking him to report his emotions is the frequently made assumption that the physiological state influences his behavioral state. The evidence of various studies would probably suggest that such an explanation is not valid. It is possible that the hormone is acting directly on the CNS, for despite the blood-brain barrier, there is evidence in animals that small amounts of the hormone can pass into the brain. Indeed, such an explanation may be involved in the process of arousal seen with the injections of the hormone. In studying psychiatric disorders, the major problem may be to take the entire organism into account. The psychological situations which cause an arousal leading to neural and hormonal stimuli to the body resulting in hormonal stimuli to the brain are all part of the same process. In that scheme, starting from a psychological situation, the resulting physiological and hormonal changes may be important feedback to the brain about the response it has triggered. This feedback may serve the purpose of altering the emotional response. Thus, one might well expect that a brain transplanted into an *in vitro* system would feel emotion if it were able to have cognitions, but that the emotional response, including the length of the experience, would be affected by compounds put into the perfusing medium.

If a cognitive response triggers a physiological response, including hormonal components, and hormonal components then influence the cognitive response, then one might be able to approach the treatment of certain types of illnesses in which such a cycle may be operative through the use of inhibitors or stimulators of hormonal action. Thus, in the simplest model, if E is produced in response to an emotion labeled as anxiety and the E then feeds back to increase the feeling of anxiety, drugs which inhibit the effect of E might affect the course of the anxiety.

There are a number of ways of testing such an approach. Several investigators, including Ax (1953) and Wolf and Wolff (1947) have suggested that there may be differences in the pattern of autonomic response to fear and anger, although the traditional view had been that there were no such differences. Ax has suggested that fear responses would be similar to the autonomic pattern after an injection of E while the autonomic responses seen in anger would be similar to a mixture of the patterns seen after E and NE. Unfortunately, as has been the case in many such experiments, there has been no investigation of the level of the excreted catechols in those same paradigms. However, it would be worthwhile to see whether drugs which block various aspects of the CA response influence the subjective experience reported by the subjects.

B. Adrenal Medullary Secretion

There have been a great number of studies in which investigators have determined the relative amounts of E and NE in the urine in response to stress and other behavioral conditions. This area has been extensively reviewed (von Euler, 1956, 1964; Breggin, 1964; Malmejac, 1964; Levi, 1966; Melmon, 1968; Mason, 1968) and we will provide only a few examples of the wealth of data from human studies.

The adrenal medulla's response to stress is characterized by a rapid secretion of E and NE into the circulation; the materials are picked up by various organs, including the brain, metabolized, and excreted primarily in the urine. Measurement of the small amount of CA present in the blood or plasma is very difficult (Udenfriend, 1962, 1969; Anton and Sayre, 1962; Welch and Welch, 1969; O'Hanlon et al., 1970).

Studies on blood CA may require as much as 10–25 ml of blood, a volume unsuitable for many types of psychological assessment studies. The problem is further complicated by the presence of substances in the blood which interfere with the CA assays. Many of the early studies did not resolve adequately the compounds of interest from these unwanted materials. While it is easier to measure CA in the urine, collection of adequate urine volumes limits the time points at which one may obtain measurements, and affords only a gross measure of CA in relation to the behavioral event under analysis. Ideally, one would hope to sample small amounts of blood plasma at close intervals to obtain a picture of the response to varying behavioral situations and the differing patterns of response.

In evaluating changes in urinary CA, it should be borne in mind that E, NE, and DA are all secreted into the urine. However, only E is primarily derived from the adrenal gland. The remaining amines are primarily a reflection of CA formed in adrenergic neurons throughout the body. The amount of NE secreted is affected by muscular exertion and other processes (Hollister and Moore, 1970). There is essentially no information on DA secreted in the urine and what influences it.

Over 90% of the CA secreted into the blood is metabolized before it reaches the urine. Despite this fact, most investigators measure only the unchanged (nonmetabolized) urinary CA, thus ignoring by far the largest component of the total urinary amine pool. One may postulate that there may be situations in which the metabolism of the compounds by liver and peripheral tissues is changed, thus altering the relative amount of unmetabolized amine excreted in the urine. In some studies, vanillylmandelic acid (VMA), one of the several CA metabolites, has been measured. Since VMA represents a final common pathway in the metabolism of both E and NE (Figs. 5 and 6), measurement of this compound provides no information as to the relative contribution of either amine to the VMA pool.

The normal excretion values of E at rest are about 2-3 ng/min, while the NE secretion is about 10 ng/min (a nanogram is 10^{-9} gram).

von Euler, who discovered NE, has performed investigations ranging from biochemical to psychological and has been a constant innovator. He has studied the effects of a variety of stresses, including aviation stress and movies of various types. The conclusions of his group conform with those of the studies of Elmadjian et al. (1957) and represent an effort of the greatest importance (von Euler and Lundberg, 1954; Levi, 1965, 1969).

The studies of Elmadjian et al. (1957) represent classical investigations of the secretion of these compounds. These investigators studied the secretion of compounds in a variety of situations and found that, in situations involving tense, anxious, but passive emotional displays, there is an increase in E secretion with a normal secretion of NE. In contrast, active, aggressive, emotional displays are related to an increased secretion of NE without any change in E. The studies were performed on persons involved in a variety of athletic competitions, as well as on psychiatric patients.

Although most of the studies referred to have been concerned with adrenal medullary secretion in humans, the studies of Mason (1968) using monkeys have been of particular importance. This series of studies has given insight into the notion that E secretion may be increased in times of novelty and uncertainty. NE secretion is increased when conditions are familiar and stereotyped or unpleasant.

There have been a number of studies which emphasized psychological processes in humans. For example, an increased secretion of E has been noted during sensory deprivation and the increase related to a change in time sense (Mendelson *et al.*, 1960). The study of Tolson *et al.* (1965) demonstrated that the levels of CA were increased on first admission to a psychiatric hospital, and subsequently decreased. Their data also suggest some of the hazards in conducting endocrine studies in a new environment, and point out the "first day" effect. A variety of other stresses have also been investigated. Silverman and Cohen (1960) and Goodall (1962) demonstrated that individuals who were subject to blackout due to centrifugation stress produced more E and had more anxiety, while those with high tolerance to centrifugation stress secreted relatively more NE and demonstrated more aggressive affect.

A variety of studies has correlated the amounts of hormones secreted to performance in psychologically stressful situations. For example, Franken-haeuser *et al.* (1968) found that subjects with high CA excretion rates performed better under specified conditions. In a series of studies these investigators have shown that subjects who secrete relatively more E tend to perform better in terms of speed, accuracy, and endurance, when working under conditions of low or moderate stimulation, while the opposite tendency occurs under conditions of high stimulation.

Potentially, an area of great interest involves studies of CA excretion in children. There have been surprisingly few studies in this area which could profit from further genetic, developmental, psychological, and sociological studies. Frankenhaeuser and Johansson (to be published) have summarized the available literature. Their data along with that of Lambert *et al.* (1969) suggest that there may be marked differences in CA excretion in children of different tempera-ments and upbringing. Some of the suggestive findings include the possibility that: boys in the 11 to 12 age group may secrete more CA; children who secrete more E may be judged as being quicker and livelier, more decided, open, curious, playful, and candid; in an active test situation, some children will have an increase and others a decrease in E output; those with increased E output perform better; there may be a positive correlation between CA output and intelligence in girls but not in boys; boys who secrete more E may be less aggressive; parental attitudes may alter amine excretion patterns. As can be seen, research in this area should prove extremely fruitful.

The work on adrenal medullary secretion represents an area involving biogenic amines and behavior in which there is increasing emphasis on subtle measurements of behavior. Hopefully, with better assay procedures, this will result in extensive detailing of the kinetic processes involving these hormones and their relation to behavior.

IV. BRAIN CATECHOLAMINES, INDOLEAMINES, AND BEHAVIOR

A. Animal Studies

1. Some General Comments

The early findings bringing together the separate observations that reserpine produced behavioral depression and also depleted brain 5-HT and NE have served as the initial tremors resulting in an avalanche of publications, new drugs, new theories, and activating old and new controversies concerning the behavioral function of the biogenic amines. It would be extremely difficult, if not impossible, to survey all of the literature and to air the numerous hypotheses which relate to work in this area. Rather, we have tried to organize our thoughts about specific areas which we feel illustrate a possible association between neurochemical processes and behavioral acts in the organism. We hope to give a critical, albeit biased, discussion of research areas which are just beginning to be understood, to show where the biogenic amines may or may not relate, and to indicate possible directions for future investigation.

2. Locomotor Activity and Gross Motor Function

Prior to the neurochemical discoveries of the early 1950's, several investigators had noticed the prominent central stimulatory effects of various sympathomimetic amines. As early as 1913, when Airila reported that ephedrine awakened narcotized animals, it was proposed that these drugs, related to "sympathin," could activate the brain and cause an increase in motor activity. Following a remarkably complete description of the CNS effects of amphetamine in human patients being treated for narcolepsy (Nathanson, 1937), the motor stimulant effects of amphetamine were documented in many species. By 1962, the relationship between the mechanism of amphetamine-induced motor stimulation and brain CA was being investigated in earnest. Van Rossum et al. (1962) observed that reserpine did not reduce the locomotor stimulant activity of amphetamine injection in mice (despite the marked reduction in brain NE levels and the overt depression seen prior to amphetamine injection) and postulated that the sympathomimetic amine directly stimulated adrenergic receptors in the brain. Subsequently, Smith (1963, 1965) observed similar effects and reached the same conclusions. Other investigators studying the same drug interactions in rats came to different conclusions, however, and postulated that CA were responsible for amphetamine's stimulatory effects, even after reserpine (Stolk and Rech, 1967).

With the introduction of α MT, a specific depletor of tissue CA (Table II; Weissman *et al.,* 1966), it was possible to test whether or not CA were important in the locomotor stimulant effects of amphetamine. The initial studies by Weissman and co-workers clearly indicated that α MT almost completely blocked the stimulant effects of amphetamine. Sulser *et al.* (1968) attempted to elucidate the relative roles of CA storage and biosynthesis in the motor stimulant response to amphetamine and to combined treatment with desmethylimipramine (DMI) and tetrabenazine. It was postulated that the latter drug combination evoked the release of stored CA in brain (due to tetrabenazine's effects) and blocked its reconcentration in adrenergic neurons following release (due to DMI's action on the nerve cell membrane). Blockade of NE synthesis by α MT abolished the central stimulatory action of amphetamine, but did not affect that due to tetrabenazine-desmethylimipramine treatment. In contrast, depletion of NE stores with α MT (Table I) prevented the stimulation caused by tetrabenazine plus DMI, but not that due to amphetamine. Sulser interpreted this data to show that the central actions of amphetamine required the uninterrupted synthesis of brain NE, whereas the rapid release of granular amine stores, and not synthesis, was involved in the motor stimulation elicited by the tetrabenazine-desmethylimipramine treatment. A further elaboration on the interactions between amphetamine and α MT extended the findings of the above studies to show that even very low doses of α MT would partially antagonize the locomotor stimulant effects of amphetamine in the intact rat. Following reserpine treatment, however, the same low doese of α MT completely blocked amphetamine's effects (Stolk and Rech, 1970). These data show quite conclusively that (1) CA are involved in the locomotor stimulant responses to various drugs, and (2) that CA biosynthesis specifically is related to the motor stimulant effects of amphetamine, even after reserpine treatment.

The above studies concentrated on the relationship between amphetamine-stimulated motor activity and CA. Whereas it is valid to interpret amphetamine's stimulant effects in terms of an action on brain CA, it is by no means true that all drugs which increase motor behavior do so through an effect on CA metabolism. More important are questions concerning the locus in the brain of amphetamine's effects, and the relationship of brain CA to the general level of activity.

Few studies have been directed toward localizing amphetamine's stimulant actions in a particular brain area. Some early work in this area postulated that amphetamine exerted its activating effects through an action on the brain stem (Bradley and Elkes, 1957; Carlsson *et al.,* 1957b). More recently, Javoy and co-workers (1968) demonstrated that relatively low doses of the sympathomimetic amine increased the rate of NE synthesis and turnover in the mesencephalon. Although these data support the activation of noradrenergic neurons in the brain stem by amphetamine, other brain areas were not studied. As an ancillary note, amphetamine's motor stimulant properties are antagonized significantly by an inhibitor of DβO (Maj and Przegalinski, 1967). This finding indicates that DA, which is highly concentrated in the basal ganglia, does not appear to be involved in this effect of the sympathomimetic amine. Since a specific type of motor behavior (to be discussed below) is associated with striatal DA, and since DA in the basal ganglia will be shown to be important for normal coordinated motor function, these findings eliminate a prominent possible site of action in the stimulant actions of amphetamine presently under consideration.

Several lines of evidence point out the importance of brain CA in the maintenance of normal activity. Apart from the expected depression induced in animals treated with reserpine, tetrabenazine, and other depressant drugs, including those which do not cause depletion of brain NE and DA stores, changes in motor activity have been observed after extremely low doses of α MT (Dominic and Moore, 1969; Stolk and Rech, 1970). Thus, doses of α MT alone which cause no discernible effects on the gross behavior of the animal or on conditioned behavioral tasks (see below) cause an inhibition of motor activity related to the dose of α MT injected. Other studies suggest that this effect of α MT is related specifically to NE and not to DA (Rech *et al.*, 1968). The activity depressant effects of α MT can be reversed by DOPA again implicating the participation of CA in the maintenance of normal activity. Also of interest in this respect is the finding that α MT has sedative, but not other overt depressant effects when given to humans (Sjoerdsma *et al.*, 1965; Charalampous and Brown, 1967).

A recent study has reported an association between brain NE metabolism and the activity level in rats (Stone and DiCara, 1969). In this report, there was an inverse correlation between the levels of ^{3}H-NE remaining in the brain 1 hour after intraventricular injection of the amine and the animals' previously determined level of activity. These data indicate a very subtle relationship between activity and brain NE metabolism, and suggest that increased turnover of NE in the brain (resulting in lower levels of ^{3}H-NE at a given time after injection) is correlated with a relatively active basal state.

Another type of motor behavior, specifically related to DA in the basal ganglia, has been documented by Randrup, Munkvad, and co-workers. A peculiar type of motor phenomenon, characterized by intense grooming, compulsive gnawing, backpeddling, tremor, and circling movements was described first by Ehrich and Krumbhaar (1937) and named amphetamine-stereotyped behavior by Quinton and Halliwell (1963). Although initially observed after the injection of amphetamine, other compounds, specifically DOPA, have been shown to elicit this behavior in rats (Randrup and Munkvad, 1966). Several species are known to exhibit stereotyped behavior of this type, with each species showing a characteristic motor pattern (Randrup and Munkvad, 1967). Subsequent studies demonstrated that DA, but not NE, in the basal ganglia was responsible for the effect. Elicitation of the phenomenon by direct chemical stimulation is localized to the dorsal part of the caudate nucleus and globus pallidum, and can be blocked by striatal or cortical lesions as well as by chlorpromazine and other phenothiazines (Munkvad *et al.*, 1968).

Work emanating from the laboratory of Snyder has made a substantial contribution to understanding the underlying biochemical mechanisms of motor behavior and of the role of CA in behavior. Coyle and Snyder (1969) first demonstrated that the two stereoisomers of amphetamine (the *d*- and *l*- forms) had a differential effect upon CA biochemistry. The *d*-isomer, or *d*-amphetamine, was found to be a potent inhibitor of CA uptake in all brain regions, as indicated in Fig. 10. The *l*-form, or *l*-amphetamine, however, was 10 times less potent than *d*-amphetamine in inhibiting uptake in all brain areas except the corpus striatum (basal ganglia), where both stereoisomers were approximately equipotent. Their attention next focused upon the motor behavioral differences between *d*- and *l*-amphetamine (Taylor and Synder, 1971). There is a substantial difference between the two amphetamine isomers and their effect in stimulating locomotion, the *d*-isomer being 10 times more potent than *l*-amphetamine. With respect to stereotyped motor behavior (the gnawing-biting-jumping syndrome described in the previous paragraph), however, both stereoisomers were equipotent. Taylor and Snyder have provided compelling evidence that locomotor stimulation to *d*-amphetamine is related to presumptive increased turnover and a demonstrated decreased uptake of NE in all brain regions. *l*-Amphetamine, on the other hand, did not affect NE metabolism outside of the basal ganglia. Stereotyped behavior was accompanied by metabolic changes in the basal ganglia that were produced by both *d*- and *l*-amphetamine. These data are interpreted as evidence for the biochemical and pharmacological differentiation of behavioral effects attributed to the two isomers of amphetamine. It is readily apparent that whole-brain NE metabolism, locomotor stimulation, and *d*-amphetamine are related intimately, as are basal ganglia DA metabolism, stereotyped behavior and *d*- or *l*-amphetamine; both relationships are separable from one another on behavioral and biochemical grounds. Thus, NE appears to be related to "normal" locomotor stimulation, while DA in the basal ganglia is associated specifically with the ganwing-biting-jumping sterotypy.

Another relationship between striatal DA and motor function has been intensively investigated during the past 10 years. Both clinical and experimental observations on the side effects of various drugs used in the psychiatric treatment of mental disorders revealed that many compounds which shared the common effect of antagonizing the actions of CA caused the appearance of a hypokinetic-hypertonic syndrome Many investigators noticed the correlation between reserpine's effects on DA in the basal ganglia and the appearance of impaired motor function. Other drugs, most notably members of the phenothiazine family, caused similar motor disturbances. In light of the proposed mechanism of action of these compounds, such observations served to focus attention on the relationship betwen the observed motor impairment and diminished levels of CA in the brain. DOPA administration was shown to alleviate the hypokinetic-hypertonic syndrome in both experimental animals and man. These data immediately focused attention upon DA in the basal ganglia. Several groups of clinical investigators interested in Parkinson's disease, a process affecting the extrapyramidal motor system, began to look for alterations in DA content and metabolism in their patients. The findings, summarized by Hornykiewicz (1966) showed that patients suffering from Parkinsonism had diminished urinary DA excretion, decreased DA levels in the basal ganglia, and very low levels of a DA metabolite, HVA (Fig. 5) in the brain. The next logical step in the pharmacological treatment of these patients was to try to increase the levels of DA in the brain. In many cases, DOPA administration was found to be beneficial and has become the drug of choice in treating these patients.

3. "Stress" and Biogenic Amine Involvement

The term "stress" is so ambiguous that it precludes an accurate definition. The amibiguity of the term is compounded further by personalized interpretations of "stress" and "stressful" situations. A limited number of studies have been conducted in which biochemical parameters have been investigated and, while some of the studies have been relatively nonspecific, a wide range of physiological mechanisms with which to begin a systematic study of behavioral processes is becoming more apparent. The present section of this review will summarize briefly the response of biogenic amine-containing systems to stimuli falling under the category of "stress." In later sections, data from more behavior-specific studies will be considered.

Many procedures are known to cause significant alterations in brain biogenic amine content. Among such manipulations are cold-water swimming, environmental hypo- and hyperthermia, electric shock, and the social environment in which the animal exists. The qualitative and quantitative effects of the aforementioned variables, as well as several others, are summarized in Table IX.

The mechanisms involved in either raising or lowering cellular stores of the biogenic amines have been investigated in some depth. A consideration of possible causative events, as derived from Fig. 7 or from the section on enzyme regulation, invites a deceptively simple task of elucidating between (1) an alteration in degradative metabolic activity, (2) changes in synthesis, or (3) a combination of both. However, in practice, such elucidation has proved difficult.

**TABLE IX. Representative Effects of
Various Stressors on Brain Biogenic Amine Concentrations**

Procedure	Effect on			Reference
	NE	*DA*	*5-HT*	
Cold-water swimming	↓ (26%)	—	↑ (15%)	Barchas and Freedman, 1963
	↓ (13%)	—	—	Stone, 1970
Electric footshock	↓ (depend on intensity)	—	0	Maynert and Levi, 1964
	↓ (20%)	—	—	Javoy *et al.*, 1968
	↓ (15%)	—	—	Thierry *et al.*, 1968a
	↓ (10-30%)	↓ (8%)	0	Bliss *et al.*, 1969
Immobilization	↓ (13%)	0	↑ (10%)	Bliss and Zwanziger, 1966
	0	↑ (25%)	↑ (5%)	Welch and Welch, 1968a
	↑ (20%)	0	↑ (23%)	Welch and Welch, 1968b

Electric shock has received the most attention with regard to "stress" and its metabolic effects, and also provides a convenient bridge between the biochemical and psychological literatures.

Footshock, in nearly all instances where tested, causes an acceleration of NE, DA, and 5-HT turnover rates in (rat) brain (e.g., Bliss *et al.*, 1968; Javoy *et al.*, 1968; Thierry *et al.*, 1968a,b). The extent of these changes is dependent upon the brain area investigated. For instance, Javoy *et al.* (1968) observed that telencephalic NE turnover increases by 160% as the result of shock, whereas acceleration of brain stem turnover is but 29%. Since the only amine whose concentration (as opposed to turnover rate) is affected by the shock is NE, it has been suggested that synthesis of DA and 5-HT, but not of NE is capable of increasing sufficiently to compensate for increased utilization. Data collected in our laboratory (Stolk *et al.*, in press) are consistent with this interpretation. Evidence against a dysequilibrium between synthesis and destruction of NE, however, has been presented by Thierry *et al.* (1968a). Thierry demonstrated that changes in NE content and turnover after footshock are not complementary. Thus, NE concentration is decreased by a moderate shock intensity (0.8 MA), but not by high shock levels (1.6 or 3.0 MA); on the other hand, NE turnover, using intracisternally injected ^{3}H-NE as a marker, increased *only* during presentation of *high* intensity shock (i.e., those not affecting NE content).

That NE synthesis is indeed increased during footshock, at least under certain circumstances, has been established by using radiolabeled tyrosine, the immediate amino acid precursor of the CA (Fig. 3). The proportion of total brain NE that is radioactive after tyrosine treatment is found to be greater in rats receiving footshock than in control animals, a change that can occur only if TH activity increases as a result of the "stress." *In vitro* brain TH activity has also been shown to be elevated by prior electroconvulsive shock exposure (Musacchio *et al.*, 1969), a procedure known to enhance brain NE turnover in rats (Kety *et al.*, 1967). More recently, Thierry *et al.* (1970) presented evidence that the increased synthesis and utilization of brain NE during periods of electric footshock involve the so-called "labile" stores within noradrenergic neurons. Thierry's group found that rats exposed to shock beginning within 5 minutes of an intracisternal injection of ^{3}H-tyrosine have lower levels of ^{3}H-NE (synthesized from the labeled precursor) than controls. Rats submitted to footshock beginning more than 5 minutes after the labeled tyrosine injection no longer revealed a decrease in ^{3}H-NE. As in their previous study (Thierry *et al.*, 1968a; see preceding paragraph), the intensity of shock employed (1.6 MA) had no effect on endogenous NE content. Thierry and his associates argue that the decreased amounts of ^{3}H-NE in the brain stem shortly after tyrosine injection support their contention that synthesis feeds NE into a small store within the neuron that (1) has a relatively rapid rate of turnover, and (2) is exquisitely sensitive to release. The failure to observe decreases in ^{3}H-NE content at longer time intervals after tyrosine injection is thought to reflect the relatively slow equilibration of newly synthesized NE with the total cellular content of the amine. Thus, the equilibration rate for the "labile" store of NE is equivalent to the synthesis rate, while the equilibration of the quantitatively larger stored amine with the small "labile" fraction is measurably slower. This concept is qualitatively similar to that diagramed in Fig. 12. Although the results described above constitute evidence for a "labile" brain NE store directly associated with synthesis, as shown to exist unequivocally in peripheral adrenergic structures (Kopin *et al.*, 1968), several equally acceptable interpretations of these data need to be evaluated before a "two-pool" hypothesis in brain is adopted.

Efforts to assess the route by which catabolism is enhanced secondary to electric shock have yielded inconclusive results. Based on the model of brain adrenergic neuronal function depicted in Fig. 7, it has become popular to associate "stress"-induced increases in apparent nerve cell activity with enhanced release of NE into the synaptic cleft, where it may activate the postsynaptic receptor. One would expect, therefore, that normetanephrine levels increase during shock due to the higher concentration in the synaptic cleft. The evidence substantiating this functional model is minimal, however. Thierry *et al.* (1968a) have described greater than normal normetanephrine formation following footshock. On the other hand, both Bliss *et al.* (1968) and Taylor and Laverty (1969) failed to observe an increase in the COMT-derived metabolite after shock. Additionally, Stolk *et al.* (in press) found that shock may even decrease normetanephrine production under certain circumstances, a finding consistent with that observed in self-stimulation experiments by Stein and Wise (1969; see below). Thus, no consistent alteration in the pattern of NE metabolism after footshock has been described. This fact may necessitate construction of a more flexible model of brain adrenergic physiology than that currently assumed in Fig. 7.

The effects of shock on biogenic amine metabolism reflect the complexity of these neurotransmittor systems and the difficulties encountered outside of the test tube. Nevertheless, it is obvious that this particular "stress" evokes profound changes in all three of the biogenic amine-containing systems in question. Biochemical studies of shock-contingent behaviors by and large have not been approached in as much detail as the studies described in the preceding paragraphs, for obvious technical reasons. To what extent the biochemical response to shock alone is modified by discrete response patterns surrounding shock presentation will bear considerable influence on subsequent animal and human investigations.

The effect of environmental temperature on biogenic amine metabolism constitutes another area where "stress" has been demonstrated to have prominent biochemical effects. While not classically as closely associated with behavior as electric shock, temperature-dependent alterations in amine bio-chemistry provide another vehicle for studying the response characteristics of the challenged organism. Thermoregulation and the possible role of NE and 5-HT in the hypothalamus has been richly documented in the physiological literature (cf. Giarman et al., 1968). The metabolic response of NE-containing neurons in brain in environmental hyper- and hypothermia, though similar to the response to electric shock, has a discrete regional localization. Using ^{3}H-NE injected intracisternally, Simmonds and Iversen (1969) and Simmonds (1969) showed a marked increase of NE turnover in the hypothalamus of rats at temperatures of both 9° and 32°C relative to normal (24°C) conditions. The increased utilization was present only in the hypothalamus, and was independent of rectal temperature. Synthesis and degradation of NE in brain were not evaluated separately, although an earlier report by Gordon et al. (1966a) showed that peripheral CA synthesis increases both after exercise or cold exposure.

A series of investigations by Aghajanian and his associates have elegantly verified the discrete physiological and anatomical relationships between the raphe nuclei and brain 5-HT metabolism (Aghajanian et al., 1967). The raphe nuclei are the origin of most serotonergic neurons present in brain (see Fig. 2). In an extension of their previous studies, Weiss and Aghajanian (1971) reported an intimate association between an environmental stressor, neurophysiological activation of a discrete nerve tract and an increase in brain 5-HT metabolism. Rats implanted with recording electrodes in the raphe system were placed in a 40°C incubator, which resulted in an increased nerve impulse activity in this system. Heat-induced neuronal activation in turn was accompanied by a significant elevation of forebrain 5-HIAA concentration, indicative of an increased turnover to brain 5-HT. Although body temperature rose with the incubation procedure, the observed alterations in 5-HT metabolism could be antagonized either by lesions in the raphe or by blockade of raphe neurons by LSD; the latter procedures do not affect the development of hyperthermia. Lesions outside the raphe nuclei had no effect on forebrain 5-HT metabolism, and recordings from brain areas other than the raphe did not show a clear-cut correlation between neuronal activity and body temperature. The latter study is extremely important for a number of reasons. First, it represents one of the few documented studies where activity in a specified nerve tract has been related to the mobilization of a biogenic amine known to be contained within that tract. Second, the precise anatomical localization of the response attests to the specificity of the relationship between raphe neurons and 5-HT. Last, the combination of sensory input, neuronal response, and biochemical effect is a rare instance of the desired degree of specificity searched for in studies of the relationship between behavior and biogenic amine involvement.

4. Social Environment and Biogenic Amines

The ability of an organism's social environment to effect changes in biogenic amine metabolism has presented researchers with a potentially rich area of investigation to approach an understanding of normal and abnormal behavioral adaptation. The route leading up to the present status of this field has followed a somewhat circuitous course. Before biogenic amines had been demonstrated in brain, a substantial amount of literature had been written regarding the social environment and drug action in mice, especially in reference to amphetamine. Gunn and Gurd (1940) first described the enhanced lethal and central stimulant properties of amphetamine in grouped mice as opposed to animals housed one per cage. Chance (1946, 1947) further explored this relationship, showing the positive correlation between excitation, toxicity, and group size. Moore (1963) later demonstrated that brain amine levels of grouped mice were not affected by similar doses of the sympathomimetic amine. Subsequent studies have shown that drugs with an antiadrenergic mechanism of action are capable of blocking the toxic effects of amphetamine in grouped mice; likewise, drugs potentiating CA activity enhance amphetamine's activity. These results provided a highly suggestive association of CA in socially differentiable drug effects.

The studies discussed above prompted more detailed investigation of the socially determined biochemical changes. Long-term social isolation, which results in heightened aggressivity of mice, was employed by several groups of researchers to study both brain and adrenal medullary biogenic amine involvement. The effect of isolation on CA and 5-HT function, and the relationship of these compounds to aggression, are covered by R. L. Conner in

Chapter 7. This section will focus on the social determinants of biogenic amine involvement.

Data on the effects of isolation in male mice reveal the following: (1) minimal effects on the concentration of biogenic amines in appropriate organs; (2) reproducible alterations in turnover of amines in specific brain areas and in the adrenal medulla, with isolated male mice having reduced utilization rates when compared to grouped male controls; and (3) changes in dynamic measures of biogenic amine function confined to male subjects of mouse strains that develop heightened aggression with isolation.

B. L. Welch (1967) presented an hypothesis regarding adrenal and brain stem NE metabolism and what he termed the "mean level of environmental stimulation." He noted that grouped mice that live in a high-stimulus environment have a higher basal level of peripheral and central CA release, as reflected in a relatively high turnover rate. The neurotransmitter thus released tonically onto adrenergic receptors in grouped rats was greater than in isolated rats. Welch used this approach to explain the heightened *reactivity* of isolated mice to stimulation; isolated animals accustomed to low levels of stimulation have relatively low rates of NE release in the CNS. Thus, the receptor "sees" less NE in the isolated mice than in the grouped situation. One well-documented response of low levels of input into sensor systems in the peripheral sympathetic nervous system is the development of receptor supersensitivity (see Trendelenburg, 1966). A supersensitive receptor gives a greater response to a given amount of neurotransmitter chemical than does a normal receptor—the result being an increased response. Although he specifically postulated this for the NE-containing brain stem neurons (as well as for adrenomedullary activity), Welch also projected that brain 5-HT metabolism might show similar changes.

Subsequent investigations have led to a further elaboration of this hypothesis. The effects of an acute stressor on brain amines in isolated mice is much greater than in grouped animals. Thus, acute stress causes a marked increase in the rate of fall of brain NE and DA in isolated mice treated with α MT, but not in grouped animals (Welch and Welch, 1968a,b; Littleton, 1967; Menon *et al.*, 1967). Welch and Welch summarize these data in a review article (1970) and suggest that rapid changes in MAO activity in adrenergic neurons may be associated with the observed differences in the response to stress. Thus, isolated mice subjected to an acute stress after inhibition of TH activity by α MT have an accelerated rate of reduction of brain NE and DA, whereas the grouped animals treated with α MT are not different from grouped subjects receiving α MT and then subjected to stress. It is argued that this antagonism of the "stress-induced" increase in CA depletion is due to a rapid inactivation of MAO and thus of one major route of catabolism. Similar arguments are presented for regulation of 5-HT metabolism during stress. Supporting data for this hypothesis, however, are lacking.

Axelrod *et al.* (1970a,b) and Henry *et al.* (1971) conducted an interesting series of studies using social interactions to determine changes in CA synthetic and catabolic enzymes. Male and female mice were housed either singly or in groups for a 4-month interval following weaning. Following this, several groups of mice were maintained in isolation or in groups, while the remaining animals were housed in cages with an interconnecting tube system and a separate central feeding station. Thus, mice living in the interconnected cage system were subjected to repeared confrontation as they traversed the tubes for water and food. During the 4-month, postweaning period, this work revealed a decrease in the activities of both TH and PNMT in long-term isolated mice. COMT and MAO activity, as well as NE and E levels in the adrenal medulla, were not altered. Dealing solely with isolation vs group living, these data indicate that decrease in synthesis alone accounts for the lowered utilization rates, at least in the adrenal medulla.

Following the 4-month period of differential social housing, Henry and his collaborators observed that stimulus enhancement (i.e., mice subjected to the tube-connected cages) has a different spectrum of biochemical effects. Adrenal NE and E concentrations were elevated above normal (i.e., grouped mice living in conventional cages), as were PNMT and TH activities. MAO activity, in addition, was elevated in all stimulus-enhanced groups. COMT levels remained unchanged across the various social conditions. Although some interactions were noted between prior individual or group living conditions and subsequent exposure to the interconnected cages, these results were of considerably less magnitude than those described above. The data presented in the two studies described above reveal prfound differences in adrenal medullary enzymes reponsible for the metabolism of CA. An important conceptual point pertaining to the onserved effects is that *both* increases and decreases in enzyme activity were realized within the social conditions imposed. This finding is of considerable importance for potential correlations of social hierarchy, psychopathology, and aggression with activity of biogenic amine-containing neuronal systems. A recent report by Redmond *et al.* (1971), for instance, indicates that alterations in brain CA metabolism may be of considerable importance in social interactions between primates.

5. *Conditioned Behaviors and Catecholamines*

The majority of the studies investigating the interactions between conditioned behavioral responses and brain CA have been pharmacological in nature. Almost uniformly, such studies have indicated that chemicals which deplete CA and/or 5-HT in the brain, or which antagonize the effects of the reputed neurotransmitters on appropriate brain receptors, tend to disrupt the behavior under investigation. Subsequent pharmacological manipulations of the behaviorally depressed experimental subject have been used to analyze the possible roles of CA or 5-HT in that particular behavior. Alternatively, several operant techniques allowing for the manipulation of stimulated as well as depressed responding have been utilized. Using both the depressed and the baseline performing operant subject, considerable evidence has been gathered which demonstrates the relative importance of the biogenic amines in modifying or controlling these behaviors.

Various investigators using a discriminated two-way shuttlebox avoidance procedure have depressed responding of previously trained subjects with reserpine. Attempts at correlating behavioral recovery with the return of brain amines to normal concentrations have revealed no apparent relationships. Using the model of reserpine-induced depression of shuttlebox avoidance behavior, however, Rech *et al.* (1968) devised an ingenious method to test for differences between various behaviors with regard to their possible dependence on brain CA. Groups of rats trained for two-way active avoidance, trained to walk a rotating cylinder (rotarod), or put into cages measuring spontaneous locomotor activity, were given a single dose of reserpine to depress the respective behavior being measured. The groups were tested for their susceptibility to α MT over the subsequent 4-week period, during which both behavior and brain amine levels returned to their prereserpine levels. The rationale for these studies was as follows: once brain amine stores are depleted by reserpine (Fig. 9), the only way available to maintain adrenergic function would be through the *de novo* biosynthesis of amines. If amine synthesis is in any way related to the restitution or maintenance of the studied behaviors, then interruption of CA synthesis with α MT should disrupt those behaviors dependent upon it. All three groups of subjects returned to their prereserpine levels of behavior within 5 days, although both DA and NE levels were still depressed significantly. Test injections of α MT were started on the third postreserpine day; in the case of motor activity, α MT did not cause a significant reduction in behavior on day 7 after reserpine or at any time thereafter. Similar results were obtained in the rats trained to walk the rotarod. Shuttlebox avoidance behavior, on the other hand, continued to be depressed significantly by α MT for as long as 15 days after reserpine injection. Concurrent measurements of brain CA revealed that NE levels were not lowered significantly by α MT on or past the seventh postreserpine day. DA levels, to the contrary, were reduced markedly by α MT treatment for as long as 14 days after reserpine. Rech and coworkers interpreted this data to show that rats were differentially sensitive in terms of particular behaviors to the depressant effects of α MT following reserpine administration. In addition, shuttlebox avoidance behavior appeared to be better associated with DA levels and synthesis in brain, whereas motor and rotarod performances were better correlated with NE synthesis and stores. Additional data presented by the same investigators further strengthened the associations between the various behaviors and CA biosynthesis. Only drugs that deplete CA stores (i.e., tetrabenazine; Table IV) rendered the subjects and their measured behaviors susceptible to subsequent doses of α MT, unlike other depressant drugs (fluphenazine, a phenothiazine derivative; pentobarbital; and urethane).

Other published work has shown that avoidance behavior depressed by reserpine can be reinstated transiently by drugs restoring or facilitating the release of brain CA. Rech (1964) reported that two-way active avoidance was depressed by reserpine in a dose-dependent manner. Doses without any effect on amine stores, or those causing a mild reduction of brain NE, DA, and 5-HT were not as effective, either in intensity or duration of depressed responding, in contrast to the effect produced by amounts of reserpine causing severe and prolonged depletion. Low doses of d-amphetamine were able to reverse the reserpine-induced depression of avoidance behavior. The same dosage of l-amphetamine, which has comparable peripheral affects but has different biochemical effects than d-amphetamine in the brain, did not restore behavior to criterion levels. Further refinements of this type of study were furnished by Hanson (1967), who demonstrated that a conditioned avoidance response in cats depressed by reserpine could be reinstated with d-amphetamine. On the other hand, if α MT was given after reserpine, not only was avoidance behavior further depressed, but the effects of d-amphetamine were antagonized completely. Treatment with a low dose of DOPA, the immediate precursor of DA and NE did not appreciably affect behavior depressed by reserpine plus α MT, but did reinstate the stimulant effects of amphetamine. This data, further substantiated in a subsequent publication (Hanson and Henning, 1967), indicated that CA were responsible for reinstating a conditioned avoidance response by amphetamine. Further, it appears that the newly synthesized CA are responsible for this effect of amphetamine. Other work by Seiden and co-workers indicates that DOPA treatment alone is able to partially restore a conditional avoidance response in mice, rats and cats after reserpine treatment (Seiden and Carlsson, 1963; Seiden and Hanson, 1964; Corrodi and Hanson, 1966; Seiden and Peterson, 1968a).

There is at least one instance in which a discriminated avoidance response, not previously depressed pharmacologically, has been related to CA biosynthesis. Rech (1966) and Rech and Moore (1968) using "poor performers" in a two-way shuttlebox (i.e., rats which did not learn the avoidance response), showed the low doses of d-, but not l-amphetamine caused a transitory acquisition of the conditional avoidance response which could be antagonized completely by α MT. Similar actions of amphetamine and α MT have been described in nondiscriminated avoidance procedures (Weissman et al., 1966; Rech and Stolk, 1970), indicating a similar relationship between CA biosynthesis and amphetamine's effects.

The literature on the drug interactions discussed above has appeared to indicate certain disparities with regard to newly synthesized and granular ("stored") CA and the effects of α MT. A close evaluation of these reports, however, reveals that certain psychologically defined behaviors are affected differentially by α MT and a pattern indicating some intriguing relationships has emerged. Using the evidence reported by Weissman *et al.* (1966) it can be assumed with some degree of reliability that low doses of α MT have a relatively specific effect on newly synthesized CA in that they do not measurably affect the total stores of NE and DA in the brain. When the effects of α MT on a previously established criterion or basal level of avoidance responding are examined, small doses of the CA synthesis inhibitor do not affect the particular behavior involved (i.e., Weissman *et al.*, 1966; Rech *et al.*, 1966). Large doses of α MT, or multiple small doses (to circumvent the toxic effects of large amounts of this drug; Moore *et al.*, 1967), cause a large decrease in brain CA levels as well as behavioral depression (Rech *et al.*, 1966; Schoenfeld and Seiden, 1967, 1969). Drugs which antagonize the effects of large or multiple doses of α MT treatment on brain CA levels, i.e., the MAO inhibitors, either partially antagonize or completely prevent the behavioral depression induced by the drug (Moore and Rech, 1967). This behavioral antagonism was specific in that drugs that depressed responding through mechanisms other than amine depletion were not antagonized by concurrent MAO inhibition. Thus, in these situations brain CA stores, and not amine synthesis alone, reflect the behavioral response capabilities of the animal. Indeed, as long as stores are not completely eliminated, and in spite of maximal TH inhibition due to α MT treatment, drugs that act by releasing CA from granular stores are able to reinstate the basal or criterion response level. Further, as in the previously cited instances where CA stores were first abolished with reserpine, inhibition of amine synthesis completely antagonized the restorative effects of amphetamine on these behaviors. On the other hand, stimulated behavior in which the subject is required to increase his normal level of responding appears to be predominantly related to the rate at which new CA can be synthesized. The previously discussed data of Rech (1966) on amphetamine's effects on "poor performers" in a two-way shuttlebox avoidance paradigm serve to illustrate this point. Likewise, increased responding in a nondiscriminated avoidance situation after amphetamine administration was blocked by doses of α MT which had a demonstrable inhibitory action on CA synthesis but no effect on the total stores of these amines in brain. On the basis of these data, one might further speculate as to the roles of CA in these behaviors. If the latter interpretation is valid, it would be predicted that acquisition of a particular response involving the participation of CA-containing neurons would be impaired by low doses of α MT only if some sort of activation of these neurons were involved in the "learning" procedure. Since the utilization of both NE and DA is increased even in the performance of the stable, acquired behavior (i.e., Schoenfeld and Seiden, 1969), the latter supposition becomes more relevant. Also, the effects of relatively specific drugs such as α MT need to be carefully examined under various response schedules. It would be of interest, for example, to study the effects of inhibition of CA biosynthesis on various schedules of reinforcement. Analyses of such problems should yield some valuable data on the participation of brain amines in a variety of behavioral situations.

Some indications of the relationship between specific CA (i.e., NE vs DA) and particular behaviors were presented above (Rech *et al.,* 1968). This study suggested that DA was better related than NE to a discriminated shuttlebox response in rats, whereas the reverse situation applied for spontaneous locomotor activity and rotarod performance. To date, there are only a few studies that suggest individual amines may be preferentially involved in a particular behavior. Schoenfeld and Seiden (1969) have published graphs showing the relationship between whole-brain CA levels and the effect of their depletion on a fixed-ratio or fixed-interval schedule of water reinforcement. Their data show that the percent decrease in brain DA corresponded with the behavioral decrement induced by α MT (i.e., a 10% fall in DA corresponded with a 10% decrease in response output). Brain NE levels on the other hand, bore a different relationship to responding. When the percent decrease in NE was plotted against the response decrement, the resultant line intersected the response decrement axis at about 25% (i.e., normal NE levels with 25% reduction in response output). The authors were cautious to avoid any interpretation of these results which related one or the other amine to the tested behavior, but the possibilities for further refinement are quite intriguing. As it stands, further interpretation would be premature but more extensive dissection certainly is warranted. Seiden and Petersen (1968b) reported that the reinstatement by DOPA of a discriminated avoidance response (shuttlebox) in mice treated with reserpine was partially antagonized by inhibiting DβO with disulfiram. This antagonism suggested that NE, whose formation from DA was blocked by disulfiram, was important for the reinstatement of the conditioned avoidance response. Similar findings in rats (Krantz and Seiden, 1968) also led to these conclusions, and eliminated the possibility of a species-specific effect. These data seemingly are at variance with that of Rech *et al.* (1968) who postulated that DA was more important than NE in the shuttlebox avoidance response. Once again, these findings suggest the need for further requirements in technique to answer some relatively important questions.

6. *Self-Stimulation Behavior and Brain Norepinephrine*

One behavior thus far studied in great detail has afforded some insight into the specificity of brain amines and behavior. Self-stimulation, as developed by Olds and Milner (1954), has been shown by Stein and his associates to be specifically related to the release of NE, and not DA, from a discrete neuroanatomical tract, the median forebrain bundle (MFB). The brilliant work by Olds (cf. 1962) showed that the MFB almost certainly is the principal neural pathway of the reward system in the brain. Histochemical studies revealed that the MFB is the primary diencephalic pathway of NE-containing neurons (Hillarp *et al.*, 1966) as well as the brain area with the greatest NE content (Table II). The pharmacology of the reward system, using the self-stimulation procedure is summarized well by Stein (1964, 1968). Briefly, drugs which release CA from stores in the brain facilitate self-stimulation (i.e., amphetamine and α-methyl-*meta*-tyrosine). The same is true for drugs which increase the amount of NE released by nerve stimulation (i.e., cocaine and imipramine, which block the membrane uptake system) or for amphetamine (imipramine and MAO inhibitors). Conversely, drugs that deplete brain amines (i.e., tetrabenazine, reserpine, and α MT) or antagonize their actions (i.e., chlorpromazine) depress self-stimulation and antagonize the facilitatory effects of amphetamine.

Using a series of laborious but ingenious techniques, Stein and his associates have shown that: (1) NE specifically is the amine which mediates self-stimulation responding in the MFB, (2) NE is released at specific sites in the hypothalamus and limbic system in conjunction with rewarding stimulation, but not with nonrewarding stimulation, and (3) amphetamine is able to facilitate rewarding stimulation in the MFB by causing a similar set of biochemial changes simulating those induced by self-stimulation. Stein and Wise (1969) made use of a permanent indwelling push-pull cannula to perfuse specific sites in the brain of self-stimulating subjects. This type of cannula allows one to collect compounds released from neurons in a localized area of brain tissue. Animals with these cannulae also had indwelling electrodes for stimulating the MFB or other areas, and an intraventricular cannula for introducing radiolabeled compounds into the CNS. Prior to the experimental manipulations, the rewarding value of the stimulating electrodes was determined by measuring the subject-supported rate of self-stimulation. Aside from determining whether electrode placement was in rewarding or nonrewarding areas, this procedure demonstrated that the rats were still behaviorally responsive after the various surgical lesions necessitated by the electrode and cannulae placement.

Prior to the perfusion, ^{14}C-NE or ^{3}H-NE was injected intraventricularly and allowed to equilibrate. It was assumed that the labeled NE mixed with endogenous brain stores in adrenergic neurons, as was demonstrated by Glowinski and Iversen (1966a,b). Stein and Wise found that rewarding stimulation caused a threefold increase in the efflux of radioactivity from either the rostral hypothalamus or the amygdala. When nonrewarding stimuli were given (i.e., in cortical areas), no such increase in efflux was noted. Surprisingly, thalamic and midbrain stimulation which, from preexperimental behavioral observations, may have been punishing, actually caused a decrease in the outflow of radioactivity. Chemical analyses of these perfusates revealed that the bulk of the radioactivity released by stimulation was comprised of NE metabolites, mainly O-methylated deaminated compounds (MHPG, MHPG-SO$_4$, MHMA; Fig. 5). The investigators attributed the low levels of NE collected in the perfusate as reflecting the importance of the membrane uptake system in the functioning of NE-containing neuron systems. The increased radioactivity was presumed to be due to an increased utilization of NE within the neuron, as reflected by the increase in catabolism. When these experiments were conducted in rats pretreated with an MAO inhibitor, the main alteration observed was an increase in normetanephrine, which is usually associated with an increase in NE release.

Under conditions in which the brains of the experimental animals were not stimulated, and instead, the subjects received doses of d-amphetamine which facilitated self-stimulation activity in other studies, an increased efflux of radioactivity was observed only in the amygdala. The chemical composition of the radioactivity released by amphetamine showed a large increase in the O-methylated metabolites, which is consistent with the known pharmacological effects of this drug (Fig. 10) and is explicable on the basis of an increased release of NE and inhibition of its uptake at the neuronal membrane. The high degree of localization of these effects of amphetamine is consistent with the hypothesis that the cortex and other forebrain areas are more sensitive than the brain stem to low doses of amphetamine [see Wise and Stein (1970) for supporting evidence].

In a subsequent publication, Wise and Stein (1969) devised a means of showing the selectivity of NE in maintaining and mediating self-stimulation behavior. In these experiments, animals with an intraventricular cannula and an electrode producing rewarding stimulation were tested behaviorally after inhibition of DβO by disulfiram or diethyldithiocarbamate (DDC; Table III). They found that self-stimulation rates were depressed to about 20% of normal following DDC. The intraventricular administration of l- or d,l-NE (the l-isomer is biologically active) restored behavior to pre-DDC levels. Intraventricular injection of d-NE (biologically inactive), DA, 5-HT, or intraperitoneal administration of l-NE did not affect the DDC-depressed behavior. This study supported the postulate that NE was the probable neurotransmitter responsible for mediating and maintaining self-stimulation behavior, and that 5-HT, DA, or peripheral NE (reaching the brain via the circulation) were not involved.

Similar studies devoted to the effects of amphetamines on self-stimulation were reported recently by Wise and Stein (1970). When injected after DDC, amphetamine did not alter the rate of self-stimulation. The facilitating action of amphetamine was restored shortly after the infusion of l-NE. Wise and Stein interpreted this evidence as follows: (a) amphetamine's facilitation of self-stimulation behavior is due to release of NE, probably localized specifically (with regard to this behavior) in the forebrain, and (b) *de novo* synthesis, as previously postulated, was not specifically required for amphetamine's action. Rather, amphetamine acts on a functionally available pool of NE (which presumably contains newly synthesized NE in the intact animal) in preference to a bound store of NE. The latter statement derives from the fact that the short duration (15 minutes) between DDC injection and amphetamine administration precludes extensive depletion of brain NE. In spite of this, amphetamine did not reverse the behavioral depression until after *l*-NE infusion.

Stein's group has taken the analysis one critical step further by attempting to define the neurophysiological role of NE, released by MFB stimulation, in the amygdala (Stein, 1968; Wise and Stein, 1970). They believe that the amygdala normally functions to suppress behavior and have related this to a punishment system, with fibers running from the amygdala through the periventricular and peraqueductal gray to the mesencephalic tectum and motor nuclei in the lower brain stem. This fiber system, called the periventricular system, is cholinergic (i.e., acetylcholine is the purported neurotransmitter) and has a suppressant action on behavior. By direct application of drugs into the amygdala, Margules (1968) and Stein (1968) found that *l*-NE, *d,l*-NE, and *l*-E inhibited the suppressant effects of punishment on behavior. As was true in the experiments described above, DA, *d*-NE, and various CA precursors were inactive in this regard, once again pointing to NE as the specific transmitter chemical. These data and the related hypothesis are important because they take into account the neurophysiological and pharmacological data indicating that NE has an inhibitory action on many brain neurons. In summary, the level of activity of the MFB is increased by neuronal input sinaling a forthcoming reward. The input of both rewarding and punishing stimuli jointly determine the level of activity in the MFB. Similar factors may dictate whether amphetamine will or will not be effective. That is, the drug will facilitate self-stimulation behavior if activity in the MFB is above some threshold level, but will not do so when MFB activity is below such a level, i.e., if the anticipation of reward is low, as in the case of "nonrewarding" or "punishing" electrode placement. The biochemical similarities in the behavioral effects of rewarding self-stimulation and amphetamine administration indicate that NE in the amygdala is the specific neurotransmitter involved. With specific regard to amphetamine's effects, Wise and Stein (1970) are very careful to point out that the drug appears to *facilitate* existing tendencies to perform operant responses, rather than to stimulate new behaviors.

7. Serotonin and Behavior

There is much work in the literature which indicates that brain 5-HT may have a major role in cerebral development. Most of the evidence has come from studies using infant rodents fed various amino acid-supplemented diets to produce a model phenylketonuria. From these studies (cf. McKean *et al.*, 1967), decreases in brain 5-HT levels concomitant with "phenylketogenic" diets are accompanied by deficits in performance which appear to be irreversible. While a case could be made for such an association of brain 5-HT with development and behavior, the possibilities of various effects of altered amino acid metabolism not related to 5-HT are much too numerous and complex to discuss further here.

Considerable interest has been focused on the effects of PCPA, a depletor of tissue 5-HT levels, and acquisition of avoidance behavior. Tenen (1967) demonstrated that PCPA-treated rats acquired an active avoidance response much more rapidly than did control subjects or PCPA-treated animals given 5-HTP, the immediate precursor of 5-HT (Fig. 11), which causes an increase in brain levels of the biogenic amine. The data supported the notion that 5-HT depletion increased learning of the avoidance task, but observation of the PCPA-treated rats revealed large increases in their response to shock. Measurements of pain sensitivity revealed that PCPA did lower shock threshold. Subsequent retesting of avoidance acquisition at a higher shock intensity revealed no differences in the rate at which the three groups of rats learned the avoidance response. Other measurements of shock thresholds in rats with various brain lesions (Lints and Harvey, 1969) have revealed that decreases in 5-HT, but not NE, levels are correlated with an increased sensitivity to footshock. Subsequent measures of emotional reactivity conducted by Tenen demonstrated that a preconditioned "emotional" stimulus (tone and light paired with footshock) disrupted drinking of water-deprived rats less after PCPA than in controls. Other measures of emotionality indicated that the 5-HT-depleted rats were less "emotional" than control animals, which also could be related to the improved avoidance acquisition.

Schlesinger et al. (1968) have reported similar effects of PCPA on avoidance learning at different shock intensities in Fisher rats, but could find no such relationship in Buffalo genotypes (avoidance responses were increased only at the highest shock intensity). Other evidence (Stevens et al., 1967) on enhanced rate of acquisition of brightness discrimination task after PCPA, implies that other sensory modalities are affected by 5-HT depletion. Results published by Sudak and Maas (1964), which report a positive correlation between "emotionality" and brain 5-HT levels, also agree with Tenen's data. A recent study by Robichaud and Sledge (1969) describes a greater rate of responding for a milk reward during a conditioned stimulus (CS)-paired punishment period in rats after treatment with PCPA than in the same subjects in pre- or postdrug sessions. Although these authors considered their results indicative of a change in drive level after PCPA (see below), no report has revealed evidence suggestive of an increased basal rate of responding for water or food. Stevens et al. (1969) used a similar design to test whether PCPA increases learning ability or decreases emotionality. Thirsty animals were trained to traverse an alley to obtain water. Water was then removed and a source offered through an electrified fount in all subsequent sessions. PCPA-treated rats took significantly longer to learn the passive avoidance response than did controls. Stevens and his associates interpreted this as an indication that 5-HT-depleted rats were less emotional rather than better able to acquire an avoidance response.

A number of other reports, commencing with Koe and Weissman (1966), have described a grossly observable hyperreactivity of rats to environmental stimuli following reduction of brain 5-HT levels. More discrete measures of altered reactivity (i.e., to shock) have been mentioned above. Recent investigations in our laboratory, conducted by Conner et al. (1970), have evaluated the effects of PCPA treatment on habituation to an auditory startle stimulus in the rat. In relation to the work of Aghajanian and Sheard (1968), which showed that electrical stimulation of the midbrain raphe area (the region containing most of the 5-HT-containing nerve cell bodies in the brain) causes an impairment of the normal process of habituation to repetitive auditory or tactile stimuli, Conner and his associates describe an impairment of the habituation process after PCPA treatment. This impairment was characterized as follows: (1) Administration of PCPA to rats previously habituated to an auditory startle stimulus caused a transient increase in the startle response coinciding with the time of maximal serotonin depletion in brain. The drug-treated rats subsequently "rehabituated," but were extremely sensitive to additional novel auditory cues introduced during the test session. (2) Injection of PCPA prior to starting habituation trials increased the time necessary for habituation to occur. Very subtle changes in the test environment (i.e., an increase in session duration) differentially affected the PCPA-treated rats.

A general trend running through the above studies, which describes relationships between 5-HT and various behaviors, may be discerned. In each situation, reduction of brain 5-HT with PCPA or, presumably, specific brain lesions, appears to cause an impairment in the organisms' response-suppressant mechanisms. Reduced emotional reactivity after PCPA, an effect entertained by Tenen (1967), Stevens et al. (1969), and Robichaud and Sledge (1969), could facilitate active, or retard passive, avoidance learning by reducing the probability of a competing suppressant response emerging. Thus, lowered 5-HT levels in brain may decrease the tendency of "freezing" behavior to occur. Such a change would result in a facilitation of active avoidance acquisition or retard acquisition of a passive avoidance or a punishment-suppressed response, as noted in the above references. Similarly, an impairment of normal suppressant mechanisms could be inferred from the data relating exaggerated drive behaviors to PCPA treatment. Finally, there is good neurophysiological evidence for neuron-mediated feedback suppression of sensory input (i.e., Galambos, 1956; Hernandez-Peon et al., 1956) to account for the effects of PCPA on habituation. If PCPA and the associated depletion of brain 5-HT destroy the organism's ability to "evaluate" the contextual cues of its environment, or if the drug "sets" this ability to some other hypothetical threshold level, then clearly many behaviors, whether they be acquired or innate, would be altered. To be sure, parsimony is but infrequently proved factual, and we must await further experimental evidence to more accurately assess the role of brain 5-HT in behavior.

8. Serotonin and Sleep

During the past five years, considerable effort has been directed toward understanding the relationship of neurotransmitters, particularly 5-HT, to sleep. Sleep has been investigated because it is more clearly defined than many other behaviors and has seemed to be a behavior particularly amenable to biochemical investigation. Four fundamental approaches have been used: (1) administering drugs that inhibit or augment the effects of a particular neuroregulatory agent and studying the effects on sleep and on amines; (2) measuring neuroregulator levels in various states of sleep; (3) making lesions in areas of brain and determing the effects on sleep and on amines; and (4) depriving animals of one of the stages of sleep and determining the effect on neuroregulators.

Sleep states can be divided into slow wave sleep, which constitutes about 80% of sleep time, and rapid-eye-movement sleep (REM sleep, dream sleep, D sleep, paradoxical sleep), which constitutes about 20% of sleep time. These various states have been reviewed (Dement, 1966; Hartman, 1967; Hobson, 1969). Among the characteristics of REM sleep are rapid eye movements observable through the closed eyelids and an activated electroencephalogram (EEG). REM sleep has been found in all mammals studied. Deprivation of REM sleep can be accomplished by monitoring the EEG and waking the subject when he begins to go into the state. REM sleep usually must be made up when it is lost through deprivation.

The evidence that 5-HT might be involved in sleep states has arisen largely from the brilliant work of Jouvet (1969). The evidence implicating 5-HT includes the findings that: (1) intracarotid injection of 5-HT induces EEG recordings consistent with slow wave sleep (Koella, 1968); (2) injection of PCPA, which decreases 5-HT, causes insomnia in the cat; and (3) lesions of the midline raphe system, thought to be the cells of origin of the majority of serotonergic pathways may induce insomnia.

Although this evidence has been widely accepted as demonstrating a close relationship of 5-HT to sleep, there have been a number of experiments which suggest that the relationship, if it exists, is a more complicated one, and that there may be marked species differences in the transmitters involved in sleep. There are major problems of interpretation of studies involving lesions or injection of 5-HT.

The most challenging data to reconcile with the serotonergic hypothesis relate to the effects of PCPA on sleep. The problem is complicated by marked species differences. Rechtschaffen et al. (1969) has found that in the rat, the PCPA-induced insomnia is of shorter duration than in the cat, while Wyatt

(1970), performing studies in man at much lower doses of PCPA, has found that the drug may decrease REM sleep without altering regular slow wave sleep.

The Stanford group (Dement *et al.*, 1969) has found that chronic PCPA treatment results in transitory insomnia lasting several days. During this period, there is slow wave sleep as well as REM sleep suppression and reduced brain 5-HT. Continuation of drug administration, however, results in return of slow wave sleep and REM sleep to about 75% of normal, despite continued low levels of 5-HT. When REM sleep returns, there is no REM rebound following the previous deprivation. Of particular interest is the finding that, in the 5-HT-depleted cat, some of the physiological manifestations of REM sleep occur in wakefulness as long as the 5-HT depletion is maintained.

Another approach to the study of sleep and its underlying biochemistry has been produced by deprivation of REM sleep. Several laboratories (Weiss *et al.*, 1968; Pujol *et al.*, 1968) have found evidence that rats deprived of REM sleep have an increased turnover of 5-HT. However, such a change may be quite nonspecific and related to a stress effect. Even so, such a change could be involved in the psychological changes associated with REM sleep deprivation.

Measurement of the levels of neuroregulators in stages of sleep and wakefulness (Sinha *et al.*, in press) has provided a different approach to the problems of neuroregulators and the control of sleep. The investigations of a number of laboratories (Quay, 1963; Reis *et al.*, 1968; Friedman and Walker, 1968; Scheving *et al.*, 1968; Manshardt and Wurtman, 1968), demonstrated circadian changes in the levels of neuroregulators and differences at varying times of day, and even multiple rhythms within the 24-hour period. Studies looking at the changes in several transmitters in different stages of sleep must be conducted to answer questions such as, what are the kinetics involving the neuroregulators just as an animal enters into or exits from a stage of sleep.

The data so far suggest a relationship between the neurotransmitters and sleep. Two major questions, as perceived by investigators in the field, are: (1) Which transmitter is involved in various aspects of the behavioral repertoire? (2) To what extent can various manipulations which alter neuroregulators influence the stages of sleep? Such questions have basic relevance to psychiatric illness since, in a number of severe illnesses (depression, schizophrenia), profound disturbances in sleep patterns have been demonstrated by a number of investigators.

B. Human Studies

1. *Catecholamines and Human Psychological Disorders*

Replacement therapy of a presumed neurotransmitter has been extremely effective in the treatment of Parkinson's disease. Patients suffering from this illness were shown to have a deficiency of DA in the striatum. Autopsied brains revealed DA concentrations of 0.4 μg/gm in a Parkinsonian striatum as compared to 4 μg/gm in normals (Ehringer and Hornykeiwicz, 1960). In addition to this DA deficiency, HVA levels were found to be depressed in the striatum of Parkinsonian brains (Bernheimer and Hornykiewicz, 1965). Initial attempts at replacement of brain DA by intravenous DOPA administration proved useful therapeutically, but this effect was short-lived (Birkmayer and Hornykiewicz, 1961). Hornykiewicz was uncertain as to whether increase in brain DA or NE were responsible for the transient clinical improvement in his Parkinsonian patients given intravenous DOPA, and consequently administered *threo*-dihydroxyphenylserine (DOPS), a compound which may be decarboxylated in the brain to form NE. When this compound was given to Parkinsonian patients no therapeutic effect was observed (Birkmayer and Hornykiewicz, 1962), and Hornykiewicz concluded that increased levels of brain DA were responsible for the therapeutic efficacy of L-DOPA in Parkinsonian patients. Since the discovery that L-DOPA administration produces long-lasting remission in the crippling effects of Parkinson's disease, new interest has been generated in replacement therapy as a model which may be applicable to some psychiatric disorders.

Currently the major interest in the relationship of CA to disturbed behavior has been in affective illness. Evidence supporting the relationship between CA and depression has been reviewed by Schildkraut (1965), who, with Bunney and Davis (1965), is credited with the formulation of the CA hypothesis of affective disease. Briefly, this hypothesis relates depression to a functional deficiency of NE and mania to a functional escess of this neurorehulator at certain central synapses. The data supporting this hypothesis include the following: reserpine (a drug which lowers brain CA levels) causes depression in about 20% of the people taking moderate doses; the tricyclic drugs which are effective in treating depression, block the reuptake of NE after it is released by neurons in the synaptic cleft (thus functionally increasing relative amounts of NE at the synapse); the MAO inhibitors are effective in the treatment of depression and act presumably by increasing synaptic concentration of CA; lithium carbonate, the most effective drug in the treatment of mania, has been shown to increase the reuptake process for NE, thus decreasing the amount of functionally available NE at the synaptic cleft. Each of these phenomena has multiple explanations and the evidence is far from compelling; nonetheless, the hypothesis has proved stimulating and has provided a further impetus to determine the role of CA in affective disease.

Although the preponderance of behavioral data concerning the effect of mood-altering drugs on biogenic amines support the CA hypothesis, there is sufficient evidence to challenge this concept. Wyatt (Wyatt *et al.*, 1971) has reported that levels of plasma NE and E in patients with depression were increased during their depression. Further, Dencker (Dencker *et al.*, 1966) has shown that CSF levels of MHPG were markedly increased during depression in contrast to levels obtained prior to and following the episode of depression. These data raise the issue of a possible increase rather than a decrease in brain CA of depressed patients.

An example of one research strategy to test the CA hypothesis was conducted by Bunney (Bunney *et al.*, 1971) using the precursor loading model. These investigators administered L-DOPA with and without a peripheral decarboxylase inhibitor to depressed patients. They found little antidepressant effect of L-DOPA, but in several patients with a history of mania there was evidence that the drug elicited manic behavior. This finding raises the possibility that mania may be due to a relative excess of DA, but that depression may not relate to a deficiency of dopamine. However, because there is little evidence that DOPA increases brain concentrations of NE (Everett and Borcherding, 1970), the fact that L-DOPA administration to depressed patients has not improved their clinical state may be explained on the basis that little of the L-DOPA is being converted to brain NE. These investigators (Brodie *et al.*, 1971) also made the important observation that α MPT, an inhibitor of CA synthesis, is effective in the treatment of some manic episodes. This is the best evidence to date suggesting a role for CA in mania. In addition to the use of precursor load strategy and inhibitors of those enzymes responsible for CA synthesis, other basic neuronal processes could be altered in an attempt to study the role of CA in affective disease. If an effective nontoxic inhibitor of COMT were discovered, this compound might have important antidepressant actions. Further, if a compound were found which increased storage of amines in the neuron this might enhance its ability to deposit CA at the synaptic cleft, thus overcoming a presumed deficit in depression. In the future, it is likely that hypotheses relating neuroregulators to behavior will become much more specific, involving certain areas of the brain and changes in particular processes, such as release, reuptake, or receptor-site activation.

2. Serotonin and Human Psychological Disorders

Abnormalities in synthesis, release, and metabolism of IA have been related to mental illness. Such studies have led to suggestions that some forms of depression or mania may be related to a functional decrease or increase in brain concentrations of 5-HT, respectively. This concept is referred to as the IA hypothesis of affective illness. Some forms of schizophrenia have been postulated to involve the formation of a psychotogen or alteration in IA synthesis or metabolism.

One primary area of investigation has focused on the role of 5-HT in depression, utilizing an assay for the major metabolite of 5-HT, 5-HIAA, in CSF and brain tissue. A refinement of this technique designed to measure metabolism of 5-HT has been developed utilizing the analysis of 5-HIAA in CSF following administration of probenecid (Tamarken et al., 1970). Probenecid blocks the exit of acid metabolites from the CSF; thus the rate of rise of 5-HIAA may reflect 5-HT utilization in brain.

Some investigators (Roos and Sjöström, 1969; van Praag et al., 1970) have shown that in some depressed patients there is a decrease in resting levels of 5-HIAA in the CSF and that after probencid treatment (van Praag and Korf, 1971) the rate of increase in 5-HIAA may be decreased as compared to controls. These data support the concept that 5-HT may be present in insufficient amounts or its utilization may be impaired in patients with depression.

Direct assay of 5-HT and 5-HIAA in the brains of suicide victims has been undertaken. These studies (Bourne et al., 1968) reveal a decreased level of hindbrain 5-HIAA in suicide victims as compared to controls. However, these studies are fraught with several problems: the delay in obtaining brain tissue, the difficulty in matching subjects, and the issue of the type of depression or disorder represented in the particular suicidal group.

The use of the precursor loading strategy in an attempt to increase levels of 5-HT in brain has been undertaken by several investigators. Bunney (Bunney et al., 1971) has shown that the administration of tryptophan to depressed patients is not effective as an antidepressant. Evidence supporting the IA hypothesis of affective illness has been reviewed by Glassman (1969). Preliminary data indicate that some depressed patients may benefit from the administration of 5-HTP, the immediate precursor of serotonin (Persson and Roos, 1967). Further evaluation of this compound is certainly needed.

Other studies have focused on metabolic pathways involving tryptophan which may be altered by stress (Curzon and Bridges, 1970). Given the inducability of some liver enzymes responsible for tryptophan metabolism which are activated by cortisol release, these investigators have hypothesized that a decrease in brain 5-HT under stress is related to a decrease in the availability of tryptophan for synthesis of brain 5-HT. Although this hypothesis is intriguing, further work is needed to support it. Other studies on the relationship of 5-HT to depression have been carried out by Davies and Carroll (1970), which suggest subpopulations of depressed patients with marked differences in biochemical parameters.

Several investigators have related mania to an increase of 5-HT content in brain (Glassman, 1969). Haskovek (Haskovek and Soucek, 1969) have suggested that methysergide, an inhibitor of 5-HT receptors, is effective in the treatment of mania. Further work by Itil et al. (1971) gives evidence that Cinnanserin, another 5-HT receptor-site blocker, may be effective in the treatment of mania. However, the number of patients treated in both series was small and adequate drug trials on a larger population are needed.

Another area in which 5-HT and its derivatives have been implicated is schizophrenia and the related psychoses. There have been several investigations suggesting that metabolism of 5-HT may be involved in such illness. Many hypotheses involve the possible effects of abnormally formed methylated derivatives of 5-HT as described earlier (Himwich, 1971; Morgan and Mandell, 1969). Bufotenin, for example, is a dimethylated 5-HT derivative which has been found in urine (Himwich, 1971). There is no evidence, however, that these compounds are formed, to any greater extent, in schizophrenics than in normals or that such compounds are involved in either the etiology or maintenance of any of the subgroups that make up the psychotic disorders (Sankar, 1969). There is no clear evidence of the degree to which methylated indole compounds are formed, where they are formed, or how they are metabolized.

The issue of regulation of formation of methylated compounds is of great importance. As described earlier in the chapter there are multiple controls, including enzymic activity of enzymes, involved in biogenic amine formation. An example of a general control mechanism, which may be involved in formation of methylated compounds, is the finding by Deguchi and Barchas (1971) that in methylation in which S-adenosylmethionine is the methyl donor; the S-adenosylhomocysteine which is formed may inhibit further methylation. The investigators found an enzyme which will cleave the inhibitor thereby stimulating methylation. Such studies need to be extended to human investigation and suggest investigation of the role of regulation of methylation processes.

Of particular interest are studies demonstrating that certain drugs (e.g., LSD) which cause model psychoses may alter the utilization of brain 5-HT and may be structurally related to 5-HT. Major impetus toward such a conclusion is derived from the work of Freedman (1961), demonstrating that LSD could elevate the levels of brain 5-HT. Such studies have been extended to other drugs and it has been demonstrated that LSD may inhibit 5-HT-containing neurons (Rosecrans *et al.*, 1967; Foote *et al.*, 1969; Holtzman *et al.*, 1969). Wooley (1962) pointed out that some hallucinogens may act through structural similarities to 5-HT and such relationships could be described in terms of metabolite-antimetabolite interrelationships. Other approaches to the action of hallucinogens in relation to 5-HT have included structural similarities, effects on glial cells in the brain, and effects on nucleic acids (Smythies, 1970). Hollister (1968) has reviewed a wide variety of materials related to chemical psychoses, including the comparisons between the chemical psychoses and natural psychotic states.

In relation to 5-HT and psychotic states, the laboratories of Dement and Barchas (Dement *et al.*, 1969) have described neurophysiological changes in cats treated with PCPA, which led them to suggest that some psychotic illnesses may represent a relative deficiency of 5-HT. Very few studies have been performed using PCPA to inhibit 5-HT synthesis in humans. The major investigations have been performed at the National Institutes of Health by Sjoerdsma and his group

(Sjoerdsma, 1970; Engelman *et al.*, 1967). The psychological changes in those patients have been further studied and reviewed by Carpenter (1970). Patients who had a tumor which secretes 5-HT causing the carcinoid syndrome were given the drug. Most, but not all, patients with the tumor have no psychological effects, a finding which might be expected since 5-HT has only a limited ability to cross the blood-brain barrier. When patients were treated with PCPA to relieve some of the peripheral symptoms of the excess 5-HT secretion, emotional changes were noted in a number of the patients but the changes did not fit any particular psychiatric entity. The degree of change in brain 5-HT levels in the patients is unclear. Emotional changes included anxiety, irritability, depression, social withdrawal, and lack of interest. The results indicate the need for further studies of the role of 5-HT in emotional behavior. PCPA is a drug with complicated biochemical effects and may alter brain NE utilization (Stolk *et al.*, 1969). Further studies will have to be undertaken with other compounds which may inhibit 5-HT formation (McGeer and Peters, 1969).

In models of abnormal behavior which assume a relative deficiency of 5-HT in an area of the brain and a predisposition to behavioral disorder, such a relative deficiency could be due to (1) an actual decrease in the amount of the transmitter at synapses in some area in brain, (2) an alteration in some process involving the transmitter, such as release, receptor interactions, reuptake, etc. which would cause the same relative deficiency, or (3) a formation of an abnormal metabolite of 5-HT which would act as a false transmitter, and, thus, create a relative deficiency or excess of the action of the natural transmitter.

It is clear that further studies will be necessary to delineate the effects of precursors, analogs, and inhibitors of 5-HT in the treatment of various forms of emotional disorders. More adequate ways of studying 5-HT in man need to be developed, for it is clear that there are several ways in which more information regarding 5-HT may eventually be of aid in psychological assessment.

V. MUTABILITY AND GENETIC FACTORS RELATING BIOGENIC AMINES AND BEHAVIOR

In the preceding sections of this chapter, changes in the rate of synthesis or rate of utilization of various neuroregulators have been described in relation to stress, behavioral, and environmental changes. Within that framework, a number of questions still remain to be investigated relating neuroregulatory agents to long-term emotional changes in behavior. To date, there have been no adequate studies, for example, of the effects of chronic stress on turnover or utilization of brain amines. Under these conditions, are there changes in the levels of the various enzymes or changes in the receptor which would alter the basic neurochemical response to a stressful situation or an altered environment? If one visualizes a relationship between biochemical and psychological events and assumes synaptic changes in response to a psychological event, then such changes become very important in relation to the length of time that they persist. To account for long-term emotional behaviors and alterability of behaviors, one would have to assume mutability in the processes underlying neurochemical events at the synapses. In the simplest model, we would assume that the psychological events affect the neural chemistry and the chemical change in turn affects the future psychological events. Thus, chemical changes which are permanent in nature could in effect, "lock" a certain psychological set. One might postulate such processes to be involved in very generalized anxiety states.

It has been found that acute stresses will generally increase the rate of amine turnover, and after certain types of stress, there may even be a decrease (Stolk *et al.*, in press) in turnover of amines. Such mutability, both short-term and long-term, is essential if these compounds are indeed involved in emotional behavior. It should be emphasized that this view does not negate a crucial role for psychological processes in behavior but rather suggests that there may be a very close interaction with biochemical processes. At some point in the future, analysis of either one by itself may prove inadequate for conceptualization.

The mutability of processes dealing with neuroregulatory agents involves investigation of genetic processes related to these compounds. There has been surprisingly little investigation to date at this level.

Beginning with the investigations of Maas and his group (Sudak and Maas, 1964), it has been recognized that there may be different levels of 5-HT and NE in brain in different inbred strains of mice. These findings have been extended to rat brain (Miller *et al.*, 1968). Schlesinger *et al.* (1965) demonstrated that inbred mouse strains susceptible to audiogenic seizures had lower levels of brain 5-HT and NE at 21 days of age when they are most susceptible to seizures. There are differences in brain in the rate of formation of IA, in the activity of tryptophan hydroxylase, and in the rate of utilization of 5-HT in different inbred mouse strains (Dominic, in press). Further, brain TH activity varies in different inbred mouse strains (Ciaranello *et al.*, to be published). To date, there has been limited investigation as to possible differences in enzyme activities, metabolic pathways, utilization rates, or responses to stress in different strains, and the genetic controls on those processes. The issue of metabolic pathways varying in different genetic strains has been demonstrated to have a considerable importance in terms of the steroid hormones produced by the adrenal cortex (Hamburg, 1967; Hamburg and Kessler, 1967; Hamburg and Lunde, 1967). A number of illnesses have been demonstrated in which there is a genetic difference in formation of adrenocortical hormones; several of these illnesses lead to marked behavioral change. Interestingly, compounds may have been detected in the adrenal medulla which have not been adequately studied from a physiological standpoint. We do not know the extent to which there can be minor or abnormal pathways in adrenal catechols or how controls on these pathways might be influenced genetically or altered by stress.

The review by Hamburg and Kessler (1967) describes a variety of ways in which genetic defects might change behavior. An extensive listing could be made of possible defects which could occur in relation to CA, either those secreted by the adrenal or those formed and utilized in the brain, and we will discuss only a few of these possibilities.

In terms of E or NE from the adrenal medulla, genetic processes might well control formation, release, passage across the blood-brain barrier, or metabolism of the hormones. It has been shown in the adrenal cortex that steroids are released in varying amounts in different genetic strains. Applying the same possibility to the adrenal medullary response to stress, two individuals might send the same number of nerve impulses to the adrenal medulla and yet, due to a genetic difference, one might secrete much more E than the other. If this were the case, clearly there could be different levels of behavioral changes when the E reached various target organs, including the brain. Recent work (Ciaranello *et al.*, 1972) has demonstrated that there can be twofold differences in the levels of the adrenal enzymes involved in the formation of CA in varying strains of mice, indicating that we need to know much more about genetic factors in the human. Investigation of biogenic amines in the framework of human biochemical genetics presents opportunities for deeper understanding of stress responses.

Altered patterns could also be present in terms of 5-HT or CA in the brain. Mechanisms which could be affected include the regulatory mechanisms, such as the degree to which the rate-limiting enzymes are activated to cause formation of transmitter, the rate of utilization, and metabolic pathways including the formation of abnormal metabolites. Of particular importance will be studies including regulation of normal biochemical events. One aspect of this problem involves the necessity of determining the multiple forms of the enzymes (isoenzymes) involved in formation and destruction of biogenic amines.

It is difficult at this early stage in the development of behavioral neurochemistry to give an adequate general formulation of the relationship between biochemistry and behavior. At this point, it seems reasonable to assume that biochemical and psychological processes are intimately related. Biochemical processes may well affect, for example, activity levels, emotional tones, and susceptibility to stress. Psychological processes may influence biochemical processes, for example, by producing shifts between pathways, altering utilization of transmitters, and inducing enzymic changes. Such biochemical events might lead to further psychological changes. While we do not assume that all types of emotional distress are primarily associated with biochemical abnormalities, it is true that biochemical events may profoundly alter the ability of the organism to respond to its environment. We consider it likely that some severe emotional disorders may be based upon genetically determined alterations in normal biochemical processes. These biochemical predispositions may interact in complex ways with environmental factors such as severe psychological stresses. The possible role of developmental processes in establishing "emoto-stats" which would be important in adult behavior must also be considered (Barchas, to be published).

It is too early to say what the role of biogenic amines and the various means of measuring them will be in assessing behavior. Nevertheless, it has become increasingly clear that these neuroregulatory agents are involved in basic forms of behavior and that investigation of their role in behavior is highly pertinent to a deeper understanding of behavior and severe mental illness.

Acknowledgements

Work of the authors' laboratory presented in this paper was supported by MH 13,259, MH 16,632, NASA NGR 05-020-168, and ONR N00014-67-A-0112-0027. J. B. holds NIMH Research Scientist Development Award MH 24,161.

Portions of the material presented here appeared in *Psychological Assessment,* Vol. 2, in a chapter entitled; "Neuroregulatory Agents and Psychological Assessment," edited by Paul McReynolds, published by Science and Behavior Books of Palo Alto, California, and are reprinted here with permission.

We would like to thank Mrs. Rosemary Schmele and Mrs. Judy Lookabill for their secretarial and editorial assistance and Miss Jill Leland for preparing the figures.

References

Abel, J. J., and Crawford, A. C. (1897). *Bull. Johns Hopkins Hosp.* **76**, 151.
Acheson, G. H., ed. (1966). "Second Symposium on Catecholamines," reprinted from *Pharmacol. Rev.* **18**, No. 1 (1966) published for the Amer. Soc. Pharmacol. and Exp. Ther. by Williams & Wilkins, Baltimore, Maryland.
Aghajanian, G. K., and Asher, I. M. (1971). *Science* **172**, 1159.
Aghajanian, G. K., and Bloom, F. E. (1967). *J. Pharmacol. Exp. Ther.* **156**, 23.
Aghajanian, G. K., and Sheard, M. H. (1968). *Commun. Behav. Biol.* **1**, 37.
Aghajanian, G. K., Rosecrans, J. A., and Sheard, M. H. (1967). *Science* **156**, 402.
Aghajanian, G. K., Foote, W. E., and Sheard, M. H. (1968). *Science* **161**, 706.
Airila, Y. (1913). *Arch Int. Pharmacodyn. Ther.* **23**, 453.
Alousi, A., and Weiner, N. (1966). *Proc. Nat. Acad. Sci. U.S.* **56**, 1491.
Alpers, H. S., and Shore, P. A. (1969). *Biochem. Pharmacol.* **18**, 1363.
Andén, N. -E., Dahlström, A., Fuxe, K., Larsson, K., Olson, L., and Ungerstedt, U. (1966). *Acta Physiol. Scand.* **67**, 313.
Andén, N. -E., Corrodi, H., Fuxe, K., and Hökfelt, T. (1967). *Eur. J. Pharmacol.* **2**, 59.
Anton, A. H., and Sayre, D. F. (1962). *J. Pharmacol. Exp. Ther.* **138**, 360.
Ax, A. F. (1953). *Psychosom. Med.* **15**, 434.
Axelrod, J. (1959). *Physiol. Rev.* **39**, 751.
Axelrod, J. (1962a). *J. Biol. Chem.* **237**, 1657.
Axelrod, J. (1962b). *J. Pharmacol. Exp. Ther.* **138**, 28.
Axelrod, J., and Weissbach, H. (1961). *J. Biol. Chem.* **236**, 211.
Axelrod, J., Weil-Malherbe, H., and Tomchick, R. (1959). *J. Pharmacol. Exp. Ther.* **127**, 251.
Axelrod, J., Hertting, G., and Patrick, R. W. (1961). *J. Pharmacol. Exp. Ther.* **134**, 325.
Axelrod, J., Mueller, R. A., Henry, J. P., and Stephens, P. M. (1970a). *Nature (London)* **225**, 1059.

Axelrod, J., Mueller, R, A,, and Thoenen, H. (1970b). New aspects of storage and release mechanisms of catecholamines. *Bayer Symp., 1900,* **2,** p. 212. Springer-Verlag, Berlin and New York.

Azmitia, E. C., Jr., and McEwen, B. S. (1969). *Science* **166,** 1274.

Bak, I. J., Hassler, R., and Kim, J. S. (1969). *Z. Zellforsch. Mikrosk. Anat.* **101,** 448.

Baldessarini, R. J., and Kopin, I. J. (1966). *Science* **152,** 1630.

Baldessarini, R. J., and Kopin, I. J. (1967). *J. Pharmacol. Exp. Ther.* **156,** 31.

Banks, P. (1966). *Biochem. J.* **101,** 536.

Barchas, J. D., and Freedman, D. (1963). *Biochem. Pharmacol.* **12,** 1232.

Barchas, J. D., DaCosta, F., and Spector, S. (1967). *Nature (London)* **214,** 919.

Barchas, J. D., Ciaranello, R. D., and Steinman, A. M. (1969). *Recent Advan. Biol. Psychiat.* **1,** 31.

Barchas, J. D., and Usdin, E., eds. (In press). "Serotonin and Behavior," Academic Press, New York.

Barchas, P. (to be published). *In* "Readings in Social Psychology: (R. Ofshe, ed.) Prentice-Hall, Englewood Cliffs, New Jersey.

Barger G., and Dale, H. H. (1910). *J. Physiol. (London)* **41,** 19.

Basowitz, H., Korchin, S. J., Oken, D., Goldstein, M. S., and Gussack, H. (1956). *AMA Arch. Neurol. Psychiat.* **76,** 98.

Bein, H. J. (1953). *Experientia* **9,** 107.

Bernheimer, H., and Hornykiewicz, O. (1965). *Klin. Wochenschr.* **43,** 711.

Berti, F., and Shore, P. A. (1967). *Biochem. Pharmacol.* **16,** 2091.

Bhagat, B. (1965). *J. Pharm. Pharmacol.* **17,** 191.

Birkmayer, W., and Hornykiewicz, O. (1961). *Wien. Klin. Wochenschr.* **73,** 787.

Birkmayer, W., and Hornykiewicz, O. (1962). *Arch. Psychiat. Nervenkr.* **203,** 560.

Blackburn, K. J., French, P. C., and Merrills, R. J. (1967). *Life Sci.* **6,** 1653.

Blaschko, H., and Welch, A. D. (1953). *Naunyn-Schmiedebergs Arch. Exp. Path. Pharmakol.* **219,** 17.

Bliss, E. L., and Zwanziger, J. (1966). *J. Psychiat. Res.* **4,** 189.

Bliss, E. L., Ailion, J., and Zwanziger, J. (1968). *J. Pharmacol. Exp. Ther.* **164,** 122.

Bliss, E. L., and Ailion, J. (1969). *J. Pharmacol. Exp. Ther.* **168,** 258.

Bloom, F. E., and Aghajanian, G. K. (1968). *J. Pharmacol. Exp. Ther.* **159,** 261.

Bloom, F. E., and Giarman, N. J. (1968a). *Annu. Rep. Med. Chem.* **1967,** 264-278.

Bloom, F. E., and Giarman, N. J. (1968b). *Annu. Rev. Pharmacol.* **8,** 229.

Bourne, H. R., Bunney, W. E., Jr., Colburn, R. W., Davis, J. M., Shaw, D. M., and Coppen, A. J. (1968). *Lancet* **2,** 805.

Bradley, P. B., and Elkes, J. (1957). *Brain* **80,** 77.

Breggin, P. R. (1964). *J. Nerv. Ment. Dis.* **139,** 558.

Brodie, B. B., and Shore, P. A. (1957). *Ann. N.Y. Acad. Sci.* **66,** 631.

Brodie, B. B., Comer, M. S., Costa, E., and Dlabac, A. (1966a). *J. Pharmacol. Exp. Ther.* **152,** 340.

Brodie, B. B., Costa, E., Dlabac, A., Neff, N. H., and Smookler, H. H. (1966b). *J. Pharmacol. Exp. Ther.* **154,** 493.

Brodie, H. K. H., Murphy, D. L., Goodwin, F. K., and Bunney, W. E., Jr. (1971). *Clin. Pharmacol. Ther.* **12,** 218.

Brown, C. W., and Searle, L. V. (1938). *J. Exp. Psychol.* **22,** 555.

Bulat, M., and Zivković, B. (1971). *Science* **173,** 738.

Bunney, W. E., Jr., and Davis, J. M. (1965). *Arch. Gen. Psychiat.* **13,** 483.

Bunney, W. E., Jr., Brodie, H. K. H., Murphy, D. L., and Goodwin, F. K. (1971). *Amer. J. Psychiat.* **127,** 7.

Cantril, H., and Hunt, W. A. (1932). *Amer. J. Psychol.* **44,** 300.

Carlsson, A., Rosengren, E., Bertler, A., and Nilsson, J. (1957a). In "Psychotropic Drugs" (S. Garattini and V. Ghetti, eds.), pp. 363-372. Elsevier, Amsterdam.

Carlsson, A., Lindqvist, M., and Magnusson, T. (1957b). Nature (London) 180, 1200.

Carlsson, A., Falck, B., and Hillarp, N. -Å. (1962). Acta Physiol. Scand. Suppl. 56, 196, 1.

Carlsson, A., Hillarp, N. -Å, and Waldeck, B. (1963). Acta. Physiol. Scand. Suppl. 59, 215, 1.

Carlton, P. L. (1963). Psychol. Rev. 70, 19.

Carpenter, W. (1970). Ann. Intern. Med. 73, 613.

Chance, M. R. A. (1946). J. Pharmacol. Exp. Ther. 87, 214.

Chance, M. R. A. (1947). J. Pharmacol. Exp. Ther. 89, 289.

Charalampous, K. D., and Brown, S. (1967). Psychopharmacologia 11, 422.

Chase, T. N., Breese, G. R., and Kopin, I. J. (1967). Science 157, 1461.

Chase, T. N., Katz, R. I., and Kopin, I. J. (1969). J. Neurochem. 16, 607.

Chen, K. K., and Schmidt, C. F. (1930). Medicine (Baltimore) 9, 1.

Ciaranello, R. D., and Black, I. B. (1971). Biochem. Parmacol. 20, 3529.

Ciaranello, R. D., Barchas, J. D., and Vernikos-Danellis, J. (1969a). Life Sci. 8, Pt. 1, 401.

Ciaranello, R. D., Barchas, R. E., Byers, G. S., Stemmle, D. W., and Barchas, J. D. (1969b). Nature (London) 221, 368.

Ciaranello, R. D., Barchas, R., Kessler, S., and Barchas, J. (1972). Life Sci. 11, Part I, 565.

Clark, W. G., and del Guidice, J. (1970). "Principles of Psychopharmacology." Academic Press, New York.

Clineschmidt, B. V., and Anderson, E. G. (1969). Brain Res. 16, 296.

Colburn, R. W., Goodwin, F. K., Bunney, W. E., Jr., and Davis, J. M. (1967). Nature (London) 215, 1395.

Conner, R., Stolk, J., Barchas, J., and Levine, S. (1970). Physiol. Behav. 5, 1215.

Contractor, S. F., and Jeacock, M. K., (1967). Biochem. Pharmacol. 16, 1981.

Cooper, A. J., Moir, A. T. B., and Guldberg, H. C. (1968). J. Pharm. Pharmacol. 20, 729.

Cooper, J., Bloom, F., and Roth, R. (1970). "The Biochemical Basis of Neuropharmacology." Oxford Univ. Press, London and New York.

Corrodi, H., and Fuxe, K. (1969). Eur. J. Pharmacol. 7, 56.

Corrodi, H., and Hanson, L. C. F. (1966). Psychopharmacologia 10, 116.

Costa, E., and Neff, N. H. (1966). In "Biochemistry and Pharmacology of the Basal Ganglia" (E. Costa, L. J. Cote and M. D. Yahr, eds.), 141-158, Raven, New York

Costa, E., Boullin, D. J., Hammer, W., Vogel, L., and Brodie, B. B. (1966). Pharmacol. Rev. 18, 577.

Cotzias, G. C., Van Woert, M. H., and Schiffer, L. M. (1967). New Engl. J. Med. 276, 374.

Coupland, R. E. (1953). J. Endocrinol. 9, 194.

Coyle, J. T., and Snyder, S. H. (1969). J. Pharmacol. Exp. Ther. 170, 221.

Curzon, G., and Bridges, P. K. (1970). J. Neurol. Neurosurg. Psychiat. 33, 698.

Curzon, G., Godwin-Austen, R. B., Tomlinson, E. B., and Kantamaneni, B. D. (1970). J. Neurol. Neurosrug. Psychiat. 33, 1.

Curzon, G., Gumpert, E. J. W., and Sharpe, D. M. (1971). Nature New Biol. 231, 189.

Dahlström, A. (1967). Naunyn-Schmiedebergs Arch. Pharmakol. Exp. Pathol. 257, 93.

Davies, B. M., and Carroll, B. J. (1970). Amer. Psychiat. Ass. Sci. Proc. p. 232.

Deguchi, T., and Barchas, J. D. (1971). J. Biol. Chem. 246, 3175.

Deguchi, T., and Barchas, J. D. (In press). Mol. Pharmacol.

Dement, W. (1966). In "American Handbook of Psychiatry" (S. Arieti, ed.), Vol. III, pp. 290-332. Basic Books, New York.

Dement, W., Zarcone, V., Ferguson, J., Cohen, H., Pivak, T., and Barchas, J. (1969). In "Schizophrenia—Current Concepts and Research" (D. V. Siva Sankar, ed.), pp. 775-811. PJD Publ., Hicksville, New York.

Dencker, S. J., Häggendal, J., and Malm, U. (1966). Lancet 2, 754.

Dewhurst, W. G. (1968). *Nature (London)* **219**, 306.

Dewhurst, W. G. and Marley, E. (1965a). *Brit. J. Pharmacol. Chemother.* **25**, 671.

Dewhurst, W. G., and Marley, E. (1965b). *Brit. J. Pharmacol. Chemother.* **25**, 705.

Diaz, P. M., Ngai, S. H., and Costa, E. (1968). *Advances Pharmacol.* **6**, Suppl., 75.

Dominic, J. A., and Moore, K. E. (1969). *Arch. Int. Pharmacondyn. Ther.* **178**, 166.

Dominic, J. A. (In press). *In* "Serotonin and Behavior," (J. Barchas & E. Usdin, eds.), Academic Press, New York.

Dubowitz, V., and Rogers, K. J. (1969). *Develop. Med. Child Neurol.* **11**, 730.

Eakins, K. E., Costa, E., Katz, R. L., and Reyes, C. L. (1968). *Life Sci.* **7**, 71.

Eccleston, D., Ritchie, I. M., and Roberts, M. H. T. (1970). *Nature (London)* **226**, 84.

Efron, D. H. ed. (1968). "Psychopharmacology—a Review of Progress 1957-1967," PHS Publ. No. 1836. US Govt. Printing Office, Washington, D.C.

Ehrich, W. E., and Krumbhaar, E. B. (1937). *Ann. Intern. Med.* **10**, 1874.

Ehringer, H., and Hornykiewicz, O. (1960). *Klin. Wochenschr.* **38**, 1236.

Eiduson, S., Geller, E., Yuwiler, A., and Eiduson, B. (1964). "Biochemistry and Behavior." Van Nostrand-Reinhold, Princeton, New Jersey.

Elfvin, L. -G. (1965). *J. Ultrastruct. Res.* **12**, 263.

Elfvin, L. -G. (1967). *J. Ultrastruct. Res.* **17**, 45.

Elmadjian, F., Hope, J. M., and Lamson, E. T. (1957). *J. Clin. Endrocinol. Metab.* **17**, 608.

Engelman, K., Lovenberg, W., and Sjoerdsma, A. (1967). *New Engl. J. Med.* **277**, 1103.

Erspamer, V., ed. (1966). "Handbook of Experimental Pharmacology," Vol. XIX. Springer-Verlag, Berlin and New York.

Everett, G. M., and Borcherding, J. W. (1970). *Science* **168**, 849.

Falck, B. (1962). *Acta Physiol. Scand. Suppl.* **56**, 197, 1.

Fieve, R. R., Platman, S. R., and Fleiss, J. L. (1969). *Psychopharmacologia* **15**, 425.

Foote, W. E., Sheard, M. H., and Aghajanian, G. K. (1969). *Nature (London)* **222**, 567.

Frankenhaeuser, M., and Johansson, G. (to be published). *In* "Society, Stress and Disease: Childhood and Adolescence" (L. Levi, ed.), Oxford Univ. Press, London and New York.

Frankenhaeuser, M., Mellis, I., Rissler, A., Björkvall, C., and Pátkai, P. (1968). *Psychosomat. Med.* **30**, 109.

Freedman, D. X. (1961). *J. Pharmacol. Exp. Ther.* **134**, 160.

Friedman, A. H., and Walker, C. A. (1968). *J. Physiol. (London)* **197**, 77.

Friedman, S., and Kaufman, S. (1965). *J. Biol. Chem.* **240**, 552.

Fuller, R. W., and Hunt, J. M. (1967). *Life Sci.* **6**, 1107.

Fuxe, K., and Ungerstedt, U. (1967). *J. Pharm. Pharmacol.* **19**, 335.

Fuxe, K., Hökfelt, T., Nilsson, O., and Reinius, S. (1966). *Anat. Rec.* **155**, 33.

Fuxe, K., Hökfelt, I. and Ungerstedt, U. (1968). *Advan. Pharmacol.* **6**, Pt. A, 235.

Gaddum, J. H. (1954). *Hypertension: Humoral Neurogenic Factors Ciba Found. Symp., 1953,* G. E. Wolstenholme and M. P. Cameron, eds., p. 75. Little, Brown, Boston, Massachusetts.

Galambos, R. (1956). *J. Neurophysiol.* **19**, 424.

Galzigna, L. (1970). *Nature (London)* **225**, 1060.

Garattini, S., and Shore, P. (1968). *Advan. Pharmacol.* **6A, 6B**.

Garattini, S., and Valzelli, L. (1965). 'Serotonin.' Amer. Elsevier, New York.

Geffen, L. B., and Livett, B. G. (1971). *Physiol. Rev.* **51**, 98.

Gerbode, F., and Bowers, M. (1968). *J. Neurochem.* **15**, 1053.

Giarman, N. J., and Schanberg, S. M. (1958). *Biochem. Pharmacol.* **1**, 301.

Giarman, N. J., Tanaka, C., Mooney, J., and Atkins, E. (1968). *Advan. Pharmacol.* **6A**, 307.

Glassman, A. (1969). *Psychosom. Med.* **31**, 107.

Glowinski, J., and Axelrod, J. (1965). *J. Pharmacol. Exp. Ther.* **149** 43.

Glowinski, J., and Iversen, L. L. (1966a). *J. Neurochem.* **13** 655.

Glowinski, J., and Iversen, L. L. (1966b). *Biochem. Pharmacol.* **15**, 1971.

Glowinski, J., Kopin, I. J., and Axelrod, J. (1965). *J. Neurochem.* **12**, 25.

Glowinski, J., Iversen, L. L., and Axelrod, J. (1966). *J. Pharmacol. Exp. Ther.* **151**, 385.

Goldberg, I. H., and Delbruck, A. (1959). *Fed. Proc. Fed. Amer. Soc. Exp. Biol.* **18**, 235.

Goldstein, M., Anagnoste, B., Owen, W. S., and Battista, A. F. (1967). *Experientia* **23**, 98.

Goodall, McC. (1962). *J. Clin. Invest.* **41**, 197.

Gordon, R., Spector, S., Sjoerdsma, A., and Udenfriend, S. (1966a). *J. Pharmacol. Exp. Ther.* **153**, 440.

Gordon, R., Reid, J. V. O., Sjoerdsma, A., and Udenfriend, S. (1966b). *Mol. Pharmacol.* **2**, 606.

Gottfries, C. G., Gottfries, I., and Roos, B. E. (1969). *J. Neurochem.* **16**, 1341.

Grahame-Smith, D. G. (1967). *Biochem. J.* **105** 351.

Green, J. P. (1966). *Yale J. Biol. Med.* **39**, 21.

Gunn, J. A., and Gurd, M. R. (1940). *J. Physiol. (London)* **97**, 453.

Gunne, L. M. (1962). *Acta Physiol. Scand.* **56**, 324.

Hamberger, B. (1967). *In* 'Behavior-Genetic Analysis" (J. Hirsch, ed.), pp. 154-175. McGraw-Hill, New York.

Hamburg, D. A., ed. (1970). 'Psychiatry as a Behavioral Science" (Behavioral Social Sci. Surv. Monogr. Ser.). Prentice-Hall, Englewood Cliff, New Jersey.

Hamburg, D., and Kessler, S. (1967). *Mem. Soc. Endocrinol.* **15**, 249-270.

Hamburg, D., and Lunde, D. (1967). *In* "Genetic Diversity and Human Behavior" (J. Spuhler, ed.), pp. 135-170. Aldine Press.

Hanson, L. C. F. (1967). *Psychopharmacologia* **10**, 289.

Hanson, L. C. F., and Henning, M. (1967). *Psychopharmacologia* **11**, 1.

Hartman, E. (1967). "The Biology of Dreaming," pp. 1-206. Thomas, Springfield, Illinois.

Harvey, S. C., Sulkowski, T. S. and Weenig, D. J. (1968). *Arch. Int. Pharmacodyn. Ther.* **172**, 301.

Haskovek, L. and Soucek, K. (1968). *Nature (London)* **219**, 507.

Haskovek, L., and Soucek, K. (1969). *Psychoparmacologia* **15**, 415.

Hawkins, D. R., Monroe, J. T., Sandifer, M. G., and Vernon, C. R. (1960). *Psychiat. Res. Rep. Amer. Psychiat. Ass.* **12**, 40.

Henry, J. P., Stephens, P. M., Axelrod, J., and Mueller, R. A. (1971). *Psychosomat. Med.* **33**, 227.

Hernandez-Peon, R., Scherrer, H., and Jouvet, M. (1956). *Science* **123**, 331.

Hidaka, H., Nagatsu, T., and Yagi, K. (1969a). *J. Neurochem.* **16**, 783.

Hidaka, H., Nagatsu, T., Takeya, K. Matsumoto, S., and Yagi, K. (1969b). *J. Pharmacol. Exp. Ther.* **166**, 272.

Hillarp, N.-A., Lagerstedt, S., and Nilsson, B. (1953). *Acta Physiol. Scand.* **29**, 251.

Hillarp, N.-A., Fuxe, K., and Dahlström A., (1966). *Pharm. Rev.* **18**, 727.

Himwich, H. E. (1971). ' Biochemistry, Schizophrenias and the Affective Illnesses." Williams & Wilkins, Baltimore, Maryland.

Hobson, J. A. (1969). *New Engl. J. Med.* **281**, 1468.

Hökfelt, T. (1967). *Acta Physiol. Scand.* **69**, 119.

Hökfelt, T., and McLean, J. (1950). *Acta Physiol. Scand.* **21**, 258.

Hollister, L. E. (1968). "Chemical Psychoses, LSD and Related Drugs." Thomas, Springfield, Illinois.

Hollister, L. E., and Moore, F. (1970). *Res. Commun. Chem. Pathol. Pharmacol.* **1**, 193.

Holtzman, D , Lovell, R. A. Jaffe, J. H., and Freedman, D. X. (1969). *Science* **163**, 1464.

Hornykiewicz, O. (1966). *Pharm. Rev.* **18**, 925.

Ichiyama, A., Nakamura, S., Nishizuka, Y., and Hayaishi, O. (1970). *J. Biol. Chem.* **245**, 1699.

Itil, T. M., Polvan, N., and Holden, J. M. C. (1971). *Dis. Nerv. Syst.* **32**, 193.

Iversen, L. L., and Glowinski, J. (1966). *J. Neurochem.* **13**, 671.

Javoy, F., Thierry, A. M., Kety, S. S. and Glowinski, J. (1968). *Commun. Behav. Biol.* **1**, 43.

Javoy, F., Hamon, M., and Glowinski, J. (1970). *Eur. J. Pharmacol.* **10**, 178.

Jequier, E., Lovenberg, W., and Sjoerdsma, A. (1967). *Mol. Pharmacol.* **3**, 274.

Jequier, E., Robinson, D. S. Lovenberg, W., and Sjoersdma, A. (1969). *Biochem. Pharmacol.* **18**, 1071.

Jost, A., and Roffi, J. (1958). *C. R. Acad. Sci.* **46**, 163.

Jouvet, M. (1969). *Science* **163**, 32.

Kety, S. S., and Sampson, F. E. (1967). *Neurosci. Res. Program Bull.* **5**, 1.

Kety. S. S., Javoy, F., Thierry, A. M., Julou, L., and Glowinski, J. (1967). *Proc. Nat. Acad. Sci.* **58**, 1249.

Kirpekar, S. M., and Misu, Y. (1967). *J. Physiol. (London)* **188**, 219.

Kirschner, N. (1962) *J. Biol. Chem.* **237**, 2311.

Kitabchi, A. E., and Williams, R. H. (1968). *J. Clin. Endocrinol. Metab.* **28**, 1082.

Klein, D., and Davis, J. (1969). "Diagnosis and Drug Treatment of Psychiatric Disorders" Williams & Wilkins, Baltimore, Maryland.

Kline, N. S. (1954). *Ann. N.Y. Acad. Sci.* **59** 107.

Koe, B. K., and Weissman, A. (1966). *J. Pharmacol. Exp. Ther.* **154**, 499.

Koella, W. (1968). *Neurosci. Res.* **2** 229.

Kopin, I. J., Hertting, G., and Gordon, E. K. (1962). *J. Pharmacol. Exp. Ther.* **138**, 34.

Kopin, I. J., Gordon, E. K., and Horst, W. D. (1965). *Biochem. Pharmacol.* **14**, 753.

Kopin, I. J., Breese, G. R., Krauss, K. R., and Weise, V. K. (1968). *J. Pharmacol. Exp. Ther.* **161**, 271.

Korf, J., and Sebens, J. B. (1970). *Clin. Chim. Acta* **27**, 149.

Krakoff, L. R., and Axelrod, J. (1967). *Biochem. Pharmacol.* **16**, 1384.

Krantz, K. D., and Seiden, L. S. (1968). *J. Pharm. Pharmacol.* **20**, 166.

Lambert, W. W., Johansson, G., Frankenhaeuser, M., and Klackenberg-Larsson, I. (1969). *Scand. J. Psychol.* **10**, 306.

LaMotte, R. H., Schmidt, D. E., and Ruliffson, W S. (1969). *J. Neurochem.* **16**, 725.

Levi, L. (1965). *Psychosom. Med.* **27**, 80.

Levi, L. (1966). *In* "An Introduction to Clinical Neuroendocrinology" (E. Bajusz, ed.). Karger, Basel.

Levi, L. (1969). *Psychosom. Med.* **31**, 251.

Levitt, M., Barchas, J., Creveling, C., and Udenfriend, S. (to be published). "The subcellular distribution of tyrosine hydroxylase and DOPA decarboxylase in animal tissues."

Lin, R. C., Costa, E., Neff, N. H., Wang, C. T., and Ngai, S. H. (1969a). *J. Pharmacol. Exp. Ther.* **170**, 232.

Lin, R. C., Neff, N. H., Ngai, S. H., and Costa, E. (1969b). *Life Sci.* **8**, 1077.

Lin, R. C., Ngai, S. H., and Costa, E. (1969c). *Science* **166**, 237.

Lindemann, E., and Finesinger, J. E. (1940). *Psychosom. Med.* **2**, 231.

Lints, C. E., and Harvey, J. A. (1969). *J. Comp. Physiol. Psychol.* **67**, 23.

Lipton, M. A., Gordon, R., Guroff, G., and Udenfriend, S. (1967) *Science* **156**, 248.

Littleton, J. M. (1967). *J. Pharm. Pharmacol.* **19**, 414.

Maas, J. W., and Landis, D. H. (1968). *J. Pharmacol. Exp. Ther.* **163**, 147.

McGeer, E. G., and Peters, D. A. V. (1969), *Can. J. Biochem.* **47**, 501.
McGeer, E. G., Gibson, S., Wada, J. A., and McGeer, P. L. (1967). *Can. J. Biochem.* **45**, 1943.
McGeer, P. L., and McGeer, E. G. (1964). *Biochem. Biophys. Res. Commun.* **17**, 502.
McKean, C. M., Schanberg, S. M., and Giarman, N. J. (1967), *Science* **157**, 213.
Maj, J., and Przegalinski, E. (1967). *J. Pharm. Pharmacol.* **19**, 341.
Malamed, S., Poisner, A. M., Trifaró, J. M., and Douglas, W. W. (1968). *Biochem. Pharmacol.* **17**, 241.
Malmejac, J. (1964). *Physiol. Rev.* **44**, 186.
Mandell, A. J., and Mandell, M. P. (1969). "Psychochemical Research in Man—Methods, Strategy and Theory." Academic Press, New York.
Mandell, A. J., and Morgan, M. (1971). *Nature (London)* **230**, 85.
Mandell, A. J., and Spooner, C. E. (1968). *Science* **162**, 1442.
Mann, P. G. J., and Quastel, J. H. (1940). *Biochem. J.* **34**, 414.
Manshardt, J., and Wurtman, R. J. (1968). *Nature (London)* **217**, 574.
Marañon, G. (1924). *Rev. Fr. Endocrinol.* **2**, 301.
Margules, D. L. (1968). *J. Comp. Physiol. Psychol.* **66**, 329.
Mason, J. W. (1968). *Psychosom. Med.* **30**, 631.
Maynert, E. W., and Levy, R. (1964). *J. Pharmacol. Exp. Ther.* **143**, 90.
Melmon, K. L. (1968). *In* "Textbook of Endocrinology" (R. Williams, ed.) pp. 379-403. Saunders, Philadelphia, Pennsylvania.
Mendelson, J., Kubzansky, P., Leiderman, P. H., Wexler, D., DuToit, C., and Solomon, P. (1960). *AMA Arch. Gen. Psychiat.* **2**, 147.
Menon, M. K., Dandiya, P. C., and Bapna, J. S. (1967). *Psychopharmacologia* **10**, 437.
Miller, F. P., Cox, R. H., Jr., and Maickel, R. P. (1968). *Science* **162**, 463.
Moir, A. T. B., and Eccleston, D. (1968). *J. Neurochem.* **15**, 1093.
Molinoff, P. B., Landsberg, L., and Axelrod, J. (1969). *J. Pharmacol. Exp. Ther.* **170**, 253.
Molinoff, P. B., Brimijoin, S., Weinshilboum, R., and Axelrod, J. (1970). *Proc. Nat. Acad. Sci. U.S.* **66**, 453.
Moore, K. E. (1963). *J. Pharmacol. Exp. Ther.* **142**, 6.
Moore, K. E., and Rech, R. H. (1967). *J. Pharmacol. Exp. Ther.* **156**, 70.
Moore, K. E., Wright, P. F., and Bert, J. K. (1967). *J. Pharmacol. Exp. Ther.* **155**, 506.
Morgan, M., and Mandell, A. J. (1969). *Science* **165**, 492.
Mueller, R. A., Thoenen, H., and Axelrod, J. (1969) *Science* **158**, 468.
Mueller, R. A., Thoenen, H., and Axelrod, J. (1970). *Endocrinology* **86**, 751.
Munkvad, I., Pakkenberg, H., and Randrup, A. (1968). *Brain, Behav. Evol.* **1**, 89.
Murphy, D. L., Colburn, R. W., Davis, J. M., and Bunney, W. E. Jr. (1969). *Life Science* **8**, 1187.
Musacchio, J. M., Julou, L., Kety, S. S., and Glowinski, J. (1969). *Proc. Nat. Acad. Sci. U.S.* **63**, 1117.
Nagatsu, T., Levitt, M., and Udenfriend, S. (1964). *J. Biol. Chem.* **239**, 2910.
Nathanson, M. H. (1937). *J. Amer. Med. Assoc.* **108**, 528.
Neff, N. H., and Costa, E. (1966). *Life Sci.* **5**, 951.
Neff, N. H., and Tozer, T. N. (1968). *Advan. Pharmacol.* **6A**, 97.
Neff, N. H., Tozer, T. N., and Brodie, B. B. (1967). *J. Pharmacol. Exp. Ther.* **158**, 214.
Neff, N. H., Tozer, T. N., Hammer, W., Costa, E., and Brodie, B. B. (1968). *J. Pharmacol. Exp. Ther.* **160**, 48.
Neff, N. H., Barrett, R. E., and Costa, E. (1969). *Eur. J. Pharmacol.* **5**, 348.
Noble, E. P., Wurtman, R. J., and Axelrod, J. (1967). *Life Sci.* **6**, Pt. 1, 281.
Nybäck, H., and Sedvall, G. (1968). *J. Pharmacol. Exp. Ther.* **162**, 294.

O'Hanlon, J., Campuzano, H., and Horvath, S. (1970). *Anal. Biochem.* 34, 568.

Olds, J. (1962). *Physiol. Rev.* 42, 554.

Olds, J., and Milner, P. (1954). *J. Comp. Physiol. Psychol.* 47, 419.

Oliver, G., and Schäfer, E. A. (1895). *J. Physiol. (London)* 18, 230.

Olsson, R., and Roos, B. E. (1968). *Nature (London)* 219, 502.

Paasonen, M., and Krayer, O. (1957). *Fed. Proc. Fed. Amer. Soc. Exp. Biol.* 16, 326.

Paasonen, M., and Krayer, O. (1958). *J. Pharmacol. Exp. Ther.* 123, 153.

Page, I. H. (1968). "Serotonin." New Year Book Med. Publ., Chicago, Illinois.

Pellegrino de Iraldi, A., Farini Duggan, H., and De Robertis, E. (1963). *Anat. Rec.* 145, 521.

Persson, T., and Roos, B. E. (1967). *Lancet* 2, 987.

Peters, D. A. V., McGeer, P. L., and McGeer, E. G. (1968). *J. Neurochem.* 15, 1431.

Pohorecky, L. A., Zigmond, M. J., Karten, H. J., and Wurtman, R. J. (1968). *Fed. Proc. Fed. Amer. Soc. Exp. Biol.* 27, 239.

Poisner, A. M., and Trifaró, J. M., (1967). *Mol. Pharmacol.* 3, 561.

Poisner, A. M., Trifaró, J. M., and Douglas, W. W. (1967). *Biochem. Pharmacol.* 16, 2101.

Pollin, W., and Goldin, S. (1961). *J. Psychiat. Res.* 1, 50.

Pujol, J. F., Mouret, J., Jouvet, M., and Glowinski, J. (1968). *Science* 159, 112.

Quay, W. B. (1963). *Gen. Comp. Endocrinol.* 3, 473.

Quinn, G. P., Shore, P. A., and Brodie, B. B. (1959). *J. Pharmacol. Exp. Ther.* 127, 103.

Quinton, R. M., and Halliwell, G. (1963). *Nature (London)* 200, 178.

Ragland, J. D. (1968). *Biochem. Biophys. Res. Commun.* 31, 203.

Randrup, A., and Munkvad, I. (1966). *Acta Psychiat. Neurol. Scand.* 42, 193.

Randrup, A., and Munkvad, I. (1967). *Psychopharmacologia* 11, 300.

Rech, R. H. (1964). *J. Pharmacol. Exp. Ther.* 146, 369.

Rech, R. H. (1966). *Psychopharmacologia* 9, 110.

Rech, R. H., and Moore, K. E. (1968). *Brain Res.* 8, 398.

Rech, R., and Moore, K. (1971). "An Introduction to Psychopharmacology." Raven, New York.

Rech, R. H., and Stolk, J. M. (1970). *In* "Amphetamines and Related Compounds," (E. Costa and S. Garattini, eds.), Raven, New York.

Rech, R. H., Borys, H. K., and Moore, K. E. (1966). *J. Pharmacol. Exp. Ther.* 153, 412.

Rech, R. H., Carr, L. A., and Moore, K. E. (1968). *J. Pharmacol. Exp. Ther.* 160, 326.

Rechtschaffen, A., Lovell, R., Freedman, D., Whitehead, P., and Aldrich, M. (1969). *Psychophysiology* 6, 223.

Redmond, D. E., Jr., Maas, J. W., Kling, A., and Dekirmenjian, H. (1971). *Psychosom. Med.* 33, 97.

Reid, W. D., Stefano, F. J. E., Kurzepa, S., and Brodie, B. B. (1969). *Science* 164, 437.

Reis, D. J., Weinbren, M., and Corvelli, A. (1968). *J. Pharmacol. Exp. Ther.* 164, 135.

Robichaud, R. C., and Sledge, K. L. (1969). *Life Sci.* 8, Pt. 1, 965.

Roffi, J. (1964). *J. Physiol. (London)* 56, 434.

Roos, B. E., and Sjöström, R. (1969). *Pharmacol. Clin.* , 153.

Roos, B. E., Andén, N. E., and Werdinius, B. (1964). *Int. J. Neuropharmacol.* 3, 117.

Rosecrans, J. A., Lovell, R. A., and Freedman, D. X. (1967). *Biochem. Pharmacol.* 16, 2011.

Ross, S. B., and Renyi, A. L. (1967). *Life Sci.* 6, 1407.

Ross, S. B., and Renyi, A. L. (1969). *Eur. J. Pharmacol.* 7, 270.

Roth, R. H., Stjärne, L., and von Euler, U. S. (1967). *J. Pharmacol. Exp. Ther.* 158, 373.

Rothballer, A. (1959). *Pharmacol. Rev.* 11, 494.

Sabelli, H. C. (1970). *Experientia* 26, 58.

Sabelli, H. C., Giardina, W. J., Alivisatos, S. G. A., Seth, P. K., and Ungar, F. (1969). *Nature (London)* **223**, 73.
Sankar, D. V. Siva. (1969). "Schizophrenia: Current Concepts and Research." PJD Publ., Hicksville, New York.
Schachter, S., and Singer, J. E. (1962). *Psychol. Rev.* **69**, 379.
Schachter, S., and Wheeler, L. (1962). *J. Abnorm. Soc. Psychol.* **65**, 121.
Schanberg, S. M., and Giarman, N. J. (1962). *Biochem. Pharmacol.* **11**, 187.
Schanberg, S. M., Schildkraut, J. J., and Kopin, I. J. (1967a). *Biochem. Pharmacol.* **16**, 393.
Schanberg, S. M., Schildkraut, J. J., and Kopin, I. J. (1967b). *J. Pharmacol. Exp. Ther.* **157**, 311.
Scheving, L. E., Harrison, W. H., Gordon, P., and Pauly, J. E. (1968). *Amer. J. Physiol.* **214**, 166.
Schildkraut, J. J. (1965). *Amer. J. Psychiat.* **122**, 509.
Schildkraut, J. J. (1970). "Neuropyschopharmacology and the Affective Disorders." Little, Brown, Boston, Massachusetts.
Schildkraut, J. J., and Kety, S. S. (1967). *Science* **156**, 21.
Schildkraut, J. J., Schanberg, S. M., Breese, G. R., and Kopin, I. J. (1969). *Biochem. Pharmacol.* **18**, 1971.
Schlesinger, K., Boggan, W., and Freedman, D. X. (1965). *Life Sci.* **4**, 2345.
Schlesinger, K., Schreiber, R. A., and Pryor, G. T. (1968). *Psychonom. Sci.* **11**, 225.
Schnaitman, C., Erwin, V. G., and Greenawalt, J. W. (1967). *J. Cell Biol.* **32**, 719.
Schoenfeld, R. I., and Seiden, L. S. (1967). *J. Pharm. Pharmacol.* **19**, 771.
Schoenfeld, R. I., and Seiden, L. S. (1969). *J. Pharmacol. Exp. Ther.* **167**, 319.
Sedvall, G. C., and Kopin, I. J. (1967a). *Life Sci.* **6**, 45.
Sedvall, G. C., and Kopin, I. J. (1967b). *Biochem. Pharmacol.* **16**, 39.
Sedvall, G. C., Weise, V. K., and Kopin, I. J. (1968). *J. Pharmacol. Exp. Ther.* **159**, 274.
Segawa, T., Kuruma, I., Takatsuka, K., and Takagi, H. (1968). *J. Pharm. Pharmacol.* **20**, 800.
Seiden, L. S., and Carlsson, A. (1963). *Psychopharmacologia* **4**, 418.
Seiden, L. S., and Hanson, L. C. F. (1964). *Psychopharmacologia* **6**, 239.
Seiden, L. S., and Peterson, D. D. (1968a). *J. Pharmacol. Exp. Ther.* **159**, 422.
Seiden, L. S., and Peterson, D. D. (1968b). *J. Pharmacol. Exp. Ther.* **163**, 84.
Sheard, M. H., and Aghajanian, G. K. (1968). *J. Pharmacol. Exp. Ther.* **163**, 425.
Shein, H. M., Wurtman, R. J., and Axelrod, J. (1967). *Nature (London)* **213**, 730.
Silverman, A. J., and Cohen, S. I. (1960). *Psychiat. Res. Rep. Amer. Psychiat. Ass.* **12**, 16.
Simmonds, M. D. (1969). *J. Physiol. (London)* **203**, 199.
Simmonds, M. D., and Iversen, L. L. (1969). *Science* **158**, 473.
Sinha, A. K., Henriksen, S., Dement, W. C., and Barchas, J. D. (In press). *Amer. J. Physiol.*
Sjoerdsma, A. (1970). *Ann. Int. Med.* **73**, 607.
Sjoerdsma, A., Engelman, K., Spector, S., and Udenfriend, S. (1965). *Lancet* **2**, 1092.
Smith, C. B. (1963). *J. Pharmacol. Exp. Ther.* **142**, 343.
Smith, C. B. (1965). *J. Pharmacol. Exp. Ther.* **147**, 96.
Smythies, J. (1970). *Neurosci. Res. Program Bull.* **8**, 1.
Snipes, R. L., Thoenen, H., and Tranzer, J. P. (1968). *Experientia* **24**, 1026.
Spector, S., Gordon, R., Sjoerdsma, A., and Udenfriend, S. (1967). *Mol. Pharmacol.* **3**, 549.
Squires, R. F. (1968). *Biochem. Pharmacol.* **17**, 1401.
Stein, L. (1964). *Fed. Proc. Fed. Amer. Soc. Exp. Biol.* **23**, 836.
Stein, L. (1968). *In* "Psychopharmacology, A Review of Progress, 1957-1967" (D. H. Efron, ed.), pp. 105-123. US Govt. Printing Office, Washington, D.C.

Stein, L., and Wise, C. D. (1969). *J. Comp. Physiol. Psychol.* **67**, 189
Steinman, A. M., Smerin, S. E., and Barchas, J. D. (1969). *Science* **165**, 616.
Stern, D. N., Fieve, R. R., Neff, N. H., and Costa, E. (1969). *Psychopharmacologia* **14**, 315.
Stevens, D. A., Resnick, O., and Krus, D. M. (1967). *Life Sci.* **6**, 2215.
Stevens, D. A., Fechter, L. D., and Resnick, O. (1969). *Life Sci.* **8**, 379.
Stolk, J. M., and Barchas, J. D. (to be published).
Stolk, J. M., and Rech, R. H. (1967). *J. Pharmacol. Exp. Ther.* **158**, 140.
Stolk, J. M., and Rech, R. H. (1970). *Neuropharmacology* **9**, 249.
Stolk, J. M., Barchas, J., Dement, W., and Schanberg, S. (1969). *Pharmacologist* **11**, 258.
Stolk, J. M., Conner, R. L., Levine, S., and Barchas, J. (In press).. Proc. 5th Int. Congress Pharmacol., San Francisco, July 1972.
Stone, E. A. (1970). *Life Sci.* **9**, 877.
Stone, E. A., and DiCara, L. V. (1969). *Life Sci.* **8**, Pt. 1, 433.
Sudak, H. S., and Maas, J. W. (1964). *Nature (London)* **203**, 1254.
Sulser, F., and Dingell, J. V. (1968). *Agressologie* **9**, 1.
Sulser, F., Owens, M. L., Norvich, M. R., and Dingell, J. V. (1968). *Psychopharmacologia* **12**, 322.
Sulser, F., Owens, M. L., Strada, S. J., and Dingell, J. V. (1969). *J. Pharmacol. Exp. Ther.* **168**, 272.
Tamarkin, N., Goodwin, F., and Axelrod, J. (1970). *Life Sci.* **9**, 1397.
Taylor, K. M., and Laverty, R. (1969). *J. Neurochem.* **16**, 1367.
Taylor, K. M., and Snyder, S. H. (1971). *Brain Res.* **28**, 295.
Tenen, S. S. (1967). *Psychopharmacologia* **10**, 204.
Thierry, A. M., Javoy, F., Glowinski, J., and Kety, S. S. (1968a). *J. Pharmacol. Exp. Ther.* **163**, 163.
Thierry, A. M., Fekete, M., and Glowinski, J. (1968b). *Eur. J. Pharmacol.* **4**, 384.
Thierry, A. M., Blanc, G., and Glowinski, J. (1970). *Eur. J. Pharmacol.* **10**, 139.
Thoenen, H., Mueller, R. A., and Axelrod, J. (1969). *J. Pharmacol. Exp. Ther.* **169**, 249.
Thoenen, H., Mueller, R. A., and Axelrod, J. (1970). *Biochem. Pharmacol.* **19**, 669.
Tolson, W. W., Mason, J. W., Sachar, E. J., Hamburg, D. A., Handlon, J. H., and Fishman, J. R. (1965). *J. Psychosom. Res.* **8**, 365.
Tozer, T. N., Neff, N. H., and Brodie, B. B. (1966). *J. Pharmacol. Exp. Ther.* **153**, 177.
Trendelenburg, U., (1963). *Pharmacol. Rev.* **15**, 225.
Trendelenburg, U., (1966). *Pharmacol. Rev.* **18**, 629.
Udenfriend, S. (1962). "Fluorescence Assay in Biology and Medicine, Molecular Biology Series," Vol. 1. Academic Press, New York.
Udenfriend, S. (1969). "Fluorescence Assay in Biology and Medicine, Molecular Biology Series," Vol. 2. Academic Press, New York.
Udenfriend, S., and Creveling, C. R. (1959). *J. Neurochem.* **4**, 350.
Usdin, E., and Efron, D. (1967) "Psychotropic Drugs and Related Compounds," P.H.S. Publ. No. 1589. US Govt. Printing Office, Washington, D.C.
Vane, J. R. (1960). *In* "Adrenergic Mechanisms" J. R. Vane, G. E. M. Wolstenholme, and M. O'Connor, eds.), pp. 356-372. Churchill, London.
Van Orden, L. S., III., Schafer, J.-M., and Burke, J. P. (1969). *Pharmacologist* **11**, 262.
van Praag, H. M., and Korf, J. (1971). *J. Biol. Psychiat.* **3**, 105.
van Praag, H. M., Korf, J., and Puite, J. (1970). *Nature (London)* **225**, 1259. OVan Rossum,
Van Rossum, J. M. Van Der Schoot, J. B., and Hurkmans, J. A. Th. M. (1962). *Experientia* **18**, 229.
Vernikos-Danellis, J., Ciaranello, R. D., and Barchas, J. D. (1968). *Endocrinology* **83**, 1357.
Viveros, O. H., Arqueros, L., and Kirshner, N. (1968). *Life Sci.* **7**, 609.

Vogel, W. H., Orfei, V., and Century, B. (1969). *J. Pharmacol. Exp. Ther.* **165**, 196.
Vogt, M. (1954). *J. Physiol. (London)* **123**, 451.
Vogt, M. (1968). *Advan. Pharmacol.* **6B**, 19.
von Euler, U. S. (1956). "Noradrenaline." Thomas, Springfield, Illinois.
von Euler, U. S. (1962). *In* "Perspectives in Biology" (C. F. Cori, V. G. Foglia, L. F. Leloir, and S. Ochoa, eds.), pp. 387-394. Amer. Elsevier, New York.
von Euler, U. S. (1964). *Actualites Neurophysiol.* **5**, 37.
von Euler, U. S. (1967). *In* "Neuroendocrinology" (L. Martini and W. F. Ganong, eds.), Vol. II, p. 283. Academic Press, New York.
von Euler, U. S., and Hillarp, N. -A. (1956). *Nature (London)* **177**, 44.
von Euler, U. S., and Lishajko, F. (1963). *Int. J. Neuropharmacol.* **2**, 127.
von Euler, U. S., and Lundberg, U. (1954). *J. Appl. Physiol.* **6**, 551.
Wearn, J. T., and Sturgis, C. C. (1919). *Arch. Intern. Med.* **24**, 248.
Weight, F. F., and Salmoiraghi, G. C. (1968). *Advan. Pharmacol.* **6A**, 395.
Weiner, N., and Rabadjija, M. (1968). *J. Pharmacol. Exp. Ther.* **164**, 103.
Weiner, W., Harrison, W., and Klawans, H. (1969). *Life Sci.* **8**, 971.
Weinshilboum, R., and Axelrod, J. (1970). *Endocrinology* **87**, 894.
Weiss, B. L., and Aghajanian, G. K. (1971). *Brain Res.* **26**, 26, 37.
Weiss, E., Bordwell, B., Seeger, M., Lee, J., Dement, W., and Barchas, J. (1968). *Psychophysiology,* **5**, 209.
Weissman, A., Koe, B. K., and Tenen, S. S. (1966). *J. Pharmacol. Exp. Ther.* **151**, 339.
Welch, A. S., and Welch, B. L. (1968). *Biochem. Pharmacol.* **17**, 699.
Welch, A. S., and Welch, B. L. (1969). *Anal. Biochem.* **30**, 161.
Welch, B. L. (1967). *UCLA (Univ. Calif. Los Angeles) Forum Med. Sci.* n.7, pp. 150-170.
Welch, B. L., and Welch, A. S. (1968a). *J. Pharm. Pharmacol.* **20**, 244
Welch, B. L., and Welch, A. S. (1968b). *Nature (London)* **218**, 575.
Welch, B. L., and Welch, A. S. (1970). *In* "Amphetamines and Related Compounds" (E. Costa and S. Garattini, eds.), pp. 415-446. Raven, New York.
Welsh, J. H. (1968). *Advan. Pharmacol.* **6A**, 171.
Wesemann, W. (1969). *F.E.B.S. Letters* **3**, 80.
White, T. A., Jenne, J. W., and Evans, D. A. P. (1969). *Biochem. J.* **113**, 721.
Wilk, S., Davis, K. L., and Thacker, S. B. (1971). *Anal. Biochem.* **39**, 498.
Williams, R. (1970). *J. Clin. Endocrinol. Metab.* **31**, 461.
Winter, J. C. (1969) *J. Pharmacol. Exp. Ther.* **169**, 7.
Wise, C. D., and Stein, L. (1969). *Science* **163**, 299.
Wise, C. D., and Stein, L. (1970). *In* "Amphetamines and Related Compounds" (E. Costa and S. Garattini, eds.), pp. 463-485. Raven, New York.
Wolf, S., and Wolff, H. G. (1947). *Rev. Gastroenterol.* **8**, 429.
Wooley, D. W. (1962). "The Biochemical Bases of Psychoses." Wiley, New York.
Wurtman, R. J. (1966a). "Catecholamines." Little Brown, Boston, Massachusetts.
Wurtman, R. J. (1966b). *Endocrinology* **79**, 608.
Wurtman, R. J., and Axelrod, J. (1966). *J. Biol. Chem.* **241**, 2301.
Wurtman, R. J., Axelrod, J., and Kelly, D. (1968). "The Pineal Gland." Academic Press, New York.
Wyatt, R. (1970). *Ann. Intern. Med.* **73**, 619.
Wyatt, R., Portnoy, B., Kupfer, D., Snyder, F., and Engelman, K. (1971). *Arch. Gen. Psychiat.* **24**, 65.

Author Index

Numbers in brackets refer to the pages on which the complete references are listed.

Jouvet, M., 176, [205], 309, 310, 311, [323, 324, 326]
Julou, L., 296, [324, 325]

K

Kado, R. T., 41, [61]
Kagan, J., 67, [100]
Kahwanago, I., 19, [57]
Kakiuchi, S., 51, [57]
Kalberer, W. D., 113, 114, [134]
Kalkut, M., 166, [171]
Kanematsu, S., 3, 7, [9]
Kang, L., 218, [231]
Kanchisa, T., 138, [171]
Kantamaneni, B. D., 277, [321]
Kappas, A., 23, [59]
Karczmar, A. G., 210, 212, 218, 229, [232, 233]
Karler, R., 42, [61]
Karli, P., 222, 223, [232]
Karten, H. J., 49, [59], 243, [326]
Kastin, A. J., 32, 33, [57]
Kato, G., 41, [60]
Kato, J., 18, [57], 190, [205]
Katz, B. T., 40, [57]
Katz, R. L., [322]
Kaufmann, L., 37, [60]
Kaufman, S., 37, 44, [60], 251, [322]
Kawa, A., 138, [171]
Kawakami, M., 3, 7, [9], 23, 28, 30, 31, 36, [57], 91, [100], 165, [170]
Kawamura, H., 30, [57]
Kawasaki, S., 200, [207]
Keene, W. R., 24, [59]
Keller, M. R., 39, [60]
Keller, P. J., 47, 48, [58]
Kellogg, W. N., 175, [205]
Kelly, D., 262, [329]
Kelly, J. S., 41, [57]
Kennedy, C., 40, [57]
Kenshalo, D. R., 200, [207]
Kernaghan, D., 126, [133]
Kesner, R. P., 185, [205]
Kerr, S. E., 38, [57]
Kessler, S., 317, 318, [323]
Keverne, E. B., 81, [101]
Khairallah, P. A., 41, [57]
Kim, J. S., 267, [320]
Kinsey, A. C., 63, 94, 95, 96, 97, [100]
Kinder, E. F., 114, [132]

King, B. D., 37, [57]
King, F. A., 128, [133]
King, J. A., 212, 214, [232, 233]
King, M. B., 224, 225, [232, 233]
King, R. J., 19, [57]
Kipnis, D. M., 35, [60]
Kirpekar, S. M., 246, [324]
Kirschner, N., 245, [324]
Kirschvink, J. F., 43, [62]
Kirshner, N., 246, [329]
Kirton, K. T., 78, [100]
Kislak, J. W., 228, [232]
Kiss, J., 41, [53]
Kitabchi, A. E., 252, [324]
Kitay, J. I., 36, [53]
Klackenberg-Larsson, I., 289, [324]
Klainer, L. M., 51, [57]
Klawans, H., 277, [329]
Klee, C. B., 38, 44, [57, 60]
Klein, D., 237, [324]
Klein, D. B., 177, [207]
Klein, M., 11, [132]
Kleitman, N., 176, [207]
Kline, N. S., 254, [324]
Kling, A., 300, [326]
Klippel, M., 28, [57]
Klippel, R. A., [170]
Knox, W. E., 49, [57]
Knowlton, K., 34, [52]
Kobayashi, T., 30, [57], 95, [101]
Kodet, M. J., 26, [55]
Koe, B. K., 267, 273, 274, 290, 303, 309, [324, 329]
Koella, W., 310, [324]
Koffka, K., 174, [205]
Kohler, W., 174, [205]
Koizumi, K., 47, [53]
Koller, G., 116, 117, 118, 123, [132]
Kollros, J. J., 13, [57]
Koltai, M., 31, [59], 165, [170]
Komisaruk, B. R., 28, [59], 91, [102], 165, [170]
König, J. F. R., [170]
Kooi, K. A., 185, [204]
Kopin, I. J., 246, 247, 250, 260, 264, 266, 268, 271, 272, 273, [320, 321, 323, 324, 327]
Koranyi, L., 24, 50, [57], 164, 165, [169, 170], 180, 194, 195, 196, 197, [204, 205]
Korchin, S. J., 284, [320]

Subject Index

A

Acetylcholine
  killing behavior and, 224-25
  levels, isolation and, 218
  and shock-induced fighting, 221
  utilization rate of, 215
Acetylcholinesterase, 43, 224
  thyroid and, 48
ACh, *see* Acetylcholine
ACTH
  and adrenal cortex activity, 152
  Al peptide, 143
  B peptide, 143, 156, 157
  brain, effects on, 26-27, 33-34, 39
  decapeptide1-10, 143 147-50, 156, 157, 159-60, 161, 162-63, 197-99
  feedback action of, 4-5
  heptadecapeptide1-17, 196-97
  heptapeptide4-10, 143, 144, 156, 157
  melanocytes, effect on, 196
  peptide11-24, 156, 157, 198, 199
  peptide1-24, polysynaptic reflex activity of, 197, 198
  postcopulatory release of, 78
  progesterone secretion control by, 154
  protein synthesis and, 44-45
  release, basal forebrain and, 195
  structure of, 156, 157
  temperature effect of, 24
Adaptation, 166
Addison's disease, 21, 22, 28
S-Adenosylhomocysteine, 315
S-Adenosylmethionine, 252, 315
Adrenaline, *see* Epinephrine
Adrenal gland
  activity rhythm and, 26
  adrenogenital syndrome, 31
  androgens, sex behavior and, 69

central nervous system metabolism, effect on, 39
  cortex, medullary catecholamines and, 252-53
  cortical insufficiency, 21, 28
  hyperplasia, 96
  nest building, effect on, 129
  potassium and sodium regulation by, 42
  size, population density and, 226
  stress, effect on, 214
  weight, social rank and, 227
  zona fasciculata, 227
Adrenal medulla
  catecholamine production by, 23
  chromaffin cell types of, 284
  glucocorticoid action on, 249, 253
  stress response of, 287
Adrenocorticoids
  avoidance behavior and, 191-93
  body temperature and, 24
  calcium metabolism and, 41
  catabolic, 45
  catecholamine synthesis and, 49-50
  compound S, 26
  corticosterone, 5, 20
  cortisol, 19
  cortisone, 27, 33-34, 39, 143
  deoxycorticosterone, 14, 21, 22, 26-27, 33, 39, 124
  dexamethasone, 20, 25, 153, 154-55
  glucocorticoids, 4-5, 22, 153
  hydrocortisone, 13, 14, 33-34, 165, 215
  mineralocorticoids, 153
  and muricide, 223
  receptors for, 19
  17-hydroxycorticoids, 19
Adrenocorticotropic hormone, *see* ACTH
Agression